MW00963513

Behçet's Syndrome

Yusuf Yazıcı · Hasan Yazıcı

Editors

Behçet's Syndrome

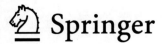 Springer

Editors
Yusuf Yazıcı, MD
New York University School of Medicine
NYU Hospital for Joint Diseases
Behçet's Syndrome Evaluation,
Treatment and Research Center
New York, New York
USA

Hasan Yazıcı, MD
Behçet's Disease Research Center
Cerrahpaşa Medical School
University of Istanbul
Aksaray, Istanbul
Turkey

ISBN 978-1-4419-5640-8   e-ISBN 978-1-4419-5641-5
DOI 10.1007/978-1-4419-5641-5
Springer New York Dordrecht Heidelberg London

Library of Congress Control Number: 2010928052

© Springer Science+Business Media, LLC 2010
All rights reserved. This work may not be translated or copied in whole or in part without the written permission of the publisher (Springer Science+Business Media, LLC, 233 Spring Street, New York, NY 10013, USA), except for brief excerpts in connection with reviews or scholarly analysis. Use in connection with any form of information storage and retrieval, electronic adaptation, computer software, or by similar or dissimilar methodology now known or hereafter developed is forbidden.
The use in this publication of trade names, trademarks, service marks, and similar terms, even if they are not identified as such, is not to be taken as an expression of opinion as to whether or not they are subject to proprietary rights.
While the advice and information in this book are believed to be true and accurate at the date of going to press, neither the authors nor the editors nor the publisher can accept any legal responsibility for any errors or omissions that may be made. The publisher makes no warranty, express or implied, with respect to the material contained herein.

Printed on acid-free paper

Springer is part of Springer Science+Business Media (www.springer.com)

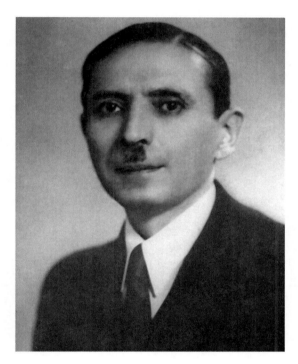

Professor Hulusi Behçet (1881–1948)

Dedication

*When I first started practicing rheumatology
about 10 years ago, I got calls from patients
saying that they had been diagnosed with
Behçet's and did some searching online and
saw that a Dr. Yazıcı had done a lot of work
and research on the subject. Then they found
another Dr. Yazıcı online working in New
York. They wondered if I was the Dr. Yazıcı
they were looking for. I would tell them that
the Dr. Yazıcı they were looking for was my
father and they would say, "Close enough,
we'll come and see you." I have tried to be
"close enough" and hope that they have
been right.*

*This book is dedicated to my wife Angie
and daughters Esra and Leyla, also
granddaughters of my coeditor; my father and
of course my mother, neither of whom I can
ever repay.*

Yusuf Yazıcı

Preface

General, or for that matter, specialized texts on Behçet's syndrome have been few. The primary aim of this book is to be a comprehensive and compact guide to help the clinicians from various disciplines, as well as the general physician to recognize and manage Behçet's. So its context is mainly clinical. On the other hand, our excellent contributors, presented, discussed, and referenced what is controversial and not known. We hope Behçet's Syndrome will also be a valuable source of ideas and a guide to the research oriented.

You will note that controversy is still a paramount theme in Behçet's syndrome, starting with the very name of this book. Beyond the title, we left the authors of each chapter free to choose naming Behçet's a disease or a syndrome. This we thought will further convey the message that there is much left to learn what Behçet's is about.

Our sincere thanks go out to everybody who helped us to put this work together. Our special thanks to the colleagues in the Department of Rheumatology at Cerrahpaşa Hospital of University of Istanbul who, most generously, not only went over the many versions of the chapters they directly contributed to but also immensely helped the editors in going over almost each and every other chapter, as well.

We also thank the American Behçet's Disease Association, Ms. Virginia Yee, the Whitsitt family for their financial support and our publishers for the initial proposal and final realization of *Behçet's Syndrome*.

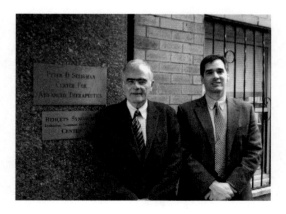

New York, NY, USA
Aksaray, Istanbul, Turkey

Yusuf Yazıcı
Hasan Yazıcı

Contents

Contributors

Ehud Baharav, MD
Department of Medicine and the Laboratory of Physiopathology of Joints and Inflammation, Felsenstein Medical Research Center, Petah Tiqva, Israel

Dongsik Bang, MD, PhD
Department of Dermatology and Cutaneous Biology Research Institute, Yonsei University College of Medicine, Seoul, Korea

Colin G. Barnes, BSc, MBBS, FRCP
Department of Rheumatology, The Royal London Hospital, London, UK
Department of Rheumatology, Queen Mary College, University of London, London, UK

Bahram Bodaghi, MD, PhD
Department of Ophthalmology, University of Paris VI, Pierre et Marie Curie, UFR Pitié-Salpêtrière, Paris, France

Kenneth T. Calamia, MD
Division of Rheumatology, Department of Internal Medicine, Mayo Clinic, Jacksonville, FL, USA

Aykut Ferhat Çelik, MD
Division of Gastroenterology, Department of Internal Medicine, University of Istanbul, Istanbul, Turkey

M. Anne Chamberlain, FRCP
Academic Department of Rehabilitation Medicine, University of Leeds, Leeds UK

Jae Hee Cheon, MD, PhD
Department of Internal Medicine, Yonsei University College of Medicine, Seoul, Korea

Cuyan Demirkesen, MD
Pathology Department, Cerrahpaşa Medical Faculty, Istanbul University,
Istanbul, Turkey

Haner Direskeneli, MD
Department of Rheumatology, Marmara University Medical Faculty,
Istanbul, Turkey

İzzet Fresko, MD
Division of Rheumatology, Department of Medicine,
Cerrahpaşa Medical Faculty, University of Istanbul, Istanbul, Turkey

Süha Göksel, MD
Pathology Department, Cerrahpaşa Medical Faculty, University of Istanbul,
Istanbul, Turkey

Ahmet Gül, MD
Division of Rheumatology, Department of Internal Medicine, University of Istanbul,
Istanbul, Turkey

Vedat Hamuryudan, MD
Division of Rheumatology, Department of Medicine, Cerrahpaşa Medical Faculty,
University of Istanbul, Istanbul, Turkey

Gülen Hatemi, MD
Division of Rheumatology, Department of Medicine, Cerrahpaşa Medical Faculty,
University of Istanbul, Istanbul, Turkey

Shunsei Hirohata, MD
Department of Rheumatology and Infectious Diseases, Kitasato University
School of Medicine, Kanagawa, Japan

Won Ho Kim, MD, PhD
Department of Internal Medicine, Yonsei University College of Medicine,
Seoul, Korea

Ina Kötter, MD
Department of Internal Medicine II (Oncology, Haematology, Immunology,
Pulmology, and Rheumatology), University Hospital, Tübingen, Germany

Ilan Krause, MD
Deptartment of Medicine, Rabin Medical Center, Beilinson Hospital,
Petah Tiqva, Israel

M. Cem Mat, MD
Department of Dermatology, Cerrahpaşa Medical Faculty, University of Istanbul,
Istanbul, Turkey

Melike Melikoğlu, MD
Division of Rheumatology, Department of Medicine, Cerrahpaşa Medical Faculty,
University of Istanbul, Istanbul, Turkey

Felix Mor, MD
Department of Medicine, Felsenstein Medical Research Center,
Petah Tiqva, Israel

Gonca Mumcu, DDS, PhD
Departments of Oral Diagnosis and Radiology, Department of Health Management,
Faculty of Health Science, Marmara University, Istanbul, Turkey

Shigeaki Ohno, MD
Department of Ocular Inflammation and Immunology, Hokkaido University
Graduate School of Medicine, Sapporo, Japan

Büge Öz, MD
Pathology Department, Cerrahpaşa Medical Faculty, University of Istanbul,
Istanbul, Turkey

Huri Özdoğan, MD
Division of Rheumatology, Department of Medicine, Cerrahpaşa Medical Faculty,
University of Istanbul, Istanbul, Turkey

Yılmaz Özyazgan, MD
Department of Ophthalmology, Cerrahpaşa Medical Faculty,
University of Istanbul, Istanbul, Turkey

Güher Saruhan-Direskeneli, MD
Department of Physiology, Istanbul Medical Faculty, University of Istanbul,
Istanbul, Turkey

Emire Seyahi, MD
Division of Rheumatology, Department of Medicine, Cerrahpaşa Medical Faculty,
University of Istanbul, Istanbul, Turkey

Aksel Siva, MD
Clinical Neuroimmunology Unit and Department of Neurology,
Cerrahpaşa Medical Faculty, University of Istanbul, Istanbul, Turkey

Abraham Weinberger, MD
The Laboratory of Physiopathology of Joints and Inflammation,
Felsenstein Medical Research Center, Petah Tiqva, Israel

Hasan Yazıcı, MD
Division of Rheumatology, Department of Medicine, Cerrahpaşa Medical Faculty,
University of Istanbul, Istanbul, Turkey

Yusuf Yazıcı, MD
Department of Medicine, Division of Rheumatology, New York University School
of Medicine, NYU Hospital for Joint Diseases, New York, NY, USA

Sebahattin Yurdakul, MD
Division of Rheumatology, Department of Medicine, Cerrahpaşa Medical Faculty,
University of Istanbul, Istanbul, Turkey

Chapter 1
Introduction: Dedicated Mondays and an *Acquaintance-Based* View of Behçet's Syndrome

Hasan Yazıcı

Keywords Diagnostic criteria • Classification criteria • Bayes theorem • Subspecialty based criteria • Seronegative spondarthritis • Disease clusters • Autoinflammatory diseases • Monday clinic

My acquaintance with Behçet's syndrome started almost 35 years ago when, after training in internal medicine and rheumatology, I came back to Istanbul from the United States, with an acquired taste to collect data along with a learned joy in teasing, discussing, and presenting what I have collected. Since 1977, a group of colleagues at the Cerrahpaşa Medical School of University of Istanbul – where Professor Hulusi Behçet had initially described the syndrome – have been dedicatedly trying to manage the care of, now up to some 8,000, patients with Behçet's syndrome. This is our multidisciplinary (rheumatologists, dermatologists, ophthalmologists regularly and neurologists, vascular surgeons, and pathologists as needed) and dedicated Monday clinic where we tend to see about 60–80 patients every week. We feel privileged to listen to their problems, advise and prescribe the necessary, and collect data. Our privilege turns into pride when we remember that more than a half of the, about two dozen, controlled clinical drug trials in Behçet's syndrome have been conducted in this unit (see Chap.19). I am indebted to all of my dedicated Monday colleagues, as well as other world experts who have contributed to the fine book at hand. Their views in their respective chapters are, by necessity, evidence-based. I like to think, on the other hand, having been invited to write an introductory chapter by a co-editor, who is also my son, entitles me, even if briefly to side step evidence and enjoy acquaintance.

I have to admit that the first ever scientific talk I attended on Behçet's syndrome was not at home in Istanbul but in Toronto in 1973 [1] by Desmond O'Duffy. As a first year rheumatology fellow at Creighton University, Omaha, Nebraska, I carefully listened to Dr. O'Duffy from the Mayo Clinic present his diagnostic criteria based on a couple of dozen patients. I was up once he finished and said

H. Yazıcı
Behçet's Disease Research Unit, University of Istanbul, Istanbul, Turkey
e-mail: hasan@yazici.net

Y. Yazıcı and H. Yazıcı (eds.), *Behçet's Syndrome*,
DOI 10.1007/978-1-4419-5641-5_1, © Springer Science+Business Media, LLC 2010

"Your criteria might indeed work but we first have to test whether these criteria can tell Behçet's from in grown toe nails." There were some gasps and hisses and then somebody from the back of the room in a very distinct English accent said: "The gentleman from Omaha is begging the issue. One has to start somewhere." That was the totality and the end of the formal discussion.

Fifteen years later in an after dinner talk in our apartment in Istanbul Dr. Colin Barnes, the author of the next chapter, suddenly said "Hasan, I see you keep using the O'Duffy criteria in your papers. You now have several hundred patients attending your clinic. Why don't you formulate your own criteria?" I replied "You see I have reason to suspect Dr. O'Duffy reviews everything I send to better journals," and added: "Furthermore, many years ago when I had expressed my rather blunt views about these criteria I was promptly silenced by this English physician." There was a big laughter "Hasan we did not know each other then. I was that Englishman" With this, and the expert help of Professor Alan Silman, started our international effort to formulate the now widely used ISBD criteria [2] (see Chap. 2).

On the other hand, criteria for Behçet's are still a hot issue. At every international meeting of ISBD there are almost always big egos and debates for change and improvement. Rather recently, it dawned on me that perhaps we all had the wrong approach to formulating such criteria. The sophisticated view for some years has been that all disease criteria at hand including those for Behçet's have been classification rather than diagnostic criteria [3]. They are good to describe groups of patients, hence better suited for research purposes, rather than to make a diagnostic decision in an individual patient. Diagnostic criteria, on the other hand, are what are required for this decision.

But how does one make strictly diagnostic criteria? Or even better, do we know of any good diagnostic, as distinct from classification criteria for any disease of unknown etiology and nonspecific pathology? I venture, no. The cerebral and, therefore, the arithmetic process are identical. Both depend on the Bayes theorem which says that posttest odds of a disease is the product of the pretest odds multiplied by the likelihood ratio ($PosTO = PreTO \times LR$) [4]. When it comes to classification or diagnosis of a disease the PreTO is the frequency of the disease in the setting of the criteria are applied and the LR is derived directly from the sensitivity and the specificity of the criteria at hand. I propose that diagnostic and classification criteria form a continuum [4,5] and there are two considerations that determine whether a set of criteria are diagnostic or classification and these are: (a) what one wants to do with the diagnosis at hand and (b) the frequency of the condition being sought (the pretest odds) [5]. The higher this frequency the more a set of criteria becomes diagnostic. On the other hand, in many instances criteria that are not specific enough can be used for diagnosis as well. For example, in an epidemic of swine flu physicians with good conscience can declare any cold as the flu and prescribe oseltamivir for the patient, knowing that they will also be giving oseltamivir to many more number of patients who do not have the flu.

I think it is time we reconsider our continuous effort to make "universal" classification/diagnostic criteria for identifying rare conditions such as Behçet's or Wegener's [4]. I also envisage that subspecialty tailored criteria will have the potential to be much more specific and sensitive in that (a) the PreO will remarkably increase and (b) the number of conditions that come into the differential diagnosis will decrease. To give an example to back up the first point, we do know that the frequency of Behçet's is at least 1,000-fold more in Japan as compared to that in North America. On the other hand, if you go to a dedicated uveitis clinic in either country you will see that the proportion of Behçet patients seen differs only by several fold, 2.5 % in North America [6] and 6.2% in Japan [7]. Furthermore, the clinical prediction rules for an gastroenterologist to tell Behçet's from inflammatory bowel disease – one of the very few conditions that Behçet's has to be separated from in a gastroenterology practice – (see Chap. 10) are very different from a rheumatologist trying to the same among a more exhaustive list of connective tissue diseases and vasculitides. This is exactly why I say criteria should be tailored to the practice setting.

Another important aspect of my acquaintance with Behçet's syndrome is whether it is a seronegative spondarthritis, another subject of considerable debate. Every seasoned rheumatologist knows that Behçet's had been included among the seronegative spondarthritides in the seminal paper by Moll et al. back in 1974 [8]. While it certainly is true that articular, eye, genital, and skin mucosa disease are also seen as Behçet's, it takes only a few dedicated Mondays in Istanbul to realize that there are some very important differences in the kind of involvement one sees in this condition as compared to ankylosing spondylitis or Reiter's disease. The blinding nature of the eye disease, the lack of sacroiliitis, the presence of genital ulcers in the absence of urinary tract infection, among others, are all very different. To top it all, there is the HLA B51 rather than the HLA B27 connection. These points were, in fact, what had made up my docent's thesis in 1977 entitled "Is Behçet's disease a spondarthritis?" [9] The answer was no as most students of Behçet's syndrome currently accept.

The issue of whether Behçet's syndrome belongs to the spondarthritides has recently rekindled. Following the initial work of our Israeli colleagues [10] and having the advantage of seeing a considerably greater number of patients, we repeated their factor analysis work [11] seeking clusters of disease expression in Behçet's syndrome. We came up with five factors which explained 70% of the symptom matrix we started with. Much to our satisfaction one cluster was the arthritis and acne cluster. A few years before and in a different group of patients, we had indeed shown that those Behçet patients with arthritis had more acne [12]. The arthritis of Behçet's was perhaps akin to a reactive arthritis some classify within the seronegative spondarthritis. Two further observations turned out to be supportive: (1) We grew bacteria from the pustular lesions [13]. (2) There was increased enthesitis among patients with acne and arthritis as compared to those without [14]. Are we now saying that Behçet's is part of the seronegative spondarthritides as was recently suggested [15]? Not really. What we are saying is that Behçet's syndrome has a subgroup, a subphenotype, that shows – and only some of – these features. Another such group is made up of those patients with dural sinus thrombi/deep vein thrombosis/superficial vein thrombosis [16,17]. Or more broadly we consider it perhaps more productive to be a splitter rather than a lumper [18] in our effort to better understand the yet enigmatic disease mechanism (s).

Splitting versus lumping around Behçet's syndrome is not confined to the issue of its being or not being a seronegative spondarthritis. For many years, Behçet's has been considered as an autoimmune disease like systemic lupus or rheumatoid arthritis with the primary aberration in the T and/or B cell repertoire. After many and very qualified efforts no single or a reproducible group of immunologic aberrations could be pinpointed. This led to a slow but a firm getting away from the autoimmune disease concept and for the last 2 decades it is in vogue to classify it with the vasculitides, more of a morphological rather than a functional approach. More recent is the effort to lump Behçet's with the autoinflammatory diseases [19]. One can make a long list of how Behçet's syndrome differs from this group starting with the fact that autoinflammatory diseases are mainly pediatric conditions with a well defined, mostly monogenic transmission. On the other hand, one can consider this lumping as healthy in that it will surely stimulate splitters to collect more specific, hence useful data [20].

To me another important consideration in the unknown pathogenesis is how/why atherosclerosis is not appreciably increased in this condition [21]. Perhaps the main issue is the predominance of vascular inflammation being on the venous side. After all, the pulmonary arterial tree – the site of most deadly disease in BS – is structurally much like a venous tree. On the other hand, I continue to be surprised how little we know about venous endothelium or for that matter the actual thickness of venous walls in health and disease. This line of inquiry, I dare say, might prove to be fruitful in deciphering Behçet's syndrome. These days we can do much more than what we were able to do for disease management when we first started our Monday clinics. The visual loss came down to 10–20 % [22,23] from around 75% [24]. With prompt recognition and treatment pulmonary aneurysms are less fatal [25]. The management of skin-mucosa lesions is quite gratifying. We might even be doing somewhat better in managing central nervous system disease [26] even though formal clinical trials to this end are certainly needed. On the other hand the management of thrombophilia, which afflicts at least one-third of the patients, is still most wanting. Perhaps addressing the basic science aspects of venous endothelium will eventually give us clues.

A dear mentor of mine, Paul D. Saville, an osteoporosis expert, once said that I should pay regular and certainly high tribute to Professor Hulusi Behçet for providing me the foundations of a career long vocation. With my son – who graciously invited me to be the co-editor of his book – running a Behçet's clinic in Manhattan of all places, with several hundred patients certainly tells me how correct my mentor had been in many ways. The same tribute also goes to Berrin, my co-editor's mother, for tolerating my, do I dare say, intellectual whims for 45 years and for not shying away our son from the same.

References

1. O'Duffy JD (1974) Suggested criteria for diagnosis of Behçet's disease. J Rheumatol 1(Suppl 1):Abstr. 32:18
2. International Study Group for Behçet's Disease (1990) Criteria for diagnosis of Behçet's disease. Lancet 335:1078–1080
3. Hunder GG (1998) The use and misuse of classification and diagnostic criteria for complex diseases. Ann Intern Med 129:417–418

4. Yazici H, Seyahi E, Yurdakul S (2008) Behçet's syndrome is not so rare: why do we need to know? Arthritis Rheum 58:3640–3643
5. Yazici H (2009) Diagnostic versus classification criteria: a continuum. Bull NYU Hosp Jt Dis 67(2):206–208
6. Rodriguez A, Calonge M, Pedroza-Seres M et al (1996) Referral patterns of uveitis in a tertiary eye care center. Arch Ophthalmol 114:593–599
7. Goto H, Mochizuki M, Yamaki K et al (2007) Epidemiological survey of intraocular inflammation in Japan. Jpn J Ophthalmol 51:41–44
8. Moll JM, Haslock I, Macrae IF et al (1974) Associations between ankylosing spondylitis, psoraitic arthritis, Rieter's disease, the inestinal arthropathies and Behçet's syndrome. Medicine (Baltimore) 53:343–364
9. Yazici H (1978) Behçet hastalığı seronegatif spondartritlerden midir? Dozent's thesis, University of Istanbul
10. Krause I, Leibovici L, Guedj D et al (1999) Disease patterns of patients with Behçet's disease demonstrated by factor analysis. Clin Exp Rheumatol 17:347–350
11. Tunc R, Keyman E, Melikoglu M et al (2002) Target organ associations in Turkish patients with Behçet's disease: a cross sectional study by exploratory factor analysis. J Rheumatol 29:2393–2396
12. Diri E, Mat C, Hamuryudan V et al (2001) Papulopustular skin lesions are seen more frequently in patients with Behçet's syndrome who have arthritis: a controlled and masked study. Ann Rheum Dis 60:1074–1076
13. Hatemi G, Bahar H, Uysal S et al (2004) The pustular skin lesions in Behçet's syndrome are not sterile. Ann Rheum Dis 63:1450–1452
14. Hatemi G, Fresko I, Tascilar K, Yazici H (2008) Enthesopathy is increased among Behçet's syndrome patients with acne and arthritis: an ultrasonographic study. Arthritis Rheum 58:1539–1545
15. Priori R, Ceccarelli F et al (2009) Do Behçet's syndrome patients with acne and arthritis comprise a true subset? Comment on the article by Hatemi et al. Arthritis Rheum 60:1201–1202
16. Tunc R, Saip S, Siva A, Yazici H (2004) Cerebral venous thrombosis is associated with major vessel disease in Behçet's syndrome. Ann Rheum Dis 63:1693–1694
17. Yazici H, Fresko I, Yurdakul S (2007) Behçet's syndrome: disease manifestations, management, and advances in treatment. Nat Clin Pract Rheumatol 3:148–155
18. McKusick VA (2005) The Gordon Wilson Lecture: the clinical legacy of Jonathan Hutchinson (1828–1913): syndromology and dysmorphology meet genomics. Trans Am Clin Climatol Assoc 116:15–38
19. Gül A (2005) Behçet's disease as an autoinflammatory disorder. Curr Drug Targets Inflamm Allergy 4:81–83
20. Yazici H, Fresko I (2005) Behçet's disease and other autoinflammatory conditions: what's in a name? Clin Exp Rheumatol 23(4 Suppl 38):S1–S2
21. Seyahi E, Ugurlu S, Cumali R et al (2008) Atherosclerosis in Behçet's syndrome. Semin Arthritis Rheum 38:1–12
22. Kural-Seyahi E, Fresko I, Seyahi N et al (2003) The long-term mortality and morbidity of Behçet syndrome: a 2-decade outcome survey of 387 patients followedat a dedicated center. Medicine (Baltimore) 82:60–76
23. Cho YJ, Kim WK, Lee JH et al (2008) Visual prognosis and risk factors for korean patients with Behçet uveitis. Ophthalmologica 222:344–350
24. Benezra D, Cohen E (1986) Treatment and visual prognosis in Behçet's disease. Br J Ophthalmol 70:589–592
25. Hamuryudan V, Er T, Seyahi E et al (2004) Pulmonary artery aneurysms in Behçet syndrome. Am J Med 117:867–870
26. Kurtuncu M, Tuzun E, Mutlu M et al (2008) Clinical patterns and course of neuro-Behçet's disease: analysis of 354 patients comparing cases presented before and after 1990. Clin Exp Rheumatol 26(4 Suppl 50):17

Chapter 2
History and Diagnosis

Colin G. Barnes

Keywords Aphthous ulceration • Behçet's disease • Behçet's syndrome • Classification • Diagnostic criteria • Pathergy • Vasculitis • Vasculopathy

Introduction

The eponymous name of Behçet's Syndrome (BS) was derived from the description of the "Triple Symptom Complex" by Professor Hulusi Behçet [1–3]. He described the association of oral and genital ulceration with uveitis and considered this to be of possible viral aetiology.

Biographies of Hulusi Behçet (1889–1948), written by Professor Türkan Saylan, have been published in the proceedings of an International Conference on Behçet's Disease held in Istanbul in 1977 [4], and in the Yonsei Medical Journal (1997) [5] the latter demonstrating the great interest in the condition in Korea. Professor Nihat Dilşen also wrote a short biography, and reviewed the development of knowledge of the syndrome between the fifth century BC and 1996, in the proceedings of the 7th International Conference on Behçet's Disease, Tunis [6].

Behçet was born in Istanbul but educated in Damascus where his family lived, and then studied medicine at the Turkish Gülhane Military Medical Academy qualifying at the age of 21 years. Subsequently he specialised in dermatology and venereology and during the first World War served at the Edirne Military Hospital. He gained post-graduate experience in Budapest and Berlin and returned to Istanbul to practise dermatology and venereology. After the formation of the University of Istanbul in 1933 he became its first Professor of Dermatology and was responsible for the development of the Department of Dermatology. He was a prolific writer and enthusiastic teacher; he retired in 1947 and died a year later.

C.G. Barnes
Formerly of the Department of Rheumatology, The Royal London Hospital, London, E1 1BB, UK
and
Department of Rheumatology, Barts and The London School of Medicine,
Queen Mary University of London, London, UK
e-mail: cgbarnes@btinternet.com

Y. Yazıcı and H. Yazıcı (eds.), *Behçet's Syndrome*,
DOI 10.1007/978-1-4419-5641-5_2, © Springer Science+Business Media, LLC 2010

He described three patients the first of whom he is said to have met in 1924–1925. These patients had the three principal features of aphthous ulceration and genital ulceration with inflammatory eye disease. However, although he described this as a "triple symptom complex," and one can comment that he described many signs in his patients and not only their symptoms, he did also record erythema nodosum in one patient and acneiform lesions on the back of another. Behçet himself, therefore, described the four major features of the condition (orogenital ulceration, inflammatory eye disease and skin lesions). It is somewhat surprising that, as a dermatologist, he did not include skin lesions as the fourth feature of the syndrome he was describing. It is also surprising that he did not comprehensively refer to previous descriptions of similar patients, including some in the German dermatological literature having worked in Berlin and known to speak good German, in his own publications. He does refer to Lipschutz who had described what was considered to be viral diseases of the skin and one of Behçet's patients had consulted Fuchs in Vienna, both of whom may have described the same syndrome in 1927 and 1926, respectively [7, 8].

The development of knowledge of BS, especially in the last 30 years, demonstrates that it has a different meaning to different interested groups. To the patient it is a problem which may last throughout life although there are records of self-limiting disease; to the physician it may be included in the differential diagnosis of occasional patients although large numbers of patients may be seen in some parts of the world; to the laboratory scientist it may be regarded as a model of disease expression involving inflammation and disturbances of immunity of uncertain aetiology.

Early Descriptions of the Syndrome

Like many diseases with eponymous names, Behçet was not the first to describe this association of clinical features. The first account probably dates back to Hippocrates in the 5th century BC. In *Epidimion,* Book 3, Case 7 (translated by Adams 1849 [9]) aphthous ulceration, genital ulceration and iridocyclitis are described. Additionally, reference was made to skin lesions – boils, sepsis, and "ecthymata". Feigenbaum (1956) [10] commented that from this description it could be suggested that the condition was endemic, and possibly of epidemic proportions, in ancient Greece.

Our Chinese colleagues also record a description of a disease known as *Huo Ho Bing* by a Dr. Zhong Jing Zhang, c. 200 AD, which included pharyngeal ulcers, genital ulcers, eye redness and pus formation (skin) (Ohno, personal communication). From Europe and Japan in the late 19th century and early 20th century came descriptions of what would probably now be regarded as Behçet's Syndrome (Table 1.1) [7, 8, 11–19]. Very small numbers of patients were described, for example a single case report from Adamantiades (who, in a subsequent paper, referred to Behçet's Syndrome), with uveitis with or without hypopyon, and combinations of oral and genital ulceration and skin lesions. In some of these early

Table 2.1 Descriptions of possible Behçet's Syndrome before 1937

Speciality	Authors	Country	Year	Reference
Ophthalmology	Gilbert	Germany	1920	[11]
	Shigeta	Japan	1924	[12]
	Fuchs	Austria	1926	[8]
	Adamantiades	Greece	1931	[13, 14]
	Dascolopoulos	Greece	1932	[15]
Internal Medicine	Chauffard et al.	France	1923	[16]
Dermatology	Neumann	Germany	1894	[17]
	Planner and Remenovsky	Germany	1923	[18]
	Lipschutz	Austria	1924	[7]
	Whitwell	United Kingdom	1934	[19]

reports other clinical features, later accepted as integral manifestations of Behçet's Syndrome, were also described including phlebitis, hydroarthrosis of the knees, and deep vein thrombosis [13].

Development of the Full Clinical Description of the Syndrome

Since the original description by Behçet the syndrome has developed such that the initial three manifestations have been further described in detail, skin manifestations have been included as the fourth major feature, and other features have been added as "minor" manifestations. These have been regarded as "minor" solely on the basis of occurring in <50% of patients and not as an indication of their clinical severity (Table 2.2). Vasculitis has been listed as a "minor" feature in the sense that it presents as a clinical feature, such as thrombophlebitis or aneurysm formation, although the condition is now regarded as being a systemic vasculitis, or vasculopathy, which is considered below. The approximate percentage prevalence of the manifestations listed in Table 2.2 is derived from various surveys including that of the International Study Group for Behçet's Disease [20–23] but it must be emphasised that this varies in different parts of the world.

Aphthous Ulceration

Oral ulceration has been found to occur in 98% of patients with BS. The lesions are painful and may be major, minor or herpetiform types of ulceration as also occurs in benign Recurrent Oral Ulceration (ROU) [24, 25]. Ulceration may be preceded by the formation of a tender submucosal nodule. Major ulceration leads to mucosal scarring. Although the more serious forms of orogenital ulceration may raise the suspicion of BS it has been accepted that there is no diagnostically "typical Behçet's ulcer".

Table 2.2 Manifestations of Behçet's Syndrome [20–23] with approximate % prevalences

Major	(%)	Minor	(%)
Recurrent oral ulceration	98	Arthritis (arthralgia)	45
Recurrent genital ulceration	80	Vasculitis	16
Inflammatory eye disease	50	Large vessel vasculitis	
Uveitis ± hypopyon		Aneurysm formation	
Retinal vasculitis		Arterial/venous thrombosis	
Skin lesions	80	Gastrointestinal lesions	0–25
Erythema nodosum	47	Cardiovascular lesions	
Folliculitis/acneiform lesions	71	Neurological lesions	5–25
Skin ulceration		Pleuropulmonary lesions	
Hyperirritability – pathergy	60	Epididymitis	8
		Family history	20

Mouth ulceration is the earliest manifestation of BS in the majority of patients and may be the presenting feature to the physician. In that oral ulceration may occur in up to 20% of western populations [26], and is the most common feature of BS, it is necessary that other features are present in order to contemplate a diagnosis of BS (see below), Similarly BS may commence with other features; 2–3% patients never develop oral ulceration. In other respects, the features of the syndrome are not significantly different between those with or without ulceration [27]. In paediatric BS in Korea it was found that all patients had oral ulceration and the authors recommended that aphthous ulceration in childhood required careful long-term follow-up [28].

It has been demonstrated in case studies that oral ulceration in BS is recurrent. In classification of the syndrome it has been arbitrarily accepted that recurrence is defined as occurring at least three times in one 12-month period [21–23].

Genital ulceration is regarded as following the same pattern as oral ulceration with respect to pain, initial tender nodule formation, major, minor and herpetiform types, recurrence and scarring [29]. Scarring of scrotal lesions is considered specific for BS.

Eye Manifestations [30–33]

The original description was of iritis/iridocyclitis with hypopyon to which has been added retinal vasculitis. The latter may lead to macular oedema, retinal haemorrhages and exudates, occlusion of retinal vessels both arteries and veins, vitreous haemorrhage and optic atrophy. Loss of visual acuity and complete blindness is, therefore, not uncommon although prognosis has been much improved by developments in treatment [34–36].

Skin Lesions

The skin lesions described in the early case reports, including by Behçet himself, were erythema nodosum and acneiform lesions [37]. These, with pustule formation and skin ulceration and scarring, have continued to be the principal reported lesions [38–40]. It is emphasised that to be significant in diagnostic terms acneiform lesions are more relevant when present in patients beyond puberty, in patients who are not taking systemic corticosteroid medication and, importantly, when present on the arms and legs – uncommon sites for common acne. It has also been shown that these acneiform lesions are not sterile and are often present in combination with arthritis [41]. However, as it became evident that BS should be classified as a vasculitis, or vasculopathy, the skin manifestations of superficial thrombophlebitis, papulopustular lesions, skin ulceration (non-genital), erythema nodosum and erythema multiforme-like lesions have been emphasised. Histological examination of mucocutaneous lesions may reveal a leucocytoplastic vasculitis with neutrophilia, extravasation of erythrocytes and fibrinoid necrosis [42–44].

Pathergy Test

The pathergy test, a hypersensitivity reaction to a sterile needle prick producing an erythematous papule, pustule or ulcer after 48 hours, was probably first described by Blobner [45] and Jensen [46]. Some investigators have claimed that the intradermal injection of 0.1 ml physiological saline produces a more reproducible response. However, this has fallen from popularity and simple, sterile, subdermal needle pricks are now used. This reaction was thought to be specific to BS and was found to be positive in the majority of patients. However the pathergy test:

- differs in the frequency of positivity in different countries being most common in Japan and Turkey and rare in western Europe [47–49],
- is more strongly positive in male patients [50],
- is more frequently positive in an individual patient if multiple needle pricks are applied some sites being positive and others negative [51],
- is more frequently positive if blunt, rather than sharp, needles are used [52],
- may be aborted if an antibiotic cream is applied after, or the skin is surgically scrubbed before, the needle prick [51, 53],
- is recorded as declining in frequency over the years,
- has been found occasionally in non-BS cases, for example in approximately 10% of patients with Crohn's disease and 7% of patients with ulcerative colitis [54, 55] and
- may be present in first degree relatives of patients with BS [56, 57].

The cutaneous response to the intradermal injection of monosodium urate crystals appears to be different from the pathergy reaction [58].

Nevertheless a positive pathergy reaction has been included in several diagnostic criteria schemes and in the Classification of Behçet's Disease by the International Study Group (see below).

Joints

Arthralgia and inflammatory synovitis have become accepted features of BS the latter occurring in approximately 45% of patients. Although arthralgia was reported in early descriptions the first report of joint swelling was probably in the 1930s. A synovitis was subsequently confirmed both clinically and histologically. It has been agreed universally that the knees are the most commonly affected joints followed by the ankles, wrists, elbows, small joints of the hands and wrists, shoulders, feet and hips. The arthritis has been variably described as monarticular, pauciarticular, polyarticular affecting an average of 5+ joints per patient, episodic and self-limiting [59–67].

Synovial pathology has been shown to be an acute neutrophilic inflammation with little, if any, synovial surface cell hyperplasia, plasma cell infiltration or lymphoid foci. It, therefore, resembles acute granulation tissue [68, 69] and differs from the more common inflammatory arthropathies characterised by rheumatoid synovitis. Rheumatoid factor test has always been found to be negative.

Initially it was thought that the synovitis was not destructive but later in a minority of cases erosive joint damage was reported clinically, radiologically and histologically [61, 69–73].

Additionally, occasional cases of avascular necrosis of the femoral head have been reported in patients not being treated with corticosteroids, presumably on the basis of a vasculitis (see below).

The presence of an associated sacroiliitis, and fully established ankylosing spondylitis, has been a question of considerable debate over the years. Sacroiliitis was described in up to 65% of patients in some series and it was suggested that the arthritis of BS should be grouped with the seronegative spondarthritides [74, 75]. However, although this suggestion raised the awareness of BS in rheumatological circles, it has not been supported by subsequent studies in which it has been demonstrated that sacroiliitis does not occur more frequently in BS than in normal subjects in the same population [76, 77]. The arthritis of BS, therefore, does not fall into the classification of seronegative spondarthritides (Table 2.3) as is discussed more fully in Chap. 9.

Vasculitis/Vasculopathy

Clinically the effects of vasculopathy have been detected as superficial (subcutaneous) thrombophlebitis, deep vein thrombosis, arterial occlusion or aneurysm formation and vena caval occlusion [78]. In 1977, of 1731 Japanese patients 133 (7.7%) had clinical evidence of vascular lesions. These affected both arteries and veins of all

Table 2.3 Comparison of the arthritis of Behçet's Syndrome with seronegative spondarthritides

	Behçet's Syndrome	Seronegative spondarthritis
Vasculitis	+++	–
Pauciarticular – large joints	++	++
Asymmetry	±	++
Spine/heel involvement	±	++
Sacroiliitis	–	+++
Family aggregation	±	+++
Skin lesions	Erythema nodosum, acneiform lesions, thrombophlebitis	Psoriasis
HLA	B5(51)	B27

sizes with a 20% mortality. Histological examination of large vessels revealed thickening of the media, fragmentation of the elastica and perivascular round cell infiltration around the vasa vasorum [79–81].

By 1993, similar clinical findings were reported from China, Saudi Arabia, Turkey and Tunisia, and vasculitis was proposed as the underlying pathology of the syndrome [82–86].

Behçet's Syndrome is now usually classified as a *vasculitis* which usually means injury or destruction of blood vessels. It is probably more accurate to call this a *vasculopathy*, an abnormality of blood vessels not necessarily leading to injury, which may affect arteries and veins of all sizes and in which there is an immunologically mediated impairment of vascular endothelial function [87–91].

Pulmonary and Neurological Lesions

Vasculopathy is regarded as the cause of pulmonary and neurological lesions. In the early descriptions of patient with BS *pulmonary lesions* were rarely or never found. This has been summarised by Dilşen et al. [92] who noted that the first mention was by Dasculopoulos in 1932 [15], whereas Oshima et al., in their study of 85 Japanese patients, did not comment on pulmonary manifestations [60]. Shimizu, in his review of the syndrome at the International Symposium on Behçet's Disease in 1977, derived from Japanese studies, described two single cases with pulmonary features of tuberculosis-like shadows. One, from the United States, did not respond to anti-tuberculous treatment and the other from Japan being attributed to vascular involvement. He also included a single case of aneurysm of the pulmonary artery among the vascular lesions which may have been the same Japanese patient [79].

These early descriptions listed pleural effusion, hilar enlargement, cavitating lesions, apical fibrosis or calcified lesions, and emphysema among the findings raising a query of whether these were coincidental or real features of BS [93–95].

Vascular lesions affecting the lungs are now well described and are the cause of pleuropulmonary manifestations of BS. Pulmonary artery occlusion or aneurysm formation with, often severe, haemoptysis are rare but potentially fatal manifestations seen mainly in young male patients. Pulmonary embolisation from thrombosis of deep leg veins is not thought to occur as the thrombus is attached to the vessel wall by the inflammatory process – thus being an inflammatory thrombophlebitis rather then a phlebothrombosis caused by stagnation. Anticoagulation is, therefore, to be avoided lest this leads to fatal haemorrhage from a pulmonary artery aneurysm [96–98].

Descriptions of *neurological manifestations* date back to 1944 [99] and have included spinal cord lesions, focal brain lesions, headaches and thrombosis and occlusion of dural sinuses, all on the basis of the underlying vasculitis [100–103]. Headaches were one of the earliest reported neurological features of BS [79] which has been confirmed by more recent studies. These headaches have been detected in up to approximately 80% of patients, fulfil internationally agreed criteria for the diagnosis of migraine but are not thought to necessarily indicate neurological pathology [104, 105]. Clinically the neurological features are those of a meningo-encephalitis affecting all parts of the central nervous systems including the brain stem and spinal cord [105]. Surprisingly, in view of the pathological confirmation of a vasculitis, involvement of the peripheral nervous system (mononeuritis multiplex) is not a feature of BS.

These clinical features have been confirmed by histopathology [105], and more recently investigation by MRI has enabled lesions to be demonstrated clinically [106–109].

Gastrointestinal System

Ulcerative lesions of the gastrointestinal system have been described affecting the entire length of the gut. The lesions show a considerable geographical variation being most common in Japan and the Far East, less common in the Middle East and rare in western Europe. In Japan it is reported that ulcerative lesions of the caecum are characteristic of BS, but these may involve the entire large colon, less frequently the small intestine and occasionally the gastroduodenal mucosa and oesophagus, frequently with vasculopathy histologically [79, 110–113].

Abdominal symptoms are less specific ranging from distension to diarrhoea, and pain with reports of stenosis [114, 115], small and large intestinal perforation [116–118].

Family History, Epidemiology and Geographical Differences in Prevalence

Sezer [119] was probably the first to record a family aggregation of the syndrome affecting three brothers. The early reports of a familial incidence of BS were reviewed by Lehner and Barnes [120] who listed reports of 34 families with affected siblings (of both sexes) or parent/child(ren) between 1956 and 1979. Since then this association has been accepted with further similar reports [121]. The association of BS and the histocompatibility antigen HLA B5(51) was first recognised by Ohno in 1973 [122]. Since then the genetic linkage in, and the epidemiological basis of, BS has been studied extensively (see chaps. 3 and 14).

Reports of groups of patients with BS from many countries have served to confirm the clinical manifestations of the syndrome. At the same time these reports reveal a considerable variation in the overall prevalence of BS and of its constituent manifestations. Examples of these variations include:

(a) A high prevalence of the syndrome was reported from the Behçet's Disease Research Committee of Japan in 1977 being 62.7:1,000,000 population with the highest prevalence in the northern island of Hokkaido and lowest in the southern island of Kyushu [79]. Epidemiological surveys from other parts of the world have included Turkey (prevalence = 8–35:10,000) [123], the USA (prevalence = 1:300,000) [124] and the United Kingdom (prevalence = 0.064:10,000 in Yorkshire and 0.03:10,000 in Scotland) [125, 126]. However, only those studies from Japan and Turkey represent formal epidemiological studies.
(b) The manifestations of the syndrome have been shown to differ in frequency in different geographical regions, for example involvement of the gastrointestinal syndrome is maximal in the Far East and rare in western Europe.
(c) The sex ratio also differs geographically, being about equal in Turkey and male predominant in the United Kingdom and Japan. However most studies find that the disease is more severe in male patients and in those with a younger age of onset [127, 128].
(d) The most common age of onset is in the second and third decades of life. However, paediatric cases are well recorded [129–131] although they are uncommon, and onset after the age of 50 is also uncommon [132].
(e) There may be a considerable interval, sometimes many years, between the development of the first manifestation of the syndrome and others which enable a diagnosis to be made [62].

Aetiopathogenesis

From the early descriptions of the syndrome there has been debate on its aetiopathogenesis. The early authors, including Behçet himself, concluded that it was of viral aetiology but this was disproved over the years [119, 133–135]. Alternative theories included bacterial infection, mainly streptococcal and exposure to chemicals particularly organophosphates neither of which stood the test of time. Therefore, over the years the theories regarding aetiology have progressed through:

- infective
- exposure to chemicals
- immunological disorder
- autoimmune
- autoinflammatory.

Latterly, it has been shown that this is an immunologically mediated condition, of uncertain aetiology, in genetically susceptible individuals (see chaps. 14 and 15).

Diagnosis

From the various clinical manifestation of the syndrome it is evident that the patient may present to one of a number of medical specialities and this has been demonstrated in the literature over the past 70 years. References have already been made in this chapter to authors who are (alphabetically) chest physicians, dermatologists, epidemiologists, gastroenterologists, immunologists, internal medicine physicians, microbiologists, neurologists, ophthalmologists, oral physicians, pathologists, rheumatologists and venereologists to which must be added general practitioners (generalists) and gynaecologists.

In the absence of any specific diagnostic test for BS various physicians with a special interest in the syndrome, therefore, have thought it necessary that schemes, or criteria, for diagnosis should be defined which depend on the grouping together of sufficient features for the physician to be confident of the diagnosis. Several such schemes have been published based on the clinical experience of the authors. There have been three basic forms of such criteria:

- the division of the manifestations of BS as "major" or "minor" (Table 2.2),
- the definition of a "complete" syndrome requiring the presence of three or four of the major manifestations, or "incomplete" requiring three major or two major + two minor manifestations [79, 136, 137],
- spectral involvement dependent on the principal manifestations present, for example mucocutaneous type, mucosal aphthosis, arthritic type, etc. [138, 139].

The first of these diagnostic criteria sets was recommended by Curth in 1946 [140] which required two or more major manifestations for diagnosis. Hewitt and colleagues [141] proposed three major manifestations, being the same three as described by Behçet himself, and recommended that all three were required for a "complete" diagnosis. Only two years later they described the diagnostic importance of skin involvement including skin hyperirritability to needle prick (pathergy test) [142].

The criteria recommended by Mason and Barnes [62], the Behçet's Disease Research Committee of Japan (1974 and 1987) [79, 136, 137], Hubault and Hamza [143], Ben Ayed and Hamza [144], O'Duffy [145] and Dilşen [146] followed (Table 2.4). The first four of these included the pathergy test as a possible major manifestation which was not included in O'Duffy's scheme. By contrast Dilşen's scheme depended on the presence of a positive pathergy test (see above), which he considered a "specific" manifestation, for the diagnosis of what he described as "definite" disease. Ben Ayed and Hamza suggested amendments to these criteria by recommending four major criteria (oral and genital ulceration, inflammatory eye disease being uveitis±hypopyon, and a positive pathergy test) relegating other cutaneous manifestations to the minor category with arthritis and thrombophlebitis.

Table 2.4 Schemes of diagnostic criteria (modified from Br J Rheumatol 1992;31:300, with permission)

	Mason and Barnes [62]	Behçet's disease research committee of Japan 1974 and 1987 [79, 137]	O'Duffy [145]	Cheng and Zhang [147]	Dilsen et al. 1986 [146]
Manifestations of disease					
Oral ulceration	Major	Major	Major	Major	Major
Genital ulceration	Major	Major	Major	Major	Major
Eye lesions	Major	Major	Major	Major	Major
Uveitis ± hypopyon	●	●	●	●	●
Iridocyclitis	●	●			
Chorioretinitis	●	●			●
Corneal ulceration	●				
Retrobulbar neuritis	●				
Skin lesions	Major	Major	Major	Major	Major
Pustules	●				
Ulceration	●				
Erythema nodosum	●	●	●	●	●
Erythema multiforme	●			●	
Subcutaneous thrombophlebitis		●		●	Major
Hyperirritability (pathergy)	●	●		●	Specific
Folliculitis/acneiform lesions		●		●	
Arthritis/arthralgia	Minor	Minor	Minor	Minor	Minor
Gastrointestinal ulceration	Minor	Minor	Minor	Minor	Minor
Ileocaecal lesions	●	●			
Colitis			●		

(continued)

Table 2.4 (continued)

	Mason and Barnes [62]	Behçet's disease research committee of Japan 1974 and 1987 [79, 137]	O'Duffy [145]	Cheng and Zhang [147]	Dilsen et al. 1986 [146]
Vasculitis/thrombophlebitis	Minor	Minor	Minor	Minor	
Large vessel arteritis			•	•	
CNS lesions	Minor	Minor	Minor	Minor	
CVS lesions	Minor				
Epididymitis	Minor	Minor		Minor	Minor
Pulmonary – haemoptysis/fibrosis				Minor	Minor
Renal – ulceration/haematuria				Minor	
Family history	Minor				Minor
DIAGNOSIS REQUIRES	3 major or 2 major + 2 minor	C – 4 major, 1 – 3 major or 2 major + 2 minor	Oral or genital ulceration + 2 other major	C – 3 major or 2 major + 2 minor, 1 – 2 major or 1 major + 2 minor	*Definite:* pathergy(+) and 2 major or 1 major and 1 minor or pathergy (–) and 3 major or 2 major and 2 minor

C complete form of disease, *I* incomplete form of disease, • manifestations described by authors

BS was being studied in China at about the same time and when there was little communication between Chinese physicians and those in other parts of the world. Our Chinese colleagues also produced diagnostic criteria in which they accepted only three, not four, major features as described by Behçet himself, their scheme otherwise being almost identical to those of Mason and Barnes and from Japan (Table 2.4) [147].

In 1993 Davatchi and colleagues produced Iranian diagnostic criteria, based on their high case load, both in a traditional form and as a "diagnostic tree," and validated these against a panel of patients derived from several Asian countries [148, 149].

The International Study Group for Behçet's Disease meanwhile had undertaken an international survey of the incidence of clinical manifestations of BS leading to the formulation of International Criteria [21–23]. This served three purposes:

1. Data regarding the *frequency of clinical manifestations* was derived from 914 patients from seven countries which were submitted by colleagues experienced in the diagnosis, study and treatment of the syndrome. The specificity and sensitivity of each manifestation was calculated.
2. The *performance of the existing schemes of diagnostic criteria* in use in 1989 was calculated for sensitivity and specificity. This showed a high specificity (≥90%) for the major manifestations, thrombophlebitis, arterial occlusion and/or aneurysm formation, CNS involvement and epididymitis (100%).
3. A *new set of criteria was derived*, which required the presence of oral ulcers (present in 98% of patients) as a common clinical feature (Table 2.5). Although these were initially called diagnostic criteria it was rapidly realised that these served as classification criteria. In discussion at the fifth International Conference on Behçet's Disease, Mayo Clinic, 1989, at which these results were presented it was recorded that "it was recommended that these (criteria) be known as "classification" criteria since they are more useful in ensuring the uniformity of groups of patients for clinical and laboratory studies, and for teaching purposes, than they are for diagnosing the individual case" [23].

This, therefore, follows the pattern of classification criteria for rheumatoid arthritis [150], systemic lupus erythematous [151], ankylosing spondylitis [152] and osteoarthritis [153].

These criteria (Table 2.5) were further validated by assessing the sensitivity in a new set of 300 patients from seven countries, sensitivity being determined against 62 control patients from China and performed well [154].

In formulating Iranian diagnostic criteria in 1993 further evaluation of the performance of diagnostic criteria schemes was again performed including that of the International Criteria. Although the earlier schemes did not perform as well in that study, it is regrettable that the International Criteria for Classification were included as diagnostic criteria since, as mentioned above, they serve a different function – for the classification of groups of patients and should not be used for the diagnosis of the individual patient [149, 155].

Table 2.5 International criteria for classification of Behçet's Disease [21, 22]

Recurrent oral ulceration
Minor aphthous, major aphthous or herpetiform ulceration observed by a physician or reported reliably by patient
Recurrent at least three times in one 12-month period
Plus 2 of:
Recurrent genital ulceration
Recurrent genital aphthous ulceration or scarring, especially males, observed by physician or reliably reported by patient
Eye lesions
Anterior uveitis
Posterior uveitis
Cells in vitreous on slit lamp examination
or
Retinal Vasculitis observed by qualified physician (ophthalmologist)
Skin lesions
Erythema nodosum-like lesions observed by physician or reliably reported by patient
Pseudo folliculitis
Papulopustular lesions
or
Acneiform nodules consistent with Behçet's disease – observed by a physician and in post-adolescent patients not receiving corticosteroids
Positive pathergy test
An erythematous papule, >2 mm, at the prick site after the application of a sterile needle, 20–22 gauge, which obliquely penetrated avascular skin to a depth of 5 mm; read by a physician at 48 hours

Note: Findings are applicable if no other clinical explanation is present

One, therefore, still needs to ask the question "how does one diagnose BS in the individual patient in the routine clinical situation"? The Hippocratic method of grouping together sufficient features to make a diagnosis has always been, and remains, the only way of making a diagnosis. However, the former diagnostic criteria have probably outlived their usefulness as a greater understanding and awareness of the syndrome has developed over the years.

A high "*index of suspicion*," and *guidelines to diagnosis* for the less experienced physician, suggest that a diagnosis of BS should be contemplated when two or three manifestations occur, such as:

- painful recurrent mouth ulcers and genital ulcers, or
- painful recurrent mouth ulcers and an inflamed eye, or
- painful recurrent mouth ulcers, genital ulcers and an inflamed eye, or
- painful recurrent mouth ulcers, genital ulcers and inflamed joints, or
- painful recurrent mouth ulcers, genital ulcers and skin lesions, or
- inflamed eye(s) and joints and skin manifestations, or
- inflamed eye(s), thrombophlebitis and skin manifestations, or
- painful recurrent mouth ulcers, an inflamed eye and a positive family history [156].

This should lead to the referral of the patient to a physician with a greater knowledge and experience of the syndrome. Specialist, or referral, clinics have been developed in those countries where there is a sufficiently high prevalence of the syndrome, such as in Turkey (Istanbul, Ankara), Iran (Tehran) and USA (New York) while in other centres patients are seen in the routine clinics of those physicians with a special interest and experience in the subject.

The same clinical manifestations may also occur in other conditions which, therefore, are included in the differential diagnosis of BS. These include Reiter's syndrome, seronegative arthropathies, inflammatory bowel disease, sarcoidosis, other vasculitides, multiple sclerosis and pulmonary embolism (Table 2.6) many of which have only been described in detail since 1937 [157].

Treatment

The treatment of BS has developed rapidly in recent years. Double blind controlled clinical trials are few and include trials of colchicine [158], and azathioprine [33], Initial treatments were entirely symptomatic and although these remain important, for example topical steroid applications for ulceration, suppressive treatment for serious eye or vascular involvement includes systemic corticosteroids, immunosuppressive agents and anti-TNFα preparations [41, 159]. This is summarised in Table 2.7.

Disease or Syndrome?

The name of the condition has been agreed internationally as being attributed to Behçet. It is recognised that a small minority of our colleagues prefer the addition of the name of Adamantiades who did describe a case before Behçet; but then so did a number of other workers from several different countries. What is more contentious is whether the title should be Behçet's Disease or Syndrome and it will be seen from the list of references in this book that both titles are in common use and may be considered to be interchangeable. However, what are the reasons behind this difference in nomenclature? The definitions of the words are:

- disease – a disorder of structure or function in a human, animal or plant, especially one that produces specific symptoms or that affects a specific part,
- syndrome – a group of symptoms or signs which consistently occur together.

Those who prefer the title "disease" do so as they regard it as a unified condition – a specific disease – with a wide spectrum of manifestations albeit, at present, of unknown aetiology. Certainly Behçet's Disease does not fulfil Koch's postulates. The use of the term Behçet's Disease was proposed by Lee [160] based on a review of the titles of published works and a survey of the opinions of 22 colleagues.

Table 2.6 Highlights of the clinical manifestations of Behçet's Syndrome and differential diagnosis (from Rheumatology 1999;38:1171, with permission) [157]

Manifestation		Differential diagnosis
Mouth ulcers	Majority similar to common aphthous ulcers regarding appearance, localization and discomfort/pain; more frequent and frequently multiple; may scar	
Genital ulcers	Most commonly scrotal or vulval, painful, recurrent and usually with scarring, Urethral discharge and penile lesions very rare	Reiter's syndrome – painless ulceration
Skin	Acneiform lesions as common acne in appearance and histology but also at uncommon sites such as the extremities	Reiter's syndrome. Seronegative arthropathies
	Not psoriasis	Inflammatory bowel disease
Eyes	Panuveitis and retinal vasculitis, usually bilateral occurring within about 2 yr of the onset of the disease	Sarcoidosis
	Conjunctivitis and sicca syndrome most unusual	
Joints	Monarthritis in 50%, otherwise oligoarticular or polyarticular involving relatively few joints; may be symmetrical; knees most frequently; intermittent resolving in 2–4 weeks or chronic and continuous; not involving sacroiliac joints or spine; deformity and erosions rare, synovial fluid usually inflammatory with good mucin clot	Inflammatory arthropathies
Peripheral arterial and venous disease	Subclinical peripheral large vein disease uncommon, usually involves large segments with skip areas without embolization; arteritis with occlusion and/or pseudo-aneurysms; microaneurysms of the polyarteritic type very uncommon	Other vasculitides
Neurological involvement	Peripheral neuropathy and isolated cerebellar involvement very unusual, headaches with dural sinus thrombosis; vascular central nervous system lesions including transverse myelitis-type manifestation	MS
	Multiple sclerosis with aphthous ulcers a problem but no plaques on magnetic resonance imaging	
Pulmonary involvement	Haemoptysis associated with pulmonary arterial aneurysm; pulmonary artery occlusion; pleural involvement uncommon; interstitial involvement very rare	Pulmonary embolism. Any cause of haemoptysis
Gastrointestinal involvement	Severe abdominal pain; ulcerative lesions at any level but mainly in the ileocaecal region; mild gastrointestinal symptoms should not be associated with Behçet's syndrome	Inflammatory bowel ase
Cardiac disease	Pericarditis, valve lesions and coronary artery involvement uncommon; rarely intracardiac thrombi	Valve lesions in seronegative arthropathies

Table 2.7 Outline of drug treatment of Behçet's Syndrome (from Rheumatology 2006;45:246, with permission) [159]

Manifestation	Mild	Severe
Mucocutaneous		
Mouth ulceration	Mouth washes	Thalidomide
	Topical steroids	Azathioprine
		Infliximab/etanercept
Genital ulceration	Topical steroids	Colchicine in females
		Thalidomide
		Azathioprine
		Infliximab
Erythema nodosum		Colchicine
		Corticosteroids
Acne		Local corticosteroid/antibiotic applications (in combination
Arthritis/arthralgia	Simple and non-steroidal anti-inflammatory analgesics	Colchicine,corticosteroids, azathioprine, interferon-α
Ocular involvement		
Anterior uveitis	Topical steroids	Azathioprine
Panuveitis, posterior uveitis		Oral cyclosporine A
		Corticosteroids
		Interferon-α
		Infliximab
Retinal vasculitis		Azathioprine
		Oral cyclosporine A
		Pulsed IV/oral corticosteroids
		Interferon-α
		Infliximab
Vasculitis		
Thrombophlebitis	Symptomatic treatment	Azathioprine
		Low dose aspirin
Arteritis		Pulsed IV/oral corticosteroids
		Pulsed IV/oral cyclophosphamide
		Azathioprine
		Infliximab
Neurological involvement		
Dural sinus thrombosis		Corticosteroids
Parenchymal disease		Pulsed IV cyclophosphamide or oral azathioprine plus pulsed IV/oral corticosteroids
		Infliximab
Gastrointestinal lesions		
Small/large bowel ulceration		Sulphasalazine, azathioprine, infliximab

The latter did reveal a majority (64%) in favour of the title Behçet's Disease. Lee expressed a concern that even those particularly interested in the condition did not have an agreed diagnostic terminology.

On the other hand, there are many who prefer the term syndrome, at least until even more knowledge has been gained about the aetiopathogenesis, on the basis that one cannot be entirely certain that it is a single disease process. That view was stated in 1979 [120] and even now, 30 years later and with a huge explosion of available research data, this still cannot be answered. The aetiopathogenesis remains unknown, no specific diagnostic test is available, and there is a considerable variation in frequency and prevalence of the syndrome and of its constituent manifestations in different parts of the world. It is not transmissible to unaffected people and, despite the genetic links and familial groupings that have been established, it is not predictable in affected families. Additionally there have been described clusters of associated features – acneiform lesions and arthritis/enthesitis; superficial thrombophlebitis is usually found with large vein thrombosis which clusters with dural vein thrombosis – raising a question of the uniformity of the "disease" [41]. This is not an entirely new concept since Lehner described a "spectral involvement or classification" of BS:

- *Mucosal aphthosis (M-C) type* – oral and genital ulceration ± skin lesions
- *Arthritic type* – joint involvement plus ≥ M-C features
- *Neurological type* – brain involvement plus some or all of the M-C and arthritis features
- *Ocular type* – uveitis plus some or all of the M-C, arthritic and neurological features

Lehner related different immunological findings to the different classification groups, which was before the recognition of a vasculopathy [138, 139, 161].

The terminology currently used by some colleagues – neuro-Behçet, oculo-Behçet, entero-Behçet, vasculo-Behçet – serves to emphasise the principal clinical problem affecting the patient without implying a sub-section of the syndrome.

Thus, the condition is an association of clinical and laboratory manifestations such that the pattern is recognised by experienced physicians as being "Behçet's Syndrome".

International Liaison

A multidisciplinary International Symposium on Behçet's Disease was held in Rome in December 1964. Eight papers were presented including a review of the syndrome, the authors and discussants coming from Germany, Italy, Japan, Turkey and the United Kingdom including Sezer [119], Strachan and Wigzell [59] who had contributed to the early literature on the condition. At this meeting Marchionini presented a paper on the "Dermatological View of Morbus Hulusi Behçet" [162]. He reflected that he had been present in Istanbul when "this syndrome was publicly named." He died before the resulting monograph was published which was dedicated to him [163].

Thirteen years later, as part of the Istanbul Medical Convention, a second International Symposium on Behçet's Disease was organised by Dilşen at which it was decided to hold a regular series of international conferences the next to be in Tokyo. These were initially held every four years but as the size of these conferences increased, both in terms of the number of participants and abstracts submitted, the interval between conferences was reduced to every three and then two years, and this continues. Proceedings reports of the first to tenth conferences (1964–2002) were published [163–172] but thereafter this was discontinued on the basis that the most important research results were published in peer reviewed journals (Table 2.8).

At the Istanbul Symposium (1977) it was decided to start an International Study Group on Behçet's Disease members of which were those particularly interested in, and researching into, Behçet's syndrome. The aim of this group was to maintain communications and contribute to multicentre research. This group continued, being more formally organised after the London conference (1985), intending to be a small number of colleagues working together. However, it became progressively larger as multidisciplinary interest and research developed and an increasing number of colleagues sought membership. Therefore, at the International Conference in Tunis (1996) it was decided to explore the possibility of starting an *International Society for Behçet's Disease (ISBD)* to succeed the Study Group and open membership to all who are interested in the syndrome. Further progress was made in Reggio Emilia, Italy (1998) and the society was formally founded at the International Conference in Seoul, Korea, in 2000 its constitutional *aim* being "to advance the knowledge of the aetiology, pathogenesis, diagnosis, natural history, clinical features, treatment and management of Behçet's Disease." The details of the ISBD may be found on its website – http://www.behcet.ws. Every two years, International Conferences continue under the auspices of the ISBD the next being scheduled to be held in London in July 2010.

Table 2.8 International conferences on Behçet's Disease

International conferences on Behçet's Disease			Reference to publication
1st	1964	Rome	[163]
2nd	1977	Istanbul	[164]
3rd	1981	Tokyo	[165]
4th	1985	London	[166]
5th	1989	Mayo Clinic, USA	[167]
6th	1993	Paris	[168]
7th	1996	Tunis	[169]
8th	1998	Reggio Emilia, Italy	[170]
9th	2000	Seoul	[171]
10th	2002	Berlin	[172]
11th	2004	Antalya, Turkey	
12th	2006	Lisbon	
13th	2008	Portschach, Austria	
14th	2010	London	

At a *national* level, and in liaison with the ISBD, through national organisations in medical/scientific disciplines (internal medicine, dermatology, rheumatology, ophthalmology, STD clinics, gynaecology, oral medicine, neurology, gastroenterology, immunology, etc.), groups dedicated to Behçet's Syndrome have been formed in Korea, Japan (governmental) and the United Kingdom (UK Forum on BS).

Similarly patient orientated organisations have been formed in Japan, Turkey, the United Kingdom and the USA and organise their own international conferences alongside the medical/scientific conferences.

References

1. Behçet H (1937) Uber rezidiverende, aphthose, durch ein Virus verursachte Gescgwure am Mund, am Auge und an den Genitalen. Derm Woch 105:1152–1157
2. Behçet H (1938) Considerations sue les lesions aphtheuses de la bouche et des parties genitals, ainsi que sur les manifestations oculaires d'origine probablement virutique et observations concernant leur foyer d'infection. Bull Soc Fr Dermatol Syphiligr 45:420–433
3. Behçet H (1940) Some observations on the clinical picture of the so-called triple symptom complex. Dermatologica 81:73–78
4. Saylan T (1979) Commemorative lecture for Professor Dr. Hulusi Behçet. In: Dilşen N, Konice M, Övül C (eds) Behçet's disease: proceedings of an international symposium on Behçet's disease, Istanbul 29–30 September 1977, International congress series no. 467. Excerpta Medica, Amsterdam, pp 1–5
5. Saylan T (1997) Life story of Dr. Hulusi Behçet. Yonsei Med J 38:327–332
6. Dilsen N (1997) History and Development of Behçet's Disease. In: Hamza M (ed) Behçet's Disease; proceeding of the seventh international conference on Behçet's Disease held at Tunis 10–11 October 1996. Pub Adhoua, Tunis, pp 15–21. ISBN 9973-17-850-5
7. Lipschutz B (1927) Ulcus vulvae acutum. In: Jadassohn J (ed) Handbuch der Haut- und Geschlechtskrankheiten, vol 21. Julius Springer, Berlin, p 392
8. Fuchs A (1926) Ueber chronische multiple Knotenbildung am Körper mit häufig rezidivierender eitriger Iritis und Skleritis. Deutsche Med Woch 36: 1502–1505
9. Adams F (1849) The genuine works of Hippocrates, translated from the Greek. The Sydenham Society, London, pp 403–404
10. Feigenbaum A (1956) Description of Behçet's syndrome in the Hippocratic third book of endemic diseases. Br J Ophthalmol 40:355–357
11. Gilbert W (1920) Arch Augenheik 86:50–51
12. Shigeta T (1924) Recurrent iritis with hypopyon and its pathological findings. Acta Soc Ophthmol Jap 28:516
13. Adamantiades B (1931) Sur un cas d'iritis à hyopyon récidivante. Ann Ocul 168:271
14. Adamantiades B, Lorando N (1949) Sur le syndrome complexe de l'uveite recidivante ou soi-disant syndrome complexe de Behçet. Presse Med 57:501–503
15. Dascalopoulos N (1932) Sur deux cas d'uveite recidivante. Ann Ocul 169:387–393
16. Chauffard A, Brodin P, Wolf M (1923) Stomatite et vulvite aphtheuses suivies de troubles dementiels passagers. Bull Mem Soc Med Hop Paris 47:841–844
17. Neumann 1894: quoted by Wien MS, Perstein HO (1932) Ulcus vulvae acutum associated with lesions of the mouth. JAMA 98:461–466
18. Planner H, Remenovsky F (1922) Beitrage zur Kenntis der ulcerationen am ausseren weiblichen Genitale. Arch Dermatol Syph (Berlin) 111:162–188
19. Whitwell GPB (1934) Recurrent buccal and vulval ulcers with associated embolic phenomena in skin and eyes. Br J Dermatol 46:414–419
20. Chajek T, Fainaru M (1975) Behçet's disease. Report of 41 cases and a review of the literature. Medicine (Baltimore) 54:179–196

21. International Study Group for Behçet's Disease (1990) Criteria for diagnosis of Behçet's Disease. Lancet 335:1078–1080
22. International Study Group for Behçet's Disease (1992) Evaluation of diagnostic ("classification") criteria in Behçet's disease – towards internationally agreed criteria. Br J Rheumatol 31:299–308
23. International Study Group for Behçet's Disease (1991) Evaluation of diagnostic ("classification") criteria in Behçet's Disease – towards internationally agreed criteria. In: O'Duffy JD, Kokmen E (eds) Behçet's Disease: basic and clinical aspects. Marcel Dekker, New York, pp 11–39
24. Cooke BED (1979) Oral ulceration in Behçet's syndrome. In: Lehner T, Barnes CG (eds) Behçet's Syndrome: clinical and immunological features. Academic, London, pp 143–149
25. Lehner T (1967) Behçet's syndrome and autoimmunity. Br med J 1:465–467
26. Sircus W, Church R, Kelleher J (1957) Recurrent aphthous ulceration of the mouth. Q J Med 26:235–249
27. Konice M, Dilsen N, Aral O (1979) The preaphthous phase of Behçet's disease. In: Dilsen N, Konice M, Övül C (eds) Behçet's disease: proceedings of an international symposium on Behçet's disease, Istanbul 29–30 September 1977, International congress series no. 467. Excerpta Medica, Amsterdam, pp 199–203
28. Kim DK, Chang SN, Bang D et al (1994) Clinical analysis of 40 cases of childhood-onset Behçet's disease. Pediatr Dermatol 11:95–101
29. Dunlop EMC (1979) Genital and other manifestations of Behçet's disease seen in venereological practice. In: Lehner T, Barnes CG (eds) Behçet's Syndrome: clinical and immunological features. Academic, London, pp 159–175
30. Dinning WJ (1986) An overview of ocular manifestations. In: Lehner T, Barnes CG (eds) Recent advances in Behçet's Disease, Royal Society of Medicine Services international congress and symposium series no. 103. Royal Society of Medicine, London, pp 227–233
31. Kansu T, Kadayifcilar S (2005) Visual aspects of Behçet's disease. Curr Neurol Neurosci Rep 5:382–388
32. Kitaichi N, Miyazaki A, Iwata D et al (2007) Ocular features of Behçet's disease: an international collaborative study. Br J Ophthalmol 91:1573–1574
33. Kacmaz RO, Kempen JH, Newcomb C et al (2008) Ocular inflammation in Behçet's disease: incidence of ocular complications and of loss of visual acuity. Am J Ophthalmol 146:828–836
34. Yazici H, Pazerli H, Barnes CG et al (1990) A controlled trial of azathioprine in Behçet's syndrome. N Engl J Med 322:281–285
35. Hamuryudan V, Ozyazgan Y, Fresko I et al (2002) Interferon-alfa combined with azathioprine for the uveitis of Behçet's disease: an open study. Isr Med Assoc J 4:928–930
36. Krause L, Altenburg A, Pleyer U et al (2008) Longterm visual prognosis of patients with ocular Adamantiades-Behçet's disease treated with interferon-alpha-2a. J Rheumatol 35:896–903
37. Nazzaro P (1966) Cutaneous manifestations of Behçet's disease; clinical and histopathological findings. In: Monacelli M, Nazzaro P (eds) Behçet's disease. Karger, Basel, pp 15–41
38. Chun SI, Su WP, Lee S et al (1989) Erythema nodosum-like lesions in Behçet's syndrome: a histopathologic study of 30 cases. J Cutan Pathol 16:259–265
39. Lee ES, Bang D, Lee S (1997) Dermatologic manifestations of Behçet's disease. Yonsei Med J 38:380–389
40. Alpsoy E, Zouboulis CC, Ehrlich GE (2007) Mucocutaneous lesions of Behçet's disease. Yonsei Med J 48:573–585
41. Yazici H, Fresco I, Yurdakul S (2007) Behçet's syndrome: disease manifestations, management, and advances in treatment. Nat Clin Pract Rheumatol 3:148–155
42. Kienbaum S, Zouboulis CC, Waibel M et al (1993) Chemotactic neutrophilic vasculitis: a new histological pattern of vasculitis found in mucocutaneous lesions of patients with Adamantiades-Behçet's disease. In: Wechsler B, Godeau P (eds) Behçet's disease, International congress series 1037. Excerpta Medica, Amsterdam, pp 337–341

43. Kienbaum S, Zouboulis CC, Waibel M et al (1993) Papulopustular skin lesions in Adamantiades-Behçet's disease show a similar histopathological pattern as the classical mucocutaneous manifestations. In: Wechsler B, Godeau P (eds) Behçet's disease, International congress series 1037. Excerpta Medica, Amsterdam, pp 331–336

44. Melikoglu M, Kural-Seyahi E, Tascilar K et al (2008) The unique features of Vasculitis in Behçet's Syndrome. Clin Rev Allergy Immunol 35:40–46

45. Blobner F (1937) Zur rezidivierenden hypopyon-iritis. Zeitschrift Augenheik 91:129–139

46. Jensen T (1941) Sur les ulcerations aphtheuses de la muqueues de la bouche et de la peau geni-tale combines avec les symptoms oculaires (Syndrome de Behçet). Acta Dermatol Venereol 22:64–79

47. Yazici H, Tüzün Y, Pazarli H et al (1980) The combined use of HLA-B5 and the pathergy test as diagnostic markers of Behçet's disease in Turkey. J Rheumatol 7:206–210

48. Davies PG, Fordham JN, Kirwan JR et al (1984) The pathergy test and Behçet's syndrome in Britain. Ann Rheum Dis 43:70–73

49. Yazici H, Chamberlain MA, Tüzün Y et al (1984) A comparative study of the pathergy reaction among Turkish and British patients with Behçet's disease. Ann Rheum Dis 43:74–75

50. Yazici H, Tüzün Y, Tanman S et al (1985) Male patients with Behçet's syndrome have stronger pathergy reactions. Clin Exp Rheumatol 3:137–141

51. Suzuki K, Mizuno N (1982) Intracutaneous test with physiological saline in Behçet's disease. In: Inaba G (ed) Behçet's disease: pathogenetic mechanism and clinical future, Japanese Medical Research Foundation publication no. 18. University of Tokyo Press, Tokyo, pp 333–342

52. Dilsen N, Konice M, Aral O et al (1993) Comparative study of the skin pathergy test with blunt and sharp needles in Behçet's disease: confirmed specificity but decreased sensitivity with sharp needles. Ann Rheum Dis 52:823–825

53. Fresko I, Yazici H, Bayramicli M et al (1993) Effect of surgical cleaning of the skin on the pathergy phenomenon in Behçet's syndrome. Ann Rheum Dis 52:619–620

54. Hatemi I, Hatemi G, Celik AF et al (2008) Frequency of pathergy phenomenon and other features of Behçet's syndrome among patients with inflammatory bowel disease. Clin Exp Rheumatol 26:591–595

55. Dilsen N, Konice M, Aral O et al (1986) Standardization and evaluation of the skin pathergy test in Behçet's disease and controls. In: Lehner T, Barnes CG (eds) Recent advances in Behçet's disease, Royal Society of Medicine Services international congress and symposium series no. 103. Royal Society of Medicine, London, pp 169–172

56. Aral O, Dilsen N, Konice M et al (1986) Positive skin pathergy reactivity as a genetic marker of Behçet's disease. In: Lehner T, Barnes CG (eds) Recent advances in Behçet's disease, Royal Society of Medicine Services international congress and symposium series no. 103. Royal Society of Medicine, London, pp 173–175

57. Dilsen N, Konice M, Aral O et al (1993) Important implications of skin pathergy test in Behçet's disease. In: Wechsler B, Godeau P (eds) Behçet's disease, International congress series 1037. Excerpta Medica, Amsterdam, pp 229–233

58. Cakir N, Yazici H, Chamberlain MA et al (1991) Response to intradermal injection of mono-sodium urate crystals in Behçet's syndrome. Ann Rheum Dis 50:634–636

59. Strachan RW, Wigzell FW (1963) Polyarthritis in Behçet's multiple symptom complex. Ann Rheum Dis 22:26–35

60. Oshima Y, Shimizu T, Yokohari R et al (1963) Clinical studies on Behçet's syndrome. Ann Rheum Dis 22:36–45

61. Mason RM, Barnes CG (1968) Behçet-Syndrom mit Arthritis. Schweiz Med Wochenschr 98:665–671

62. Mason RM, Barnes CG (1969) Behçet's syndrome with arthritis. Ann Rheum Dis 28:95–103

63. Nasr F (1969) Les manifestations articulaires de la maladie de Behçet. Rev Rheum 36:81–83

64. Bisson M, Amor B, Kahan A et al (1971) Les manifestations articulaires de l'aphthose (syndrome de Behçet). Sem Hôp Paris 47:2024–2033

65. Dilsen N, Konice M, Övül C (1979) Arthritis patterns in Behçet's disease. In: Dilşen N, Konice M, Övül C (eds) Behçet's disease: proceedings of an international symposium on Behçet's disease, Istanbul 29–30 September 1977, International congress series no. 467. Excerpta Medica, Amsterdam, pp 145–153

66. Yurdakul S, Yazici H, Tüzün Y et al (1983) The arthritis of Behçet's disease: a prospective study. Ann Rheum Dis 42:505–515

67. Dawes PT, Raman D, Haslock I (1983) Acute synovial rupture in Behçet's syndrome. Ann Rheum Dis 42:591–592

68. Hashimoto T, Shimizu T (1975) Immunohistopathological studies on arthritis in Behçet's syndrome. Scand J Rheumatol 4(Suppl 8):36–38

69. Vernon-Roberts B, Barnes CG, Revell PA (1978) Synovial pathology in Behçet's syndrome. Ann Rheum Dis 37:139–145

70. Ben-Dov I, Zimmerman J (1982) Deforming arthritis of the hands in Behçet's disease. J Rheumatol 9:617–618

71. Currey HLF, Elson RA, Mason M (1968) Surgical treatment of manubrio-sternal pain in Behçet's syndrome. J Bone Joint Surg 50B:836–840

72. Takeuchi A, Mori M, Hashimoto A (1984) Radiographic abnormalities in patients with Behçet's disease. Clin Exp Rheumatol 2:259–262

73. Jawad ASM, Goodwill CJ (1986) Behçet's disease with erosive arthritis. Ann Rheum Dis 45:961–962

74. Dilşen N, Konice M, Aral O (1986) Why Behçet's disease should be accepted as a seronegative arthritis. In: Lehner T, Barnes CG (eds) Recent advances in Behçet's disease, Royal Society of Medicine Services international congress and symposium series no. 103. Royal Society of Medicine, London, pp 281–284

75. Moll JMH, Haslock MD, Macrae IF et al (1974) Associations between ankylosing spondylitis, psoriatic arthritis, Reiter's disease, the intestinal arthropathies, and Behçet's syndrome. Medicine 53:343–364

76. Yazici H, Turunc M, Özdoğan H et al (1987) Observer variation in grading sacroiliac radiographs might be a cause of "sacroiliitis" reported in certain disease states. Ann Rheum Dis 46:139–145

77. Chamberlain MA, Robertson RJH (1993) A controlled study of sacroiliitis in Behçet's disease. Br J Rheumatol 32:693–698

78. Scavo D, Cramarossa L (1966) Discussion. In: Monacelli M, Nazzaro P (eds) Behçet's disease. Karger, Basel, pp 137–138

79. Shimizu T (1979) Clinicopathological studies on Behçet's disease. In: Dilsen N, Konice M, Övül C (eds) Behçet's disease: proceedings of an international symposium on Behçet's disease, Istanbul 29–30 September 1977, International congress series no. 467. Excerpta Medica, Amsterdam, pp 9–43

80. Shimizu T (1977) Vascular lesions of Behçet's disease. Cardioangiology 1:124

81. Shimizu T (1977) Behçet's disease: a systemic inflammatory disease. In: Shiokawa Y (ed) Vascular lesions of collagen diseases and related conditions. Tokyo University Press, Tokyo, pp 201–211

82. Bayraktar Y, Balkanci F, Demirkazik F et al (1993) Type of vessel involvement in patients with Behçet's disease. In: Wechsler B, Godeau P (eds) Behçet's disease, International congress series 1037. Excerpta Medica, Amsterdam, pp 331–336

83. Hamza M (1993) Angio Behçet. In: Wechsler B, Godeau P (eds) Behçet's Disease, International congress series 1037. Excerpta Medica, Amsterdam, pp 523–526

84. Dong Y, Liu J (1993) Vasculo-Behçet's disease. In: Wechsler B, Godeau P (eds) Behçet's disease, International congress series 1037. Excerpta Medica, Amsterdam, pp 527–530

85. El-Ramahi KM, Al-Dalaan A, Al-Balaa S et al (1993) Vascular involvement in Behçet's disease. In: Wechsler B, Godeau P (eds) Behçet's disease, International congress series 1037. Excerpta Medica, Amsterdam, pp 531–536

86. Demirkazik FB, Balkanci F, Cekirge S et al (1993) Vascular involvement in Behçet's disease. In: Wechsler B, Godeau P (eds) Behçet's Disease, International Congress Series 1037. Excerpta Medica, Amsterdam, pp 537–540

87. Yazici H, Yurdakul S, Hamuryudan V et al (2003) The vasculitides: Behçet's syndrome. In: Hochberg MC, Silman AJ, Smolen JS, Weinblatt ME, Weisman MH (eds) Rheumatology, 3rd edn. Elsevier, Barcelona, pp 1665–1669

88. Lehner T (2000) Immunopathogenesis of Behçet's disease. In: Bang D, Lee E-S, Lee S (eds) Behçet's disease: proceedings of the international conference on Behçet's disease, held in Seoul, Korea, May 27–29, 2000. Design Mecca, Seoul, pp 3–18. ISBN 89-951655-1-0

89. Haskard DO, Chambers JC, Kooner JS (2000) Impaired vascular endothelial function in Behçet's syndrome can be restored by Vitamin C. In: Bang D, Lee E-S, Lee S (eds) Behçet's disease: proceedings of the international conference on Behçet's disease, held in Seoul, Korea, May 27–29, 2000. Design Mecca, Seoul, p 229. ISBN 89-951655-1-0

90. Chambers JC, Haskard DO, Kooner JS (2001) Vascular endothelial function and oxidative stress mechanisms in patients with Behçet's syndrome. J Am Coll Cardiol 37:517–520

91. Kaiser EDE, Ozyazgan Y, Rao NA (2003) Immunohistopathology of Behçet's disease. In: Zierhut M, Ohno S (eds) Immunology of Behçet's disease. Swets & Zeitlinger, Lisse, pp 47–55

92. Dilsen N, Konice M, Gazioğlu K et al (1979) Pleuropulmonary manifestations in Behçet's disease. In: Dilsen N, Konice M, Övül C (eds) Behçet's disease: proceedings of an international symposium on Behçet's disease, Istanbul 29–30 September 1977, International congress series no. 467. Excerpta Medica, Amsterdam, pp 163–1703

93. Okamoto S, Kimura T, Masugi Y et al (1969) A case report of Behçet's syndrome which showed a massive haemoptysis. J Jap Soc Intern Med 58:1268

94. Petty TL, Scoggin CH, Good JT (1977) Recurrent pneumonia in Behçet's syndrome. JAMA 238:2529–2530

95. Efthimiou J, Spiro SG (1986) Pulmonary involvement in Behçet's syndrome. In: Lehner T, Barnes CG (eds) Recent advances in Behçet's disease, Royal Society of Medicine Services international congress and symposium series no. 103. Royal Society of Medicine, London, pp 261–266

96. Erkan F, Gül A, Tasali E (2001) Pulmonary manifestations of Behçet's disease. Thorax 56:572–578

97. Hamuryudan V, Er T, Seyahi E et al (2004) Pulmonary artery aneurysms in Behçet's syndrome. Am J Med 117:867–870

98. Yazici H, Esen F (2008) Mortality in Behçet's syndrome. Clin Exp Rheumatol 26(Suppl 51): S138–S140

99. Berlin C (1944) Behçet's syndrome with involvement of central nervous system: report of a case of necropsy. Arch Dermatol Syph 49:227

100. Evans AD, Pallis CA, Spillane JD (1957) Involvement of the nervous system in Behçet's syndrome; report of three cases and isolation of virus. Lancet 273:349–453

101. Rubinstein LJ, Urich H (1963) Meningoencephalitis of Behçet's disease: case report with pathological findings Brain 86:151–160

102. Pallis CA (1966) Behçet's disease and the nervous system. Trans St Johns Hosp Dermatol Soc 52:201–206

103. Pallis CA, Fudge BJ (1956) The neurological complications of Behçet's syndrome. AMA Arch Neurol Psyhchiatry 75:1–14

104. Al-Araji A, Sharquie K, Al-Rawi Z (2003) Prevalence and patterns of neurological involvement in Behçet's disease: a prospective study from Iraq. J Neurol Neurosurg Psychiatry 74:608–613

105. Kidd D (2006) The prevalence of headache in Behçet's syndrome. Rheumatology (Oxford) 45:621–623

106. Fukuda Y, Hayashi H, Kuwara N (1982) Pathological studies on neuro-Behçet's disease. In: Inaba G (ed) Behçet's disease: pathogenetic mechanism and clinical future, Japanese Medical Research Foundation publication no. 18. University of Tokyo Press, Tokyo, pp 137–143

107. Al-Araji A, Kidd DP (2009) Neuro-Behçet's disease: epidemiology, clinical characteristics, and management. Lancet Neurol 8:192–204

108. Khosravi F, Samangooei Sh (2000) The long term clinical outcome of central nervous system involvement in Behçet's disease. In: Bang D, Lee E-S, Lee S (eds) Behçet's disease: proceed-

ings of the international conference on Behçet's disease, held in Seoul, Korea, May 27–29, 2000. Design Mecca, Seoul, pp 302–306. ISBN 89-951655-1-0

109. Emmi L, Salvati G, Li Gobbi F et al (2000) A SPECT study protocol for the evaluation of cerebral blood flow alterations in Behçet's disease. In: Bang D, Lee E-S, Lee S (eds) Behçet's disease: proceedings of the international conference on Behçet's Disease, held in Seoul, Korea, May 27–29, 2000. Design Mecca, Seoul, pp 307–311. ISBN 89-951655-1-0

110. Boe J, Dalgaard JB, Scott D (1958) Mucocutaneous-ocular syndrome with intestinal involvement; a clinical and pathological study of four fatal cases. Am J Med 25:857–867

111. O'Duffy JD, Carney JA, Deodhar S (1971) Behçet's disease. Report of 10 cases, 3 with new manifestations. Ann Intern Med 75:561–570

112. Fukuda Y, Watanabe I (1979) Pathological studies on intestinal Behçet's (entero-Behçet's) disease. In: Dilsen N, Konice M, Övül C (eds) Behçet's disease: proceedings of an international symposium on Behçet's disease, Istanbul 29–30 September 1977, International congress series no. 467. Excerpta Medica, Amsterdam, pp 90–103

113. Sladen GE, Lehner T (1979) Gastrointestinal disorders in Behçet's syndrome and a comparison with recurrent oral ulcers. In: Lehner T, Barnes CG (eds) Behçet's syndrome: clinical and immunological features. Academic, London, pp 151–158

114. Hamza M (1988) Pharyngeal stenosis in Behçet's disease. Clin Exp Rheumatol 6:139–140

115. Houman MH, Ben Ghorbel I, Lamloum M (2002) Esophageal involvement in Behçet's disease. Yonsei Med J 43:457–460

116. Taylor CB, Low N, Raj S et al (1997) Behçet's syndrome progressing to gastrointestinal perforation in a West African male. Br J Rheumatol 36:498–501

117. Dowling CM, Hill ADK, Malone C et al (2008) Colonic perforation in Behçet's syndrome. World J Gastroenterol 14:6578–6580

118. Ebert EC (2009) Gastrointestinal manifestations of Behçet's disease. Dig Dis Sci 54(2):201–207

119. Sezer FN (1956) The isolation of a virus as the cause of Behçet's diseases. Am J Ophthalmol 36:301–315

120. Lehner T, Barnes CG (1979) Criteria for diagnosis and classification of Behçet's syndrome. In: Lehner T, Barnes CG (eds) Behçet's syndrome: clinical and immunological features. Academic, London, pp 1–9

121. Dilsen N, Konice M, Övül C et al (1982) A preliminary family study on Behçet's disease in Turkey. In: Inaba G (ed) Behçet's disease: pathogenetic mechanism and clinical future, Japanese Medical Research Foundation publication no. 18. University of Tokyo Press, Tokyo, pp 103–111

122. Ohno S, Aoki K, Sugiura S et al (1973) HL-A5 and Behçet's disease. Lancet 2:1383–1384

123. Yurdakul S, Günaydin I, Tüzün Y et al (1988) The prevalence of Behçet's syndrome in a rural area of northern Turkey. J Rheumatol 15:820–822

124. O'Duffy JD (1978) Summary of international symposium on Behçet's disease. J Rheumatol 5:229–233

125. Chamberlain MA (1977) Behçet's syndrome in 32 patients in Yorkshire. Ann Rheum Dis 36:491–499

126. Jankowski J, Crombie I, Jankowski R (1992) Behçet's syndrome in Scotland. Postgrad Med J 68:566–570

127. O'Neill TW, Silman AJ, Rigby AS, et al. (1993) Sex and regional differences in clinical manifestations of Behçet's disease. Br J Rheumatol 32(Suppl 1) p85

128. Yazici H, Tüzün Y, Pazarli H et al (1984) Influence of age of onset and patient's sex on the prevalence and severity of manifestations of Behçet's syndrome. Ann Rheum Dis 43: 783–789

129. Hamza M (1993) Juvenile Behçet's disease. In: Wechsler B, Godeau P (eds) Behçet's disease, International congress series 1037. Excerpta Medica, Amsterdam, pp 377–380

130. Shafaie N, Shahram F, Davatcghi F et al (1993) Behçet's disease in children. In: Wechsler B, Godeau P (eds) Behçet's disease, International congress series 1037. Excerpta Medica, Amsterdam, pp 381–383

131. Koné-Paut I, Bernard J-L (1993) Behçet's disease in children: a French nationwide survey. In: Wechsler B, Godeau P (eds) Behçet's disease, International congress series 1037. Excerpta Medica, Amsterdam, pp 385–389

132. Zouboulis CC, Kötter I, Djawari D et al (1997) Epidemiological features of Adamantiades-Behçet's disease in Germany and in Europe. Yonsei Med J 38:411–422

133. Sezer FN (1966) Discussion. In: Monacelli M, Nazzaro P (eds) Behçet's disease. Karger, Basel, p 139

134. Dudgeon JA (1961) Virological aspects of Behçet's disease. Proc R Soc Med 54:104–106

135. Dowling GB (1961) Behçet's disease. Proc R Soc Med 54:101–104

136. Mizushima Y (1991) Behçet's disease. Curr Opin Rheumatol 3:32–35

137. Mizushima Y (1988) Recent research into Behçet's disease in Japan. Int J Tissue React 10:59–65

138. Lehner T (1977) Oral ulceration and Behçet's syndrome. Gut 18:491–511

139. Lehner T, Batchelor JR (1979) Classification and an immunogenetic basis of Behçet's syndrome. In: Lehner T, Barnes CG (eds) Behçet's syndrome: clinical and immunological features. Academic, London, pp 14–32

140. Curth HO (1946) Recurrent genito-oral aphthosis with hypopyon (Behçet's syndrome). Arch Dermatol 54:179–196

141. Hewitt J, Escande JP, Laurent P et al (1969) Critères de prevision du syndrome de Behçet. Bull Soc Fr Dermatol Syphiligr 76:565–568

142. Hewitt J, Escande JP, Manesse S (1971) Révision des critères diagnostiques du syndrome de Behçet. Presse Med 79:901

143. Hubault A, Hamza M (1974) La maladie de Behçet en 1974. L'Actualité Rhumatologique. Expansion Scientifique, Paris, pp 43–55

144. Ben Ayed H, Hamza M (1976) La Maladie de Behçet: Les critères du diagnostique. Imprimerie Officielle, Tunis, pp 81–84

145. O'Duffy JD (1974) Suggested criteria for diagnosis of Behçet's disease. J Rheumatol 1(Suppl 1):18, abstract 32

146. Dilşen N, Konice M, Aral O (1986) Our diagnostic criteria of Behçet's disease – an overview. In: Lehner T, Barnes CG (eds) Recent advances in Behçet's disease, Royal Society of Medicine Services international congress and symposium series no. 103. Royal Society of Medicine, London, pp 177–180

147. Cheng SP, Zhang X-Q (1980) [Some special clinical manifestations of Behçet's disease – report of illustrative cases and review of literature (author's transl)] (in Chinese). Chinese J Intern Med 19:15–22

148. Davatchi F, Shahram F, Akbarian M et al (1997) APLAR validation of Behçet's disease diagnosis criteria. The Iran experience. In: Hamza M (ed) Behçet's disease; proceeding of the seventh international conference on Behçet's disease held at Tunis 10–11 October 1996. Pub Adhoua, Tunis, pp 212–216. ISBN 9973-17-850-5

149. Davatchi F, Shahram F, Akbarian M et al (1993) Accuracy of existing diagnosis criteria for Behçet's disease. In: Wechsler B, Godeau P (eds) Behçet's disease, International congress series 1037. Excerpta Medica, Amsterdam, pp 225–228

150. Arnett FC, Edworthy SM, Bloch DA et al (1988) The American Rheumatism Association 1987 revised criteria for the classification of rheumatoid arthritis. Arthritis Rheum 31:315–324

151. Tan EM, Cohen AS, Fries JF et al (1982) The 1982 revised criteria for the classification of systemic lupus erythematosus. Arthritis Rheum 25:1271–1277

152. Bennet PM, Wood PHN (1966) Recommendations – ankylosing spondylitis. In: Bennet PM, Wood PHN (eds) Population studies of the rheumatic diseases, International congress series no. 148. Excerpta Medica, Amsterdam, pp 456–457

153. Altman R, Asch E, Bloch D et al (1986) Development of criteria for the classification and reporting of osteoarthritis. Arthritis Rheum 29:1039–1049

154. O'Neill TW, Rigby AS, Silman AJ et al (1994) Validation of the International Study Group criteria for Behçet's disease. Br J Rheumatol 33:115–117

155. Silman AJ, Rooney BK (1998) Classification of Behçet's disease. In: Bang D, Lee E-S, Lee S (eds) Behçet's Disease: proceedings of the 8th international conference on Behçet's disease, held in Reggio Emilia, Italy, October 7–9, 1998. Design Mecca, Seoul, pp 573–575. ISBN 89-951655-1-0
156. Behçet's Syndrome Society. http://www.behçets.org.uk
157. Barnes CG, Yazici H (1999) Behçet's syndrome. Rheumatology 38:1171–1176
158. Yurdakul S, Mat C, Tüzün Y et al (2001) A double-blind trial of colchicine in Behçet's syndrome. Arthritis Rheum 44(11):2686–2692
159. Barnes CG (2006) Treatment of Behçet's syndrome. Rheumatology (Oxford) 45:245–247
160. Lee S (2000) Behçet's disease or Behçet's syndrome – considerations for the unified diagnosis related terminology. In: Bang D, Lee E-S, Lee S (eds) Behçet's Disease: proceedings of the international conference on Behçet's disease, held in Seoul, Korea, May 27–29, 2000. Design Mecca, Seoul, pp 573–575. ISBN 89-951655-1-0
161. Lehner T (1968) Recurrent oral ulcers and Behçet's syndrome: pathological, immunological and clinical study. MD Thesis, University of London
162. Marchionini A, Müller E (1966) The dermatological view of Morbus Hulusi Behçet. In: Monacelli M, Nazzaro P (eds) Behçet's disease. Basel, Karger, pp 6–14
163. Monacelli M, Nazzaro P (eds) (1966) Behçet's disease. Basel, Karger
164. Dilsen N, Konice M, Övül C (eds) (1979) Behçet's disease: proceedings of an international symposium on Behçet's disease, Istanbul 29–30 September 1977, International congress series no. 467. Excerpta Medica, Amsterdam
165. Inaba G (ed) (1982) Behçet's disease: pathogenetic mechanism and clinical future, Japanese Medical Research Foundation publication no. 18. University of Tokyo Press, Tokyo
166. Lehner T, Barnes CG (eds) (1986) Recent advances in Behçet's disease, Royal Society of Medicine Services international congress and symposium series no. 103. Royal Society of Medicine, London
167. O'Duffy JD, Kokmen E (eds) (1991) Behçet's disease: basic and clinical aspects. Marcel Dekker, New York
168. Wechsler B, Godeau P (eds) (1993) Behçet's disease, International congress series 1037. Excerpta Medica, Amsterdam
169. Hamza M (ed) (1997) Behçet's disease; proceeding of the seventh international conference on Behçet's disease held at Tunis 10–11 October 1996. Pub Adhoua, Tunis. ISBN 9973-17-850-5
170. Bang D, Lee E-S, Lee S (eds) (1998) Behçet's disease: proceedings of the 8th international conference on Behçet's disease, held in Reggio Emilia, Italy, October 7–9, 1998. Design Mecca, Seoul. ISBN 89-951655-1-0
171. Bang D, Lee E-S, Lee S (eds) (2000) Behçet's disease: proceedings of the international conference on Behçet's disease, held in Seoul, Korea, May 27–29, 2000. Design Mecca, Seoul. ISBN 89-951655-1-0
172. Zouboulis CC (ed) (2003) Adamantiades-Behçet's disease, vol 528, Advances in experimental medicine and biology. Kluwer Academic/Plenum, New York

Chapter 3
Epidemiology of Behçet's Syndrome and Regional Differences in Disease Expression

Sebahattin Yurdakul and Yusuf Yazıcı

Keywords Arthritis • Behçet's disease • Behçet's syndrome • Disease expression • Epidemiology • Erythema nodosum • Field survey • Folliculitis • Genital ulcer • HLA-B5(51) • Oral ulceration • Pathergy test • Regional difference • Uveitis

Behçet's syndrome (BS) is more prevalent in the regions along the ancient trading route known as "Silk Road," extending from Mediterranean countries such as Turkey and Iran to the Far East including Korea and Japan (Fig. 3.1) where the prevalence of HLA-B5(51) is relatively high, compared to the rest of the globe. This suggests that the possible causative agent(s), including genetic factors such as HLA-B51, spread along this route [1].

Epidemiology of Behçet's Syndrome in Turkey

There were five field surveys about the frequency of BS conducted in different regions between 1981and 2004 [2–6] (Table 3.1). These were cross-sectional, population-based multidisciplinary surveys and their methodologies were quite similar. As the disease is rare in childhood, the age of the screened population was 10 years or older in the villages or the cities in four surveys [2–4, 6]. The fifth survey was conducted among those older than 12 years in a randomly selected population of Istanbul [5]. In the first stage, the target population was questioned for oral ulceration at their dwelling. Then, those with oral ulcers were questioned further and screened for the other manifestations of BS at the field or at a hospital by a team of experienced physicians. While the two earlier studies [2, 3] used O'Duffy's criteria

S. Yurdakul (✉)
Department of Medicine, Division of Rheumatology, Cerrahpasa Medical Faculty, University of Istanbul, Turkey
e-mail: profsyurdakul@yahoo.com

Y. Yazıcı and H. Yazıcı (eds.), *Behçet's Syndrome*,
DOI 10.1007/978-1-4419-5641-5_3, © Springer Science+Business Media, LLC 2010

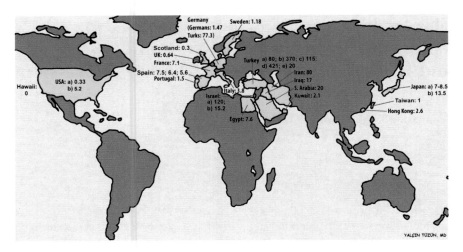

Fig. 3.1 The prevelance of Behçet's syndrome in the world (per 100.000 population). (Courtesy of Y. Tüzün)

for diagnosis [7] the later three [4–6] utilized the International Study Group (ISG) criteria after it was published in 1990 [8]. These five field studies showed that the prevalence of BS was between 20 and 421 among 100,000 in adolescent/adult population in Turkey (Table 3.1) [2–6] giving a high rate of 115, 370, and 421 in Anatolia, the Asian part. These compared with the lower frequencies of 20 and $80/10^5$ in the European region (Thrace). On the other hand there were no patients with BS among 47,000 children in another field survey [9] whereas the prevalence of juvenile chronic arthritis was $64/10^5$ and that of familial Mediterranean fever $28/10^5$ [9]. These figures nicely reflect the relative paucity of pediatric cases of BS in general.

Of the 19 patients with mild BS in the Camas study [3], in the northeastern part of Anatolia, none had eye involvement. This contrasted with frequencies of ~50% of eye disease in hospital-based reports (see Chap. 5). Furthermore, 18/19 patients had not previously been diagnosed with BS. Another point was that the frequency of HLA-B5 was not increased (26%) among the patients identified. This frequency was similar to the ~30% frequency in the general population of Turkey [10] and is significantly lower than the 60–80% frequency among the hospital-based patients [10] (Table 3.2). These observations suggested that the association of HLA-B5 was probably not with the disease itself but with its severity. Information about the HLA-B5 positivity was available only in one other survey which identified only four patients, three of whom were HLA B5 positive.

Contrary to what was observed in the Camas study from a rural area [3] the frequency of eye disease was reported as 44% and 28% in the field surveys coming from Ankara and Istanbul (heavily populated urban, metropolitan areas), respectively

Table 3.1 Epidemiological features of field surveys of Behçet's syndrome in Turkey

Author and year	Demirhindi, 1981 [2]	Yurdakul, 1988 [3]	Idil, 2002 [4]	Azizerli, 2003 [5]	Cakir, 2004 [6]
City, village (location)	Istanbul, Silivri, (Thrace)	Ordu, Camas, (Northeast)	Ankara, Park	Istanbul	Edirne, Havsa (Thrace)
Region	Rural	Rural	Suburban	Urban	Rural
Total population (n)	–	9,128	20,007	9,500,000	5,727
Age screened (years)	>10	≥10	>10	>12	≥10
Population screened (n)	4,960	5,131	13,894	23,986	4,861
Patients with BS (n) (M/F)	4 (–)	19 (6/13)	16 (5/11)	101 (52/49)	1 (–)
Previously diagnosed (n)	1	1	9	47	0
Prevalence per 100,000 *adults*	80	370	115	421	20
Diagnostic criteria used	O'Duffy's	O'Duffy's	ISG	ISG	ISG
Clinical features (%)					
Aphtae	100	100	100	100	+
Genital ulcer	75	74	75	70	
Folliculitis	75	95	a	40	+
Erythema nodosum	50	42	a	37	
Uveitis	50	0	44	28	
Arthritis	25	47	–	32	
Positive pathergy (n)	67 (2/3)	33 (6/18)	81 (13/16)	69 (70/101)	+
HLA-B5 (n)	75 (3/4)	26 (5/19)	–	–	–

M male, *F* female, *ISG* International Society Group for Behçet's Disease, – Not reported or not done, + Only one patient diagnosed had these lesions
a Skin disease was reported to be 50% as a combination of both erythema nodosum and folliculitis

Table 3.2 Epidemiological features of Behçet's syndrome over the world excluding Turkey

	Country, city, observation period, population	No. of patients with Behçet's syndrome (F/M)	Prevalence per 100,000 population	Aft	GU	Skin	Joint	Eye	Pathergy (%) (n)	HLA-B5 or (51)[a] % (n)
Asia										
Yamamoto, 1974 [17]	Japan	4,123	7–8.5							
Nakae, 1993 [19]	Japan, 1991	Evaluated 3,316 (1678/1638) of 16,750 total	13.5	98	73	87	57	69	44	55[a]
Mousa, 1986 [28]	Kuwait 1,374,600 Arabs 1,152,400	29 (7/22) 26 Arabs 9 Kuwaiti Arabs 17 Non-Kuwaiti Arabs	2.1 1.58 2.9	100	93	76	69	69	34	36 (5/14)
	Non-Arabs 222,200	3 Non-Arabs	1.35							
Al-Dalaan, 1997[a] [14]	Saudi Arabia, Al Qassim, surveyed 10,267 of 660,000	2 (0/2)	20						0 (0/2)	
Chen, 2001 [29]	Taiwan, 1991–1999	22	1	100	55	91	32	55	23	
Mok, 2002 [27]	China, Hong Kong, 1978–2000, 1,410,000	37 (19/18)	2.6	100	81	73	54	35	6 (2/34)	
Al-Rawi, 2003[a] [12]	Iraq, Saglawia, surveyed 14 155 (aged 16–45) of 35,125	6 (2/4)	17	100	83	50	33	40	83	
Jaber, 2002 [16]	Israel, Taibe (Arab town) surveyed 4876 (aged 10–20) of 30,000	6 (5/1)	120	100	100	67	100	67	50 (1/2)	83
Krause, 2007 [15]	Israel, Galilee, 737,000	112 (53/59) overall 46 Jewish 49 Arabs 17 Druze	15.2 8.6 26.2 146.4	100	68	41	70	53	44	81
Davatchi, 2008[a] [13]	Iran, Tehran, surveyed 10 291	7 (3/4)	80							

Europe

Chamberlain, 1977 [31]	UK, Yorkshire, 5,000,000	32 (20/12)	0.64	100	91	66	63	25		18 (5/28)
Jankowski, 1992 [30]	Scotland, 5,500,000	15 (11/4)	0.3	100	73	87	93	93		13 (2/15)
Ek, 1993 [32]	Sweden, Stockholm, 1981–1989, 345,000	12 (3/9) overall 5 (3/2) Swedish	3.5 overall 1.2 Swedish	91	83	83	58	50		80 (4/5)
Crespo, 1993 [33]	Portugal, Coimbra, 1,900,000	29 (18/11)	1.5	100	85	93	75	66	37	75[a] (15/20)
Sanchez, 1998 [37]	Spain, Seville, 1980–1998	30 (20/10)	7.5	100	90	77	30	77	7	27[a]
Gonzalez-Gay, 2000 [35]	Spain, Lugo, 1988–1997 250,000	16 (7/9)	6.4	100	88	88	56	44	19	
Graña, 2001 [36]	Spain, Galicia, 1978–2000 500,000	28	5.6							
Papoutsis, 2006 [38]	Germany, Berlin, 2005 German 2,932,755 Non German 458,589 Turks 117,624	43 122 91	1.47 26.6 77.37							
Salvarani, 2007 [34]	Italy, Reggio Emilia, 1984–2004, 486,961	18 (9/9)	3.8	100	78	100	50	56	11 (1/9)	75 (9/12)[a]

(continued)

Table 3.2 (continued)

Country, city, observation period, population	No. of patients with Behçet's syndrome (F/M)	Prevalence per 100,000 population	Aft	GU	Skin	Join	Eye	Pathergy (%) (n)	HLA-B5 or (51)[a] % (n)[b]
Mahr, 2008 [39] France, Paris, Seine–Saint-Denis County, 2003,1,094,412	79 (34/45) overall 19 European 43 North African 11 Asian (incl.Turks) 3 Sub-Saharan African 3 Noncontinental French	7.1 2.4 34.6 17.5 5.1 6.2	100	80	90	59	51	20 (16/79)	33 (20/61)
Africa									
Assaad-Khalil, 1997 [46] Egypt, Alexandria, 3,600,000	274(43/231)	7.6	92	76	39	50	76	70	58[a]
America									
Hirohata, 1975 [49] USA, Hawaii, 768,561	0	0							
O'Duffy, 1978 [50] USA, Olmsted County, MN		0.33							
Calamia, 2009 [51] USA, 1960–2005	13	5.2	100	62	85	46	62	0	0

[a]Field surveys
[b]Combination of HLA-B5 and HLA-B51

Table 3.3 Geographical differences in the features of Behçet's syndrome

Country	Behçet's syndrome (n)	Gastrointestinal involvement (%)	Pathergy positivity (%) (n)	HLA-B5 or B(51)* Behçet syndrome (BS) vs. healthy controls (HC) % (n)
Asia				
Oshima, 1963 [56]	Japan	85	58		
Nakae, 1993 [19]	Japan	3,316	15	44	55*
Tanaka, 2003 [55]	Japan	200	25		
Ohno, 1975 [75]	Japan	21			71% (15/21) BS
					31% (24/78) HC
Ohno, 1978 [76]	Japan	23			61% (14/23)* BS
					21% (118/553)* HC
Ohno, 1982 [77]	Japan	55			62% (34/55)* BS
					21% (118/553)* HC
Bang, 2001 [24]	Korea	1,527	7	15 (110/715)	
Chang, 2002 [79]	Korea	73	15	34 (25/73)	51 (37/73)* BS
Bang, 2003 [85]	Korea	1,901	3		
Al-Rawi, 1986 [61]	Iraq	60	10	71 (37/52)	62 (32/52)* BS
					29 (51/175)* HC
Shahram, 2003 [62]	Iran	4,704	7.9	58	53
Madanat, 2003 [63]	Jordan	295	12.5	51	
Hamdan, 2006 [64]	Lebanon	90	6	69 (16/23)	
Al-Dalaan, 1994 [65]	Saudi Arabia	119	4	17.5 (15/85)	72 (61/85)* BS
					26 HC
Europe				
Jankowski, 1992 [30]	Scotland	15	53		13 (2/15) BS
Chamberlain, 1977 [31]	UK	32	9		18 (5/28) BS
Dilsen, 1979 [59]	Turkey	106	0		
Yurdakul, 1996 [58]	Turkey	1,000	0.6		
Tursen, 2003 [60]	Turkey	2,313	1.4	52(1,208/2,331)	

(continued)

Table 3.3 (continued)

	Country	Behçet's syndrome (n)	Gastrointestinal involvement (%)	Pathergy positivity (%) (n)	HLA-B5 or B(51)* Behçet syndrome (BS) vs. healthy controls (HC) % (n)
Yazici, 1977 [10]	Turkey	19			84% (16/19) BS 27% (41/150) HC
Gul, 2002 [78]	Turkey	174			61% (105/174)* BS 25% (47/191)* HC
Africa					
Assaad-Khalil, 1997 [46]	Egypt	274	10	70	58*
B'chir Hamzaoui, 2006 [42]	Tunisia	519	–	51 (128/252)	35 (65/187)*
Houman, 2007 [43]	Tunisia	260	1.5	62 (108/173)	54 (60/111)* BS 26 (11/43)* HC
America					
Ward, 2003 [66]	USA	164	8		

[4, 5] Whether these findings reflect a difference in the frequency of more severe disease in the urban setting remains to be seen.

It is to be noted from Table 3.1 that the frequency of pathergy positivity also varied between the regions. This might have been due to repeated tests or different numbers of skin pricks such as one versus three and the use of needles of different sizes, respectively.

The Cerrahpaşa group investigated the prevalence of BS and familial Mediterranean fever among ethnic Armenians living in Istanbul. There were significantly more FMF and fewer BS cases as compared with frequencies reported among the ethnic Turks [11]. These preliminary observations support a greater role of genetic factors compared to environmental agents in BS.

Epidemiology of Behçet's Syndrome in the World

The prevalence of BS is less frequent in the rest of the globe (Fig. 3.1 and Table 3.3). Most of the data are mainly based on case registries, hospital records or mail questionnaires apart from three field surveys coming from Iraq [12], Iran [13], and Saudi Arabia [14].

Asia (Table 3.2)

Iraqi researchers conducted a field study in Saglawia during 1999–2000, a town with a population of 35,125. A sample of 14,155 people from the town's food registry between the ages 16 and 45 were screened. They identified six patients with BS, giving a prevalence of $17/10^5$ [12].

As musculoskeletal complaints and rheumatic disorders were screened in a field survey among a sample of 10,291 people aged over 15 years in Tehran, seven patients were diagnosed as having BS. The adjusted prevalence calculated was $80/10^5$ in Tehran, Iran. No further details were given [13].

In another population-based field survey, a sample of 10,267 among 660,000 in Al Qassim region, Saudi Arabia, was interviewed for signs and symptoms of BS. Two patients with BS were found [14]. This rate of $20/10^5$ population in Saudi Arabia is quite similar to that of $17/10^5$ reported from Iraq [12] and that of $26/10^5$ among Arabs living in Israel [15]. However it is also six times lower than those of Arabs living in an Arab town, in Taibe, Israel [16] (see below).

A high frequency of BS was reported in Taibe, an Arab community in Israel [16]. The authors surveyed the parents of children attending a pediatric center and their children aged between 10 and 20 years, and identified those with recurrent oral ulceration among 4,876 people. Six BS patients were identified giving a prevalence of $120/10^5$ [16]. Also from Israel the patient charts from three hospitals serving the majority of the population of 737,000 in the Galilee area during a 15-year period identified 112 patients with BS giving an overall frequency of $15.2/10^5$ of the population [15]. The adjusted prevalences were $8.6/10^5$ for Jews, $26.2/10^5$ for Arabs, and $146.4/10^5$ for Druzes.

In Japan, a nationwide hospital survey estimated 16,750 patients with a prevalence of $13.5/10^5$ of the general population in 1991. This was actually higher than the rate of $7-8.5/10^5$ in 1972 [17–19] *while* there is the impression that the frequency of BD might be decreasing in this country [20]. This impression is further backed up by data showing that the percentage of BS patients among uveitis cases has decreased from ~25% in 1979 [21] to ~6% in 2007 [22] in similar surveys from Japan.

Although a great number of patients with BS were reported from a nationwide multicenter survey ($n = 1,527$) [23] and another study of two university hospital records ($n = 1,901$) in Seoul [24], no formal data are available regarding the prevalence of the disease in Korea.

Behçet's syndrome was mentioned among one of five common rheumatic diseases in China [25] and Kaneko et al. cited it at a high rate of $120/10^5$ of the population in this country [26] The frequency was $2.6/10^5$ in the Hong Kong area based on hospital records of 37 patients between 1978 and 2000 [27]. Similar low rates were reported from Kuwait and Taiwan [28, 29].

Europe

The estimated prevalences of BS are variable, being low in the northern part of Europe compared to the south: 0.3 in Scotland [30], 0.64 in the UK [31], 1.2 in Sweden [32], 1.5 in Portugal [33], 3.8 in Italy [34], $5.6-7.5/10^5$ in Spain [35–37]. It was $1.47/10^5$ in Berlin, Germany among the Germans and $27/10^5$ in non-Germans [38]; however, Turks living in Berlin had a distinctly higher rate of $77/10^5$ [38]. However, this rate is still considerably lower from what has been generally reported from the surveys in Asian Turkey [3–5] (Table 3.1).

A recent cross-sectional prevalence study from France was carried out in a population of 1,094,421 of Seine–Saint-Denis County, a northern suburb of Paris in France. Information about BS was obtained from three sources: community physicians, hospitals, and the National Health Insurance database using the capture–recapture method. There was an overall prevalence of $7.1/10^5$; however, as expected, this was $2.4/10^5$ in Europeans, $17.5/10^5$ in Asians including Turks, and $35/10^5$ in North Africans living in Paris, France [39]. These findings indicate that the non-European subgroups such as those with Asian and North African descent had substantially higher prevalence rates compared to the native European population. Interestingly, age at immigration was not related to the risk of having BS. The same group had, previously, also investigated the frequencies of vasculitis including polyarteritis nodosa (PAN), microscopic polyangiitis (MPA), Wegener's granulomatosis (WG), and Churg–Strauss syndrome (CSS) using almost the same method and in the same geographic area [40]. They had found a combined rate of $9/10^5$ for all of the above listed vasculitides, with BS showing a higher frequency from each disease entity taken on its own. This work suggests that heredity is perhaps more important than environmental factors in the pathogenesis of BS but also that BS is not so rare in continental Europe where it had previously been thought to be rather rare [39–41].

Africa

Although there are a number of reports with considerable number of patients with Behçet's syndrome from North African countries [42–45], the only available formal survey information is from a report of a registry in Alexandria, Egypt [46]. This survey quotes a prevalence of a $7.6/10^5$. This figure is substantially lower than what had been found ($35/10^5$ among the immigrants from North Africa (Moroccans, Algerians, Tunisians, and Egyptians) in the recent Paris survey quoted above [39].

On the other hand, there are limited numbers of reports of a few cases from other parts of Africa. A study reported 17 patients diagnosed as BS during a 26-year period in Dakar, Senegal [47]; in another work there were eight patients of west African and Afro-Caribbean origin living in the UK [48]. This apparent relative low frequency of BS in these regions might be related to the lower frequency of HLA B51 carriers in these parts [48].

America

In 1975, a study of mail questionnaires sent to practicing physicians showed no patient with BS in Hawaii where 217,307 Japanese, a genetically susceptible population, lived. This observation suggests the importance of environmental factors compared to genetics [49]. If the Japanese rate had been applied to those migrant populations at least 15 patients should have been detected [49]. While an estimated rate of $0.33/10^5$ was reported in Olmsted County, Rochester in 1978 [50], a higher rate ($5.2/10^5$) was calculated in the same region between 1996 and 2005 [51].

The Behçet's Syndrome Evaluation, Treatment and Research Center at NYU Hospital for Joint Diseases in New York, has been collecting data on BS patients since 2005. Several interesting observations about disease manifestations have been noted. In this dedicated center 197 consecutive patients were divided into two groups, Group 1 of patients with northern European background and Group 2 with patients ethnically from areas where Behçet's prevalence is high (Turkey, Greece, Israel, Middle East, and the Far East). These groups were compared as to their demography and disease manifestations [52]. There were significantly more females (78% vs. 54%) in Group 1, made up of predominantly patients with skin-mucosa disease. About a third of patients had eye disease in both groups; interestingly there were no patients who were blind in the whole cohort. Vascular involvement was seen in three patients in Group 2 and none in Group 1. These suggest that even though most manifestations of BS were similar in frequency between the two groups some manifestations might be more severe in patients with backgrounds in BS endemic areas, like the Middle East.

There are only few case reports from South America.

Australia

Thirty-five years ago 17 patients with BS [53] were reported. Some case reports followed also suggesting a low frequency of BD on this continent.

Like in almost all conditions of uncertain etiology, it is also difficult in BS to separate environmental from genetic factors. Moreover, it is quite common that what is traditionally taken as environmental turns out to be genetic and what is genetic, environmental on closer scrutiny [54]. The higher frequency of BS among the Arabs and Druzes as compared to the ethnic Jews living in Israel can be taken as evidence for genetic factors. On the other hand, there is also the consideration that the living conditions among the Arabs and Druzes might not as good as the ethnic Jews. Similarly, the recent data from the Northern suburb of Paris at first sight indicate ethnic influences. On the other hand this area is also regularly in the international news with its rather poor living conditions.

Differing Disease Expression in Behçet's Syndrome

Gastrointestinal Involvement

Gastrointestinal disease is frequent among the patients from the Far East, especially in Japan where one-third to one-half of the patients with BS had symptoms of inflammatory bowel disease such as diarrhea, abdominal pain, and abdominal distension [55, 56]. The intestinal histo-pathology specimens show necrotic, granulomatous, or combined type inflammation [57]. This is not easy to differentiate from Crohn's disease (see Chap. 10). This is also the case for the Korean patients, though less frequently [23, 24]. Patients with BS reported from the UK and Scotland had gastrointestinal problems similar to those from Japan [30, 31] (Table 3.3).

In contrast to the high frequency of gastrointestinal involvement among the Japanese, it is rather infrequent among those from Turkey. A retrospective chart review showed that the frequency of diarrhea was quite low (0.06%) among 1,000 patients with BS in Turkey [58]. In addition, when questioned prospectively, there were not any significant differences in the frequency of diarrhea between patients with BS and the diseased controls. Furthermore, the same study showed no differences in histological abnormalities in rectal biopsies between 75 BS patients and 47 controls [57]. A low frequency of gastrointestinal problems has also been the experience of other Turkish centers [59, 60].

Similarly, gastrointestinal involvement does not seem to be prevalent in some other countries like the USA. Furthermore, this involvement is not as severe as it is reported from Japan and Korea [42, 43, 61–66] (Tables 3.2 and 3.3). However, it was recently reported that US patients may have increased numbers of patients with GI involvement [67]. In a cohort of 347 US patients with BS, GI involvement was seen in 38% [68].

Pathergy Test

The pathergy test is the hyper-reactivity of the skin to a needle prick. This curious phenomenon is almost unique to Behçet's syndrome [69–71]. While the pathergy phenomenon was reported to be present in the majority of the patients among the countries where the disease was prevalent from Turkey and Mediterranean countries to Japan, it was less common in northern European countries and the United States [72, 73] (Tables 3.2 and 3.3). Many researchers doubted its existence. Some years ago the prevalence of pathergy positivity was formally compared among patients and controls from Istanbul, Turkey (48 Turkish Behçet patients and 24 Turkish healthy controls), and Leeds, England (12 British Behçet patients and 7 British healthy controls) in a blind protocol by means of photography. In both countries, nondisposable needles of the same kind (21 G) and of the same manufacturer were used for the pathergy test. The pathergy phenomenon was positive only among the Turkish patients (28/48, 58%) [73].

A lower frequency of pathergy positivity has been reported in recent years. These observations are in parallel with a previous study. In this study, the authors showed a decreased frequency of a positive pathergy performed with disposable needles compared to nondisposable needles [74].

HLA-B5(51) Association

The strongest genetic association between BS and HLA-B5 was first reported in 1973 by Ohno et al. [75] and later with HLA-B51, a suballele of B5 [76, 77]. Since then this prominent association has been found in many other ethnic groups [10, 42, 43, 46, 61, 62, 65, 78, 79]. Around 50–80% of BS patients along the "Silk Road" carry HLA B51 where the frequency of this allele is ~25% in the general population. In regions where BS is less common, like USA and UK, the frequency of HLA B51 among the patients is ~15% and that in the general population ~2–8% [1, 30, 31, 80, 81].

Conclusions

Prominent regional differences exist in the expression of BS around the globe [82] while there is the suggestion that the condition might be getting milder in recent years [83, 84]. On the other hand most available epidemiologic data at hand are not strictly comparable. There is a list of biases including publishing, selection, information, and classification. Properly designed and conducted, population-based field surveys, preferably with international collaboration are clearly needed.

References

1. Verity DH, Marr JE, Ohno S et al (1999) Behçet's disease, the Silk Road and HLA-B51: historical and geographical perspectives. Tissue Antigens 54:213–220
2. Demirhindi O, Yazici H, Binyildiz P et al (1981) Silivri Fener koyu ve yoresinde Behçet hastaligi sikligi ve bu hastaligin toplum icinde taranabilmesinde kullanabilecek bir yontem. Cerrahpasa Tip Fak Derg 12:509–514 (in Turkish)
3. Yurdakul S, Gunaydin I, Tuzun Y et al (1988) The prevalence of Behçet's syndrome in a rural area in northern Turkey. J Rheumatol 15:820–822
4. Idil A, Gurler A, Boyvat A et al (2002) The prevalence of Behçet's disease above the age of 10 years. The results of a pilot study conducted at the Park Primary Health Care Center in Ankara, Turkey. Ophthalmic Epidemiol 9:325–331
5. Azizlerli G, Kose AA, Sarica R et al (2003) Prevalence of Behçet's disease in Istanbul, Turkey. Int J Dermatol 42:803–806
6. Cakir N, Dervis E, Benian O et al (2004) Prevalence of Behçet's disease in rural western Turkey: a preliminary report. Clin Exp Rheumatol 22(4 Suppl 34):S53–S55
7. O'Duffy JD (1974) Suggested criteria for diagnosis of Behçet's disease. J Rheumatol 1(Suppl 1):18, Abstract 32
8. International Study Group for Behçet's Disease (1990) Criteria for diagnosis of Behçet's disease. Lancet 335:1078–1080
9. Ozen S, Karaaslan Y, Ozdemir O et al (1998) Prevalence of juvenile chronic arthritis and familial Mediterranean fever in Turkey: a field study. J Rheumatol 25:2445–2449
10. Yazici H, Akokan G, Yalgin B, Muftuoglu A (1977) A high prevalence of HLA-B5 in Behçet's disease. Clin Exp Immunol 30:259–261
11. Seyahi E, Mangan MS, Oktay V, Cevirgen D, Muratyan S, Yazici H (2008) The prevalence of familial Mediterranean fever and Behçet's syndrome among Armenians living in Istanbul: preliminary results of a survey. Clin Exp Rheumatol 26(Suppl 50):Abstract A 10
12. Al-Rawi ZS, Neda AH (2003) Prevalence of Behçet's disease among Iraqis. Adv Exp Med Biol 528:37–41
13. Davatchi F, Jamshidi AR, Banihashemi AT et al (2008) WHO-ILAR COPCORD Study (Stage 1, Urban Study) in Iran. J Rheumatol 35:1384–1390
14. Al-Dalaan A, Al Ballaa S, Al Sukati M, Mousa M, Bahabri S, Biyari T (1997) The prevalence of Behçet's disease in Al Qassim region of Saudi Arabia. In: Hamza M (ed) Behçet's disease. Pub Adhoua, Tunis (Tunisia), pp 170–172
15. Krause I, Yankevich A, Fraser A, Rosner I, Mader R, Zisman D, Boulman N, Rozenbaum M, Weinberger A (2007) Prevalence and clinical aspects of Behçet's disease in the north of Israel. Clin Rheumatol 26:555–560
16. Jaber L, Milo G, Halpern GJ et al (2002) Prevalence of Behçet's disease in an Arab community in Israel. Ann Rheum Dis 61:365–366

17. Yamamoto S, Toyokawa H, Matsubara J et al (1974) A nation wide survey of Behçet's disease in Japan. Jpn J Ophthalmol 18:282–290
18. Shimizu T, Ehrlich GE, Inaba G, Hayashi K (1979) Behçet's disease (Behçet's syndrome). Semin Arthritis Rheum 8:223–260
19. Nakae K, Masaki F, Hashimoto T, Inaba G, Mochizuki M, Sakane T (1993) Recent epidemiological features of Behçet's disease in Japan. In: Wechsler B, Godeau P (eds) Behçet's disease. Excerpta Medica, Amsterdam, pp 145–151
20. Iwata D, Namba K, Kitaichi N et al (2004) Recent clinical features of Behçet's disese in Hokkaido, Japan. Clin Exp Rheumatol 22(Suppl 34):S-48
21. Mishima S, Masuda K, İzawa Y et al (1979) Behçet's disease in Japan: ophthalmologic aspects. Trans Am Ophthalmol Soc 76:225–279
22. Goto H, Mochizuki M, Yamaki K et al (2007) Epidemiological survey of intraocular inflammation in Japan. Jpn J Ophthalmol 51:41–44
23. Bang D, Yoon KH, Chung HG, Choi EH, Lee ES, Lee S (1997) Epidemiological and clinical features of Behçet's disease in Korea. Yonsei Med J 38:428–436
24. Bang D, Lee JH, Lee ES, Lee S, Choi JS, Kim YK, Cho BK, Koh JK, Won YH, Kim NI, Park SD, Ahn HJ, Lee YW, Wang HY, Lee WW, Eun HC, Song ES, Lee SW, Lee CW, Lee CJ, Park JH, Song YW, Kim ST, Kim CY, Park JK, Kwon KS (2001) Epidemiologic and clinical survey of Behçet's disease in Korea: the first multicenter study. J Korean Med Sci 16:615–618
25. Chang NC (1983) Rheumatic diseases in China. J Rheumatol 10(Suppl 10):41–44
26. Kaneko F, Nakamura K, Sato M, Tojo M, Zheng X, Zhang JZ (2003) Epidemiology of Behçet's disease in Asian countries and Japan. Adv Exp Med Biol 528:25–29
27. Mok CC, Cheung TC, Ho CT et al (2002) Behçet's disease in southern Chinese patients. J Rheumatol 29:1689–1693
28. Mousa AR, Marafie AA, Rifai KM, Dajani AI, Mukhtar MM (1986) Behçet's disease in Kuwait, Arabia: a report of 29 cases and a review. Scand J Rheumatol 15:310–332
29. Chen Y-C, Chang H-W (2001) Clinical characteristics of Behçet's disease in southern Taiwan. J Microbiol Immunol Infect 34:207–210
30. Jankowski J, Crombie I, Jankowski R (1992) Behçet's syndrome in Scotland. Postgrad Med J 68:566–570
31. Chamberlain MA (1977) Behçet's syndrome in 32 patients in Yorkshire. Ann Rheum Dis 36:491–499
32. Ek L, Hedfors E (1993) Behçet's disease: a review and a report of 12 cases from Sweden. Acta Derm Venereol 73:251–254
33. Crespo J, Ribeiro J, Jesus E, Moura A, Reis C, Porto A (1993) Behçet's disease: particular features at the central zone of Portugal. In: Wechsler B, Godeau P (eds) Behçet's disease: International Congress Series 1037. Exerpta Medica, Amsterdam, pp 207–210
34. Salvarani C, Pipitone N, Catanoso MG et al (2007) Epidemiology and clinical course of Behçet's disease in the Reggio Emilia area of Northern Italy: a seventeen-year population-based study. Arthritis Rheum 57:171–178
35. Gonzalez-Gay MA, Garcia-Porrua C, Branas F et al (2000) Epidemiologic and clinical aspects of Behçet's disease in a defined area of Northwestern Spain, 1988–1997. J Rheumatol 27:703–707
36. Graña J, Sánchez-Meizoso MO, Galdo F (2001) Epidemiological aspects of Behçet's disease in Galicia. J Rheumatol 28:2565–2566
37. Sanchez Burson J, Grandal Y, Mendoza M, Montero R, Rejon E, Marenco JL (1998) Clinical characteristics, HLA antigen and mortality in Behçet's syndrome in Spain. In: Olivieri I, Salvarani C, Cantini F (eds) 8th International Congress on Behçet's disease: program and abstracts. Prex, Milan, p 102
38. Papoutsis NG, Abdel-Naser MB, Altenburg A et al (2006) Prevalence of Adamantiades-Behçet's disease in Germany and the municipality of Berlin: results of a nationwide survey. Clin Exp Rheumatol 24(5 Suppl 42):S125
39. Mahr A, Belarbi L, Wechsler B, Jeanneret D, Dhote R, Fain O, Lhote F, Ramanoelina J, Coste J, Guillevin L (2008) Population-based prevalence study of Behçet's disease: differences by ethnic origin and low variation by age at immigration. Arthritis Rheum 58:3951–3959

40. Mahr A, Guillevin L, Poissonnet M, Ayme S (2004) Prevalences of polyarteritis nodosa, microscopic polyangiitis, Wegener's granulomatosis, and Churg–Strauss syndrome in a French urban multiethnic population in 2000: a capture–recapture estimate. Arthritis Rheum 51:92–99

41. Yazici H, Seyahi E, Yurdakul S (2008) Behçet's syndrome is not so rare: why do we need to know? Arthritis Rheum 58:3640–3643

42. B'chir Hamzaoui S, Harmel A, Bouslama K, Abdallah M, Ennafaa M, M'rad S, Ben Dridi M, le groupe tunisien d'étude sur la maladie de Behçet (2006) La maladie de Behçet en Tunisie. Étude clinique de 519 cas [Behçet's disease in Tunisia. Clinical study of 519 cases]. Rev Med Interne 27:742–750

43. Houman MH, Neffati H, Braham A, Harzallah O, Khanfir M, Miled M, Hamzaoui K (2007) Behçet's disease in Tunisia. Demographic, clinical and genetic aspects in 260 patients. Clin Exp Rheumatol 25(4 Suppl 45):S58–S64

44. Benamour S, Zeroual B, Alaoui FZ (1998) Joint manifestations in Behçet's disease. A review of 340 cases. Rev Rhum Engl Ed 65:299–307

45. Taarit CB, Ben Turki S, Ben Maïz H (2001) Rheumatologic manifestations of Behçet's disease: report of 309 cases. Rev Med Interne 22(11):1049–1055

46. Assaad-Khalil SH, Kamel FA, Ismail EA (1997) Starting a regional registry for patients with Behçet's disease in North West Nile Delta region in Egypt. In: Hamza M (ed) Behçet's disease. Pub Adhoua, Tunis (Tunisia), pp 173–176

47. Dia D, Dieng MT, Sy Ndiaye T, Fall S, Ndongo S, Diallo M, Moreira Diop T, Labou A, Ndiaye B (2003) Behçet's disease in Dakar (Senegal): epidemiological and clinical features. Dakar Med 48:64–67

48. Poon W, Verity DH, Larkin GL et al (2003) Behçet's disease in patients of West African and Afro-Caribbean origin. Br J Ophthalmol 87:876–878

49. Hirohata T, Kuratsune M, Nomura A, Jimi S (1975) Prevalence of Behçet's syndrome in Hawai. Hawaii Med J 34:244–246

50. O'Duffy JD (1978) Summary of international symposium on Behçet's disease. J Rheumatol 5:229–233

51. Calamia KT, Wilson FC, Icen M, Crowson CS, Gabriel SE, Kremers HM (2009) Epidemiology and clinical characteristics of Behçet's disease in the US: a population-based study. Arthritis Rheum 61:600–604

52. Yazici Y, Moses N (2007) Clinical manifestations and ethnic background of patients with Behçet's Syndrome in a US Cohort. Arthritis Rheum 56:S502

53. Cooper DA, Penny R (1974) Behçet's syndrome: clinical, immunological and therapeutic evaluation of 17 patients. Aust NZ J Med 4:585–596

54. Hemminki K, Bermajo LJ, Forsti A (2006) The balance between heritable and environmental aetiology of human disease. Nat Rev Genet 7:958–965

55. Tanaka C, Matsuda T, Hayashi E, Imamura Y, Ozaki S (2003) Clinical manifestations and course of 200 Japanese patients with Behçet's disease. Adv Exp Med Biol 528:77–79

56. Oshima Y, Shimizu T, Yokohari R, Matsumoto T, Kano K, Kagami T, Nagaya H (1963) Clinical studies on Behçet's syndrome. Ann Rheum Dis 22:36

57. Fukuda Y, Watanabe I (1979) Pathological studies on intestinal Behçet's (entero-Behçet's) disease. In: Dilsen N, Konice M, Ovul C (eds) Behçet's Disease, Proceedings of an International Symposium on Behçet's Disease. Excerpta Medica, Amsterdam, pp 90–95

58. Yurdakul S, Tuzuner N, Yurdakul I et al (1996) Gastrointestinal involvement in Behçet's syndrome: a controlled study. Ann Rheum Dis 55:208–210

59. Dilsen N, Konice M, Ovul C (eds) (1979) Clinical evaluation of 106 cases of Behçet's disease. Behçet's Disease. Proceedings of an international symposium on Behçet's disease. Excerpta Medica, Amsterdam, pp 124–129

60. Tursen U, Gurler A, Boyvat A (2003) Evaluation of clinical findings according to sex in 2313 Turkish patients with Behçet's disease. Int J Dermatol 42:346–351

61. Al-Rawi ZS, Sharquie KE, Khalifa SJ, Al-Hadithi FM, Munir JJ (1986) Behçet's disease in Iraqi patients. Ann Rheum Dis 45:987–990

62. Shahram F, Davatchi F, Nadji A, Jamshidi A, Chams H, Chams C, Shafaie N, Akbarian M, Gharibdoost F (2003) Recent epidemiological data on Behçet's disease in Iran: the 2001 survey. Adv Exp Med Biol 528:31–36
63. Madanat W, Sharaiha Z, Khasawneh S, Zureikat H, Fayyad F (2003) Gastro-intestinal manifestations of Behçet's disease. Adv Exp Med Biol 528:455–457
64. Hamdan A, Mansour W, Uthman I, Masri AF, Nasr F, Arayssi T (2006) Behçet's disease in Lebanon: clinical profile, severity and two-decade comparison. Clin Rheumatol 25: 364–367
65. Al-Dalaan A, al Balaa S, el Ramahi K, al-Kawi Z, Bohlega S, Bahabri S et al (1994) Behçet's disease in Saudi Arabia. J Rheumatol 21:658–661
66. Ward EM, Woodward TA, Mazlumzadeh M, Calamia KT (2003) Gastrointestinal disease in Behçet's disease. Adv Exp Med Biol 528:459–464
67. Yazici Y, Schimmel E, Swearingen CJ (2009) Behçet's syndrome in the US: Clinical characteristics, treatment and ethnic/racial differences in manifestations in 347 patients with BS. Arthritis Rheum 60 (Suppl.)
68. Kobayashi T, Kishimoto M, Tokuda Y, Schimmel E, Swearingen C, Yoshida K, Utsunomiya M, Yamamoto M, Yazici Y (2009) Disease manifestations and treatment differences among Behçet's syndrome patients in the United States and Japan. Ann Rheum Dis 68(SIII):609
69. Tuzun Y, Yazici H, Pazarli H, Yalcin B, Yurdakul S, Muftuoglu A (1979) The usefulness of the nonspecific skin hyperreactivity (the pathergy test) in Behçet's disease in Turkey. Acta Derm Venereol (Stockh) 59:77–79
70. Altac M, Tuzun Y, Yurdakul S, Binyildiz P, Yazici H (1982) The validity of the pathergy test (non-specific skin hyperreactivity) in Behçet's disease: a double blind study by independent observers. Acta Derm Venereol (Stockh) 62:158–159
71. Yazici H, Tuzun Y, Pazarli H, Yalcin B, Yurdakul S, Muftuoglu A (1980) The combined use of HLA-B5 and pathergy test as diagnostic markers of Behçet's disease in Turkey. J Rheumatol 7:206–210
72. Davies PG, Fordham JN, Kirwan JR, Barnes CG, Dinning WJ (1984) The pathergy test and Behçet's syndrome in Britain. Ann Rheum Dis 43:70–73
73. Yazici H, Chamberlain MA, Tuzun Y et al (1984) A comparative study of the pathergy among Turkish and British patients with Behçet's disease. Ann Rheum Dis 43:74–75
74. Dilsen N, Konice M, Aral O, Ocal L, Inanc M, Gul A (1993) Comparative study of the skin pathergy test with blunt and sharp needles in Behçet's disease: confirmed specificity but decreased sensitivity with sharp needles. Ann Rheum Dis 52:823–825
75. Ohno S, Aoki K, Sugiura S, Nakayama E, Itakura K, Aizawa M (1973) HL-A5 and Behçet's disease. Lancet 2:1383–1384
76. Ohno S, Asanuma T, Sugiura S et al (1978) HLA-Bw51 and Behçet's disease. JAMA 240:529
77. Ohno S, Ohguchi M, Hirose S, Matsuda H, Wakisaka A, Aizawa M (1982) Close association of HLA-Bw51 with Behçet's disease. Arch Ophthalmol 100:1455–1458
78. Gul A, Uyar FA, Inanc M, Ocal L, Barrett JH, Aral O, Konice M, Saruhan-Direskeneli G (2002) A weak association of HLA-B*2702 with Behçet's disease. Genes Immun 3:368–372
79. Chang HK, Kim JW (2002) The clinical features of Behçet's disease in Yongdong districts: analysis of a cohort followed from 1997 to 2001. J Korean Med Sci 17:784–789
80. O'Duffy JD, Taswell HF, Elveback LR (1974) HLA antigens in Behçet's disease. J Rheumatol 3:1
81. Moore SB, O'Duffy JD (1986) Lack of association between Behçet's disease and major histocompatibility complex II antigens in an ethnically diverse North American Caucasoid patient group. J Rheumatol 13:771–773
82. Lewis KA, Graham EM, Stanford MR (2007) Systematic review of ethnic variation in the phenotype of Behçet's disease. Scand J Rheumatol 36:1–6
83. Kotake S, Namba K, Higashi K, Goda C, Ariga T, Ogawa A, Ohno S (2003) The change of clinical manifestations of patients with Behçet's disease in Japan. Adv Exp Med Biol 528:83–84

84. Yoshida A, Kawashima H, Motoyama Y, Shibui H, Kaburaki T, Shimizu K, Ando K, Hijikata K, Izawa Y, Hayashi K, Numaga J, Fujino Y, Masuda K, Araie M (2004) Comparison of patients with Behçet's disease in the 1980s and 1990s. Ophthalmology 111:810–815
85. Bang D, Oh S, Lee K-H, Lee E-S, Lee S (2003) Influence of sex on patients with Behçet's disease in Korea. J Korean Med Sci 18:231–235

Chapter 4
The Mucocutaneous Manifestations and Pathergy Reaction in Behçet's Disease

M. Cem Mat, Dongsik Bang, and Melike Melikoğlu

Keywords Acneiform • Behçet's syndrome • Behçet's disease • Cutaneous lesions • Erythema nodosum • Papulopustular • Pathergy • Pseudofolliculitis

The original description of Behçet's disease (BD) in 1937 by Hulusi Behçet was a trisymptom complex of recurrent oral ulcerations, genital ulcerations, and uveitis [1]. Hulusi Behçet had also reported the presence of acneiform symptoms, folliculitis, erythema nodosum, thrombophlebitis as well as hemoptysis. It has since been recognized that BD is a systemic vasculitis, mainly involving the venous side of the circulation and affecting many organ systems [2]. The cardinal features of the disease occur on the mucous membranes and skin and in some patients the diagnosis can be made clinically only on the basis of skin/mucosa findings. Patients exhibiting the myriad of skin/mucosa symptoms all at the same time are rare. Frequent visits and close follow-up are necessary for the correct diagnosis.

Recurrent Aphthous Stomatitis

BD usually starts with mucocutaneous features and recurrent aphthous stomatitis (RAS) is the hallmark [3]. The frequency of RAS is about 97–100% in different patient series [4–6]. It represents the initial manifestation of the disease in 90% of the patients [4] and precedes the diagnosis of BD by an average of 6–7 years [4, 5, 7].

RAS presents as painful, shallow, round to oval ulcers covered with a yellowish pseudomembrane surrounded by a red border (Fig. 4.1). Although they can occur anywhere in the oral cavity, they are more frequent in buccal mucosae, tongue, mucosal surface of lips, gingiva and the soft palate [3, 8, 9].

M.C. Mat (✉)
Department of Dermatology, Istanbul University, Cerrahpaşa Medical Faculty, Istanbul, Turkey
e-mail: cemmat@superonline.com

Y. Yazıcı and H. Yazıcı (eds.), *Behçet's Syndrome*,
DOI 10.1007/978-1-4419-5641-5_4, © Springer Science+Business Media, LLC 2010

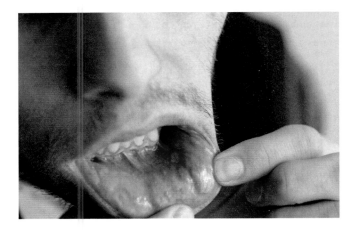

Fig. 4.1 Aphthous ulcers

Three types of aphthae occur in BD: minor aphthae, major aphthae, and herpetiform aphthae [3, 9]. More than one type of aphthae may be present at the same time. Minor aphthae is the most common type (85–99%). They are less than 10 mm in their greatest diameter and heal within 7–10 days without scarring. Major aphthous ulcers are painful, larger (range 1–3 cm in diameter), deeper, and heal more slowly and often with scarring. Herpetiform aphthae are rare [4].They are characterized by successive crops of dozens of painful ulcerations usually 1–3 mm in diameter and can, on occasion, leave scars. In contrast to minor and major ulcers, herpetiform aphthae can also involve the nonkeratinized mucosae [10].

Although aphthae are the cardinal manifestation of BD, there are varying views about their various features. While there is a consensus that a posterior localization in the oral cavity is more characteristic of aphthae associate with BD [11, 12], there is still a debate about (a) their total frequency, (b) the respective frequencies of the three main kinds, and (c) their rate of recurrence.

According to the criteria of the International Study Group (ISG), RAS with an annual recurrence rate of at least three times must be present to classify BD and 97% of the patients fulfill this requirement [13]. Although there is general agreement RAS is the most frequent relapsing lesion of BD, we still do not know if the annual relapse rate is different from what is seen in other conditions associated with RAS, such as systemic lupus erythematosus (SLE), inflammatory bowel disease (IBD), or simple RAS itself, which has an estimated rate of prevalence of up to 20% in the general population [9].

In particular, the literature regarding the frequency of major aphthae in BD is rather controversial. Our experience, based on the controlled drug trials performed in the dedicated Behçet's clinic in Istanbul, indicates that major or herpetiform oral ulcers do not frequently contribute to RAS, except for in rare cases where single-time events may occur [14–16]. In retrospective patient surveys, however, the frequency of major oral ulcers during the disease course has been reported to range from 14 to 55% [4, 17, 18]. In a study from Israel, of 35 patients with BD who reported a frequency rate of oral ulcers more than three times annually, major oral ulcers were found in 50%. This was significantly more frequent than what was observed in RAS (9%) [18].

It seems that neither gender [19] nor disease severity [18] is related to any specific clinical feature of oral ulceration in BD. Only a single study found that female patients with BD were more frequently affected with major oral ulcerations than males. No gender difference was observed among the RAS patients [17]. A recent study reported that pain scores were similar in patients with BD and RAS [19].

Oral trauma has been implicated as a predisposing factor in oral aphthae [9]. Incidental trauma such as tooth brushing, gum chewing, solid foods with sharp surfaces, malocclusion, as well as dental treatments might induce RAS [9]. We are not aware of similar work in BD. On the other hand, Sharque et al. performed oral pathergy test in BD and found that needle prick at the oral mucosa caused a positive pathergy reaction in 39/83 (47%) of patients and the positive pathergy sites tuned into typical oral ulcers in 6/39 (15%) [20].

The relationship of smoking with a lower prevalence of RAS has also been shown in BD [21, 22]. Of 47 asymptomatic current smokers with Behçet's disease who temporarily stopped smoking, 31(66%) developed oral aphthous ulcers after 1 week compared with the development of ulcers in only 25% of a control group of nonsmoking patients with Behçet's disease during that time [21].

Genital Ulcers

Genital ulceration is another major cardinal manifestation of BD. It is also the most specific (95%) as was formally quantified in the formulation of the ISG criteria [13]. Genital ulcers usually begin as a papule, pustule, or circumscribed necrosis that ulcerates within a short period. They are frequently painful, round to oval, punched out in appearance, and usually covered with yellowish fibrin or crust (Fig. 4.2a). Their borders are regular and edematous. The frequency of genital ulcers is about 50–85% in different patient series [4–6]. They usually heal within 10–30 days, if they are not secondarily infected. In a 6-week prospective study, genital scar formation was studied in 102 BD patients with genital ulcers [23]. In males, genital ulcers occured mostly on scrotum (89%), penis (%5), and femoroinguinal (%5.8) regions. Large ulcers which were equal or greater than 1 cm in diameter usually led to scarring (90%). Scaring rate of small ulcers was 49%. In females, ulcers were commonly found on both major (71%) and minor labiae (10%). Vaginal and cervical lesions were less frequent. Similarly large ulcers healed with scarring (Fig. 4.2b), while only 54% of small ulcers did so in females. The ulcers, located at the labia minor, did not result in scars similar to what is seen in oral ulcers. It is also possible that mucosal scarring can not be discerned by the naked eye.

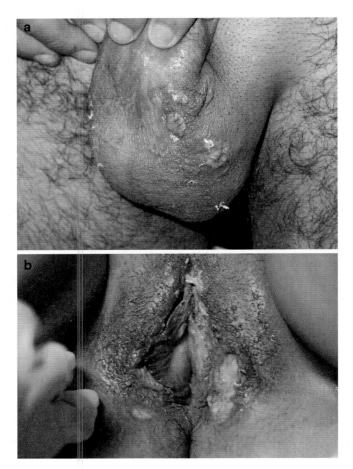

Fig. 4.2 (**a, b**) Genital ulcers

Cutaneous Lesions

The skin lesions of BD are:

1. Nodular lesions:

    (a) Erythema nodosum-like lesions
    (b) Superficial thrombophlebitis

2. Papulopustular and acneiform lesions
3. Other lesions

The skin pathergy reaction (SPR) is a unique lesion singularly reflecting the exaggerated inflammatory response in BD. As such it will be separately discussed.

Based on case studies the occurrence of cutaneous manifestations ranges from 38 to 99% in patients with BD, although regional differences exist [24–26]. Papulopustular lesions and erythema nodosum-like lesions are the most common cutaneous manifestations [24–27]. More than two types of cutaneous lesions are seen frequently in patients with BD and the most frequent combination is erythema nodosum-like lesions and papulopustular lesions, which occurs at a similar frequency in adults and children [26, 28].

The frequency and clinical pattern of cutaneous lesions in pediatric patients with Behçet's disease also varies from country to country, which is similar to adult-onset patients [28] (see also Chap. 12).

Erythema Nodosum-Like Lesions

Erythema nodosum (EN)-like lesions are characterized by the presence of red, tender, erythematous nonulcerating nodules that are 1–5 cm in diameter and frequently located on the lower extremities. They are observed in up to 50% of patients [4–6]. They tend to be symmetrical in distribution and are located particularly on the anterior tibial surface, but may also involve other sites including the face, neck, forearms, buttocks, lower part of the thighs, and ankles (Fig. 4.3a–c) [26, 29].

EN-like lesions are more frequently seen in females (70%) [30], and generally resolve within 1–6 weeks with residual pigmentation resembling bruises. EN is a reactive process that may be idiopathic or associated with a wide spectrum of diseases such as infections, drugs, sarcoidosis, IBD, and malignancy [25]. EN associated with BD can sometimes led to hyperpigmentation but morphology, in general, is not very helpful for differentiation of BD-associated lesions from the other etiologies.

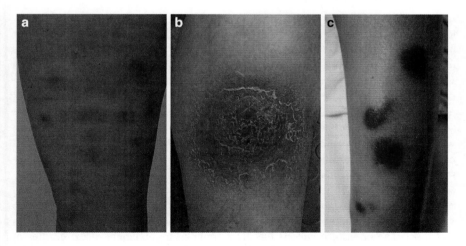

Fig. 4.3 (a–c) Clinical features of erythema nodosum-like lesions

EN-like lesions in BD are characterized histopathologically by predominant septal and lobular panniculitis in which neutrophilic vascular inflammation (neutrophilic vasculitis) is more frequently observed than in classical EN where they are conspicuously absent [29, 31]. The lesions resemble histologically to that of nodular vasculitis, but granuloma formation is rarely seen [29] (see Chap. 13).

Superficial Thrombophlebitis

Superficial thrombophlebitis (ST) is the most common type of venous involvement in BD [32]. It presents as palpable, painful subcutaneous nodules or string-like hardenings with reddening of the overlying skin. With time new nodules can appear on the same vein as old ones heal [25].

It may be difficult to differentiate ST from EN-like lesions with the naked eye. Being distinctly more common among males [32] the presence of ST indicates more severe disease. ST tends to be associated with deep venous thrombosis and dural sinus thrombosis in the central nervous system [33]. Thus it is important to differentiate ST from EN-like lesions and high-resolution ultrasonography of nodular lesions was found to be useful in this regard [34]. There, ST presented itself as hypoechoic nodules which were noncompressible with a probe, while EN-like lesions appeared as hyperechoic nodules.

Papulopustular Lesions, Pseudofolliculitis, and Acneiform Lesions

Over the last years there has been debate about the nature and frequency of papulopustular lesions of BD and the main issue seems to be whether these lesions, observed in many patients, are part of the disease spectrum. Some authors disagree with this view [35]. Furthermore, there has also been some disagreement among dermatologists regarding exact descriptive terminology, especially over what discriminated an acne lesion from folliculitis [36].

Papulopustular and acneiform lesions are frequent skin manifestations of BD, with a reported prevalence ranging from 30 to 96% [24–27]. They are characterized by follicular or nonfollicular papules and pustules which are occasionally surrounded by an erythematous halo (Fig. 4.4a–c). Acneiform lesions have polymorphic features presenting as inflammatory papules, pustules, nodules, and noninflammatory comedones and cannot be clinically differentiated from acne vulgaris even by experienced dermatologists [37]. This applies to histopathology as well [38]. The only difference is the more frequent involvement of extremities in BD-associated lesions than in acne vulgaris. In one study, the most common local-

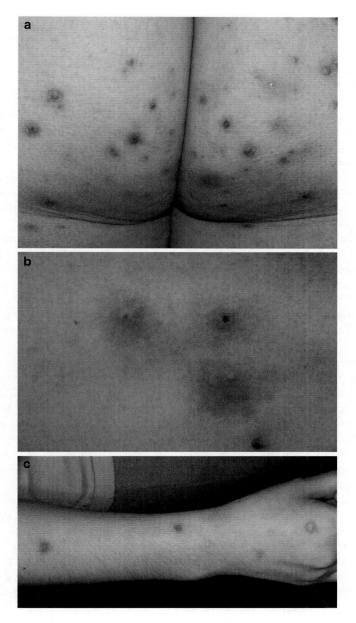

Fig. 4.4 (**a–c**) Papulopustular eruptions

ization in BD was trunk followed by extremities while face was the most common site in acne vulgaris and other dermatoses [39].

The mechanism behind the papulopustular lesions in BD is still unknown. Since the age of onset in BD is usually in the twenties and thirties, the presence of papulopustular lesions may simply be related to the persistence of acne vulgaris which is the most prevalent skin disease of the adolescent (60–70%) [40]. The ISG criteria require that the papulopustular lesions of Behçet's syndrome (BS) should present in the postadolescent period and, in the absence of steroid therapy [13]. Furthermore, acne does not always end with adolescence and is still relatively common in adulthood with 5% of males and 20% of females showing persisting lesions at the age of 25 [40, 41]. So what is observed in BD might be the reflection of persistence with some augmentation of acne vulgaris at an older age. We know that genetic predisposition is important in ordinary acne [42] but are unaware of formal studies in BD.

Sebum excretion is an androgen-driven phenomenon well known to be increased in acne vulgaris [40, 43]. In a controlled study, sebum excretion in BD patients was found to be comparable to that of acne vulgaris and was significantly greater than in healthy controls, children and patients with ankylosing spondylitis, but not different from rheumatoid arthritis [44]. Since BD runs a distinctly more severe course in the male (see Chap. 17), it can be proposed that androgens are involved in the development of papulopustular lesions of BD. Although there is no direct evidence, a study found higher androgen receptor frequency in papulopustular lesions of SPR in males compared to females, while oral and genital ulcers of the same patients had similar expression pattern [45]. On the other hand, it seems that the frequency of papulopustular lesions does not significantly differ between genders [4].

Pustules associated with BD are usually considered as noninfectious inflammatory lesions. A recent study suggested that they were not sterile [46]. The predominant bacteria were *Staphylococcus aureus* and *Prevotella spp* in pustules from BD patients while coagulase-negative staphylococci were predominant in pustules from acne patients. The presence of *Staphlyocccus aureus* in ordinary acne is known to be rare [40] while it is, by definition, a requirement for infectious folliculitis [36]. Thus it can be proposed that at least some of the follicular-based acneiform lesions of BD represent a propensity to skin infection in this syndrome. This is in line with data suggesting impaired innate immunity in BD [47] (see Chap. 14).

Papulopustular lesions of BD are not always follicle-based and acne lesions, as a rule, are always follicle-based. Some authors suggest that because of the nonspecific nature of follicular lesions, only nonfollicular lesions with histologic confirmation of vasculitis should be considered as BD-associated lesions [35, 48–50]. It should be emphasized that this differentiation is especially important in individuals not meeting full diagnostic criteria, although the proportion of such patients in BD has not been formally documented. However, it seems that clinical examination fails to differentiate nonfollicular lesions from nonspecific follicular lesions [51]. Histopathology of these lesions, even taken from carefully selected nonfollicular sites, do not always show vasculitis [52] (see Chap. 13).

Finally, several recent studies showed a strong association of papulopustular skin lesions with arthritis in BD [53] (see also Chap. 8). This might also back up the contention that these skin lesions are part of the syndrome rather than a chance finding.

Other Cutaneous Lesions

The spectrum of cutaneous lesions in BD can be expanded according to case series and case reports and many unusual manifestations were documented in patients with BD (Table 4.1) [25, 54–68].

BD may be among the conditions that may present as Sweet's syndrome [67, 68]. In a patient series, this was reported up to 4% during the disease course [69]. These lesions are usually located on the face and extremities and consist of painful inflammatory nodules and plaques (Fig. 4.5) [70]. Since there may be overlaping features between the extracutaneous manifestations of primary Sweet's syndrome and BD, such as arthritis, oral ulcerations, and uveitis, the differential diagnosis between the two may occasionally become a semantic exercise.

Extragenital skin ulcers are rare and usually located in the axillary and interdigital areas [71].

Leg ulcers in BD, which may be caused by vasculitis or deep vein thrombosis, have a chronic recurrent course and are refractory to treatment [55].

Skin Pathergy Reaction

A unifying feature of the inflammation observed in BD is the presence of the pathergy phenomenon where traumatic insult or various types of inflammatory stimuli to tissues cause an enhanced inflammatory response. In clinical practice, SPR is induced by perpendicular or oblique insertion of a 20-gauge needle into the dermis at three different sites on each forearm. Introduction of saline or other solutions/chemicals are not necessary. A positive test is defined as the development of a papule or pustule at the needle prick site at 48 h (Fig. 4.6). SPR has no association with disease activity nor any particular disease manifestation [72–74], however, it is more strongly positive among males [75].

Table 4.1 Rare cutaneous manifestations associated with Behçet's disease

Cutaneous vasculitis
Palpable purpura
Henoch–Schönlein purpura
Bullous necrotizing vasculitis
Polyarteritis-like lesions
Neutrophilic dermatoses
Sweet's syndrome-like lesions
Pyoderma gangrenosum
Neutrophilic eccrine hidradenitis
Others
Pernio-like cutaneous lesions, erythema multiforme-like lesions, subungal infarctions, hemorrhagic bullae, furuncles, abscesses, Kaposi's sarcoma, acral purpuric papulonodular lesions, necrobiosis lipoidica

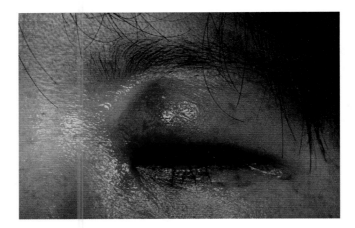

Fig. 4.5 Sweet's syndrome-like lesions

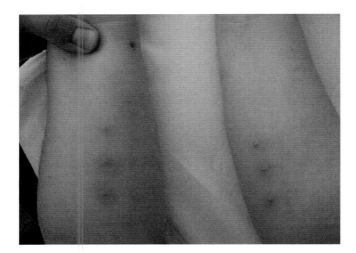

Fig. 4.6 Positive pathergy reaction

The pathergy phenomenon is not only restricted to the skin. In fact, any disruption of tissue integrity is potentially associated with an exaggerated inflammatory response in BD. In particular, the posttraumatic arterial thrombus and/or aneurysm formation following conventional angiographic interventions [76], vascular surgery [76–78], superficial thrombophlebitis induced by venipuncture, eye inflammation after intraocular corticosteroid injections [79] and anastomotic ulcers following surgical treatment of intestinal ulcer [80] are well-known examples of pathergy reactions triggered at different tissue sites. On the other hand, wound healing time is normal as shown in one study [81].

SPR is one of the most diagnostically-relevant lesions of BD included in the ISG criteria [13]. However, it has limited reproducibility and shows great geographic variation, with very low positivity rate in regions of low prevalence [6, 74]. The frequency of test positivity ranges from 30 to 70% in endemic areas [6]. An analysis of retrospective patient series indicates decreasing rates of positivity over years [6]. Increasing use of less traumatic disposable needles seems to account for this decrease [82]. Moreover, an increased positivity rate of SPR with the use of blunt needle insertion [83] and a decreased positivity rate when it is induced at surgically cleaned skin has been shown [84].

SPR induced by intradermal injection of monosodium urate (MSU) crystals has a greater sensitivity and reproducibility compared to classical pathergy test [85]. Unlike the classical pathergy reaction, MSU induce an erythematous skin lesion. The test positivity in BD is characterized by sustained erythema at 48 h which is significantly greater in diameter compared to healthy controls [74]. When Turkish BD patients were compared with the diseased controls including familial Mediterranean fever (FMF), rheumatoid arthritis, ankylosing spondylitis, and SLE patients, the test found to be 60% sensitive and 100% specific to BD. However, among the British population the MSU-induced pathergy reaction in BD had higher sensitivity (93%) than the classical pathergy reaction (28%) but lest specificity being positive in 18% of healthy controls and 25% of diseased controls including rheumatoid arthritis and ankylosing spondylitis patients [74].

SPR shows features of T cell-mediated immune responses [86–88]. A comparative study of the skin immune responses to a needle prick between normal controls and BD patients with a positive SPR revealed that, in contrast to self- limited innate inflammatory responses observed in normal skin during the initial 8 h, an exaggerated Th1-type inflammatory response developed in SPR sites by 48 h [87]. It was characterized by marked influx of mature dendritic cells, monocytes, and CD4+ T lymphocytes into the site of injury. Similarly, increases in Th1-type cytokines (IFN-gamma, IL-12 p40, IL-15) and chemokines (MIP3-alpha, IP-10, Mig, and iTac), along with adhesion molecules (ICAM-1, VCAM-1) were noted at 48 h in the skin of BD patients with SPR but not in the skin of normal controls.

On the other hand, a T cell-mediated immune response is not a consistent finding of the SPR. The presence of neutrophil-predominating inflammatory infiltrates, some of which exhibit the features of leukocytoclastic vasculitis [89, 90], and an increased presence of mast cells in skin infiltrates [91–93] has been reported. It is not clear if this may reflect different pathogenic mechanisms operating in tissue inflammation or if the exact nature of the infiltrate may depend on the timing of biopsy or the way SPR were induced, such as by histamine. However, immunohistological studies did not find an antibody-mediated or immune complex-mediated immune response associated with SPR [90].

The mechanisms underlying the exaggerated Th1-type immune response in positive SPR sites are not well understood. Immunohistological studies suggest that either an inadequate innate immune response that provokes a compensating adaptive response, or insufficient regulatory mechanisms acting upon the adaptive response may operate in this inflammatory process [86, 87] (see also Chap. 14).

It has been assumed that immune priming upon a constitutively abnormal leukocyte population is necessary for the pathergy response, as suggested by the appearance of SPR in chronic myelogenous leukemia patients undergoing immune-activating treatment with IFN-alpha [93]. On the other hand, a high positivity rate was not observed in BD patients receiving IFN-alpha treatment compared to those taking cyclosporine A, azathioprine, colchicine, or no treatment [94]. In a short-term controlled study with etanercept in BD patients, it has been shown that TNF-α blockage did not suppress SPR while it was significantly effective in controlling most of the mucocutaneous manifestations of the disease [95].

Differential Diagnosis

Differential diagnosis, although not often difficult in patients presenting with classical signs and symptoms of BD, must include many conditions that are associated with oral, genital, and skin lesions (Table 4.2).

Complex aphthosis is a severe form of RAS and is characterized by almost constant presence of oral ulcers with or without genital ulcers [10]. Complex aphtosis, consistently presenting in conjunction with genital ulcers is probably an incomplete form of BD [96, 97]. On the other hand, complex aphthosis may also associate with several other systemic diseases including ulcus vulva acutum, Reiter's syndrome, mouth and genital ulcers with inflamed cartilage (MAGIC) syndrome, autoinflammatory diseases such as the PFAPA (periodic fever, aphthous ulcers, pharyngitis, adenopathy) syndrome, and cyclic neutropenia [9, 97] (Table 4.2).

Some mucocutaneous diseases manifesting as nonaphthous oral or genital lesions may need to be differentiated from BD. In this context, patients with erythema multiforme, autoimmune bullous disease such as mucosal pemphigoid and pemphigus vulgaris, and vulvovaginal form of erosive lichen planus are particularly problematic [98]. Bullous dermatoses are blistering diseases of the mucous membranes and skin. Mucous membrane involvement is primarily of oral mucosa, but may also include conjunctiva, nasopharynx, larynx, esophagus, genitalia, and rectal mucosa. Erythema multiforme is considered to be a hypersensitivity reaction associated with certain infections and medications. It manifests as a polymorphous eruption of macules, papules, and characteristic "target" skin lesions. There is minimal mucosal involvement usually limited to oral mucosa. Erythema multiforme resolves spontaneously in 3–5 weeks without sequelae, but it may recur. Lichen planus often occurs only on cutaneous surfaces with characteristic violaceous polygonal flat-topped papules and plaques. Pruritus is often severe. Oral lichen planus classically presents as reticular or erosive lesions with radiating striae, genital lichen planus among males is visible as violaceous papules on the glans penis. In women, violaceous papules, hypertrophic lesions or erosions may occur and are located typically on the vulva.

Table 4.2 Differential diagnosis of BD

Diseases associated with ulcerative oral and/or genital mucosal lesions	Distinguishing feature from BD
Dermatological	
Complex aphthosis	Idiopathic form with recurrent oral and genital ulceration represents forme fruste of BD
Ulcus vulvae acutum	Coexisting infectious gastroenteritis
Fixed drug eruption	Localized sharply-circumscribed cutaneous drug reaction recurring in the same location
Erythema multiforme and Stevens-Johnson syndrome	Typical "target" skin lesion
Autoimmune bullous disorders	
Pemphigus	Blistering mucosal and skin lesions, erosions
Mucosal pemphigoid	
Erosive lichen planus	Itchy papulosquamous skin lesion, discrete or desquamative, oral and genital mucosa lesions.
Systemic disorders	
Inflammatory bowel disease	Genital ulcers rare, positive pathergy in 8%
Celiac disease	Response to gluten-free diet
Hematinic deficiencies (Iron, vitamin B12, folate)	Response to replacement
SLE	No genital scaring
Reiter's syndrome	
MAGIC syndrome	Relapsing polychondritis
Cyclic neutropenia	Neutropenia during episodes
Autoinflammatory diseases (FMF, PFAPA, hyper-IgD)	Onset in childhood, febrile episodes
Infectious	
Acute necrotizing ulcerative gingivostomatitis	Bacterial infection with inter-dental papilla involvement
Syphilis	Oral, genital and anal ulcers (primary, secondary, tertiary syphilis)
HIV	Usually major oral ulcers, CD4+ cell count <100
HSV	Cluster of small vesicles along the vermilion, border of the lip or genital integument
Hand, foot and mouth disease	Vesicular oral mucosal lesions, hand and foot lesions
Infectious mononucleosis	Fever, pharyngitis
Oral malignancy	Persisting ulcers for >6 weeks, red or white patches of oral mucosa, age >45, smoking

IBD has many overlapping clinical features with BD. Patients with IBD not only have RAS, but may also have EN, papulopustular lesions, arthritis, and eye inflammation such as iritis or uveitis. A study from Turkey, screening the ISG criteria among 223 patients with IBD, found oral ulcers in 20% and papulopustular lesions in 25%, positive SPR in 8%, EN in five, history of genital ulceration without observed scar in four, arthritis in five, and uveitis in two patients. There were only two patients with ulcerative colitis fulfilling ISG criteria for BD [99]. A study from the same clinic assessed the performance of ISG criteria among 302 patients with BS and 438 patients with other rheumatic conditions, mainly including IBD and FMF [100]. There were only five patients meeting ISG criteria for BD. It seems that the ISG criteria perform well to differentiate BD from IBD, although it may sometimes be challenging in an individual patient.

SLE can present with mucosal lesions that occur most frequently in oral and nasal mucosa followed by the perianal area [101]. However, genital ulceration is probably rare in SLE. A cross-sectional study including consecutive 48 female SLE patients, found no genital ulcer or scaring while the rates were 20 and 26% in female patients with BD, respectively [102].

The term autoinflammatory diseases defines a group of hereditary disorders which are characterized by recurrent episodes of inflammatory manifestations in different organs [103]. Various skin eruptions such as erythematous macules and papules, urticaria, erysipelas as well as oral ulcerations, notably in PFAPA syndrome, may be part of inflammatory episodes. However, unlike in BD, these other disease episodes are characteristically accompanied by fever.

Local Treatment of Mucocutaneous Lesions (See Chap. 19 for Systemic Treatment)

Antiseptic mouth washes, topical lidocain gels (2–5%), triamcinolon acetonid containing oral pastes are used to reduce pain and healing time of aphthae. Dexamethasone mouth washes are useful for posterior mouth ulcers. Triamcinolone acetonide (5 mg/ml) injections at the base of major aphthae can reduce healing time.

In a double-blind randomized study, sucralfate suspension was found to be effective in the treatment of oral aphthous ulcers [104]. It reduced the frequency, pain, and healing time of aphthous ulcers. Five milliliter suspension of sucralfate should be kept in the mouth for a while four times a day.

Topical antiseptics, antimicrobials, mid-potent corticosteroid ointments, and wet dressings are useful in the treatment of scrotal and labial, pubic, and inguinal ulcers.

Major ulcers located on vestibul, introitus vagina, and perineal are very painful. As these ulcers are also prone to bacterial contamination, local antiseptics and antimicrobials should be used. For severe cases mid-dose systemic steroids can be added. Thalidomide as well as immunosuppresives such as azathioprine can also be used in selected patients. These ulcers heal with scar and fibrosis formation within 3–4 weeks. Prolonged use of immunosuppresive drugs should be considered for prophylaxis.

In an open label study azitromicine decreased the number of papulopustular lesions and oral ulcers [105]. As papulopustular lesions in BD patients are not sterile [46], this line of treatment seems justified.

Neither oral pastes and losanges (including those containing interferon-alpha) nor topical cyclosporine A were shown to be effective in the treatment of oral ulcers of BD in separate double-blind placebo-controlled studies [106, 107]. In a double-blind placebo-controlled study, chromoline 4% gel was also reported to be ineffective in controlling genital ulcers [108].

In a pilot study, Lactobacillus paste was shown to be effective in controlling oral ulcers [109]. Further studies using proper controls are needed.

Finally, stasis ulcers of the legs are managed with wet dressings, Unna boots, zinc ointments containing zinc oxide, colagenase enzyme, and wound dressings. Rest and leg elevation are also useful.

References

1. Behçet H (1937) Ueber rezidivierende aphtose durch ein virus verursachte geschwuere am mund, am auge und an den genitalien. Dermatol Wochenschr 105:1152
2. Yazici H, Yurdakul S, Hamuryudan V (1998) Behçet's syndrome. In: Maddison PJ, Isenberg DA, Woo P, Glass DN (eds) Oxford textbook of rheumatology, 2nd edn. Oxford University Press, Oxford, pp 1394–1402
3. Zunt SL (2003) Recurrent aphthous stomatitis. Dermatol Clin 21:33–39
4. Gürler A, Boyvat A, Tursen U (1997) Clinical manifestations of Behçet's disease. An analysis of 2147 patients. Yonsei Med J 38:423–427
5. Alpsoy E, Dönmez L, Önder M et al (2007) Clinical features and natural course of Behçet's disease in 661 cases. a multicenter study. Br J Dermatol 157:901–906
6. Saylan T, Mat C, Fresko I, Melikoğlu M (1999) Behçet's disease in the middle-east. Clin Dermatol 17:209–223
7. Bang D, Hur W, Lee ES, Lee S (1995) Prognosis and clinical relevance of recurrent oral ulceration in Behçet's disease. J Dermatol 22:926–929
8. McCarthy MA, Garton RA, Jorizzo JL (2003) Complex aphthosis and Behçet's disease. Dermatol Clin 21:41–48
9. Rogers RS III (1997) Recurrent aphthous stomatitis in diagnosis of Behçet's disease. Yonsei Med J 38:370–379
10. Letsinger JA, MacCarty MA, Jorizzo JL (2005) Complex aphthosis: a large case series with evaluation algorithm and therapeutic ladder from topicals to thalidomide. J Am Acad Dermatol 52:500–508
11. Ifeacho SN, Malhi G, Hamburger M (2004) Recurrent aphtous stomatitis and Behçet's disease: is there a link? XI International Congress on BD. Clin Exp Rheumatol 22(4):101
12. Main DM, Chamberlain MA (1992) Clinical differentiation of oral ulceration in Behçet's disease. Br J Rheumatol 31:767–770
13. International Study Group for Behçet's Disease (1990) Criteria for diagnosis of Behçet's disease. Lancet 335:1078–1080
14. Hamuryudan V, Mat C, Saip S, Ozyazgan Y, Siva A, Yurdakul S, Zwingenberger K, Yazici H (1998) Thalidomide in the treatment of the mucocutaneous lesions of the Behçet's syndrome. A randomized, double-blind, placebo-controlled trial. Ann Intern Med 128(6):443–450
15. Melikoglu M, Fresko I, Mat C, Ozyazgan Y, Gogus F, Yurdakul S, Hamuryudan V, Yazici H (2005) Short-term trial of etanercept in Behçet's disease: a double blind, placebo controlled study. J Rheumatol 32:98–105
16. Yurdakul S, Mat C, Tüzün Y, Ozyazgan Y, Hamuryudan V, Uysal O, Senocak M, Yazici H (2001) A double-blind trial of colchicine in Behçet's syndrome. Arthritis Rheum 44(11): 2686–2692

17. Cosgun S, Seyahi E, Mat C, Yazici H (2004) Female Behçet's syndrome patients have more severe oral ulceration. XI International congress on Behçet's disease. Clin Exp Rheumatol 22:86

18. Krause I, Rosen Y, Kaplan I, Milo G, Guedj D, Molad Y, Weinberger A (1999) Recurrent aphthous stomatitis in Behçet's disease: clinical features and correlation with systemic disease expression and severity. J Oral Pathol Med 28(5):193–196

19. Mumcu G, Sur H, Inanc N, Karacayli U, Cimilli H, Sisman N, Ergun T, Direskeneli H (2009) A composite index for determining the impact of oral ulcer activity in Behçet's disease and recurrent aphthous stomatitis. J Oral Pathol Med 38(10):785–791

20. Sharquie KE, Al-Araji A, Hatem A (2002) Oral pathergy test in Behçet's disease. Br J Dermatol 146(1):168–169

21. Soy M, Erken E, Konca K, Ozbek S (2000) Smoking and Behçet's disease. Clin Rheumatol 19(6):508–509

22. Kaklamani VG, Tzonou A, Markomichelakis N, Papazoglou S, Kaklamanis PG (2003) The effect of smoking on the clinical features of Adamantiades-Behçet's disease. Adv Exp Med Biol 528:323–327

23. Mat C, Goksugur N, Ergin B, Yurdakul S, Yazici H (2006) The frequency of scarring after genital ulcers in Behçet's syndrome: a prospective study. Int J Dermatol 45:554–556

24. Bang D, Lee ES, Sohn S (2001) Behçet's disease: a guide to its clinical understanding. Springer, Heidelberg

25. Alpsoy E, Zouboulis CC, Ehrlich GE (2007) Mucocutaneous lesions of Behçet's disease. Yonsei Med J 48:573–585

26. Lee ES, Bang D, LEE S (1997) Dermatologic manifestation of Behçet's disease. Yonsei Med J 38:380–389

27. Lin P, Liang G (2006) Behçet's Disease: recommendation for clinical management of mucocutaneous lesions. J Clin Rheumatol 12:282–286

28. Kim B, LeBoit PE (2000) Histopathologic features of erythema nodosum-like lesion in Behçet's disease: a comparison with erythema nodosum focusing on the role of vasculitis. Am J Dermatopathol 22:379–390

29. Demirkesen C, Tuzuner N, Mat C, Senocak M, Buyukbabani N, Tuzun Y, Yazici H (2001) Clinicopathologic evaluation of nodular cutaneous lesions of Behçet's syndrome. Am J Clin Pathol 116:341–346

30. Yazici H, Tüzün Y, Pazarli H, Yurdakul S, Ozyazgan Y, Ozdoğan H, Serdaroğlu S, Ersanli M, Ulkü BY, Müftüoğlu AU (1984) Influence of age of onset and patient's sex on the prevalence and severity of manifestations of Behçet's syndrome. Ann Rheum Dis 43(6):783–789

31. Mat CM, Demirkesen C, Melikoglu M, Yazici H (2006) Behçet's syndrome. In: Sarzi-Puttuni P, Doria A, Girolomoni G, Kuhn A (eds) The skin and autoimmune disease. Elsevier, Amsterdam, pp 185–206

32. Kuzu MA, Ozaslan C, Köksoy C, Gürler A, Tüzüner A (1994) Vascular involvement in Behçet's disease: 8-year audit. World J Surg 18(6):948–953

33. Tunc R, Saip S, Siva A, Yazici H (2004) Cerebral venous thrombosis is associated with major vessel disease in Behçet's syndrome. Ann Rheum Dis 63(12):1693–1694

34. Kucukoglu S, Tunc R, Cetinkaya F, Demirkesen C, Mat C, Yazici H (2000) The importance of cutaneous ultrasonography on the differentiation of nodular skin lesions seen in patients with Behçet's disease. Yonsei Med J 41(3):S40

35. Jorizzo JL, Abernethy JL, White WL, Mangelsdorf HC, Zouboulis CC, Sarica R, Gaffney K, Mat C, Yazici H, al Ialaan A et al (1995) Mucocutaneous criteria for the diagnosis of Behçet's disease: an analysis of clinicopathologic data from multiple international centers. J Am Acad Dermatol 32(6):968–976

36. Luelmo-Aguilar J, Santandreu MS (2004) Folliculitis: recognition and management. Am J Clin Dermatol 5(5):301–310

37. Yazici H, Hekim N, Tüzün Y, Serdaroglu S, Kotogyan A, Öz F, Yurdakul S, Pazarlı H, Müftüoğlu A (1986) Sex factor and Behçet's syndrome. In: Lehner T, Barnes CG, (Eds) Recent advances in Behçet's Disease, Royal Society of Medicine Services, London. pp 205–206

38. Ergun T, Gurbuz O, Dogusoy G, Mat C, Yazici H (1998) Histopathologic features of the spontaneous pustular lesions of Behçet's syndrome. Int J Dermatol 37:194–196
39. Alpsoy E, Aktekin M, Er H, Durusoy C, Yilmaz E (1998) A randomized, controlled and blinded study of papulopustular lesions in Turkish Behçet's patients. Int J Dermatol 37(11):839–842
40. Kligman AM (1974) An overview of acne. J Invest Dermatol 62(3):268–287
41. Kligman AM (1991) Postadolescent acne in women. Cutis 48(1):75–77
42. Goulden V, McGeown CH, Cunliffe WJ (1999) The familial risk of adult acne: a comparison between first-degree relatives of affected and unaffected individuals. Br J Dermatol 141(2):297–300
43. Thiboutot D, Gilliland K, Light J, Lookingbill D (1999) Androgen metabolism in sebaceous glands from subjects with and without acne. Arch Dermatol 135(9):1041–1045
44. Yazici H, Mat C, Deniz S, Iscimen A, Yurdakul S, Tuzun Y, Hekim N, Yazici Y (1987) Sebum production is increased in Behçet's syndrome and even more so in rheumatoid arthritis. Clin Exp Rheumatol 5(4):371–374
45. Alpsoy E, Elpek GO, Yilmaz F, Ciftcioglu MA, Akman A, Uzun S, Karakuzu A (2005) Androgen receptor levels of oral and genital ulcers and skin pathergy test in patients with Behçet's disease. Dermatology 210(1):31–35
46. Hatemi G, Bahar H, Uysal S, Mat C, Gogus F, Masatlioglu S, Altas K, Yazici H (2004) The pustular skin lesions in Behçet's syndrome are not sterile. Ann Rheum Dis 63(11):1450–1452
47. Inanc N, Mumcu G, Birtas E, Elbir Y, Yavuz S, Ergun T, Fresko I, Direskeneli H (2005) Serum mannose-binding lectin levels are decreased in Behçet's disease and associated with disease severity. J Rheumatol 32(2):287–291
48. Alpsoy E, Uzun S, Akman A, Acar MA, Memişoglu HR, Başaran E (2003) Histological and immunofluorescence findings of non-follicular papulopustular lesions in patients with Behçet's disease. J Eur Acad Dermatol Venereol 17(5):521–524
49. Ilknur T, Pabuçcuoglu U, Akin C, Lebe B, Gunes AT (2006) Histopathologic and direct immunofluorescence findings of the papulopustular lesions in Behçet's disease. Eur J Dermatol 16(2):146–150
50. Kalkan G, Karadag AS, Astarci HM, Akbay G, Ustun H, Eksioglu M (2009) A histopathological approach: when papulopustular lesions should be in the diagnostic criteria of Behçet's disease? J Eur Acad Dermatol Venereol 23(9):1056–1060
51. Boyvat A, Heper AO, Koçyiğit P, Erekul S, Gürgey E (2006) Can specific vessel-based papulopustular lesions of Behçet's disease be differentiated from nonspecific follicular-based lesions clinically? Int J Dermatol 45(7):814–818
52. Ergun T, Gürbüz O, Dogusoy G, Mat C, Yazici H (1998) Histopathologic features of the spontaneous pustular lesions of Behçet's syndrome. Int J Dermatol 37(3):194–196
53. Diri E, Mat C, Hamuryudan V, Yurdakul S, Hizli N, Yazici H (2001) Papulopustular skin lesions are seen more frequently in patients with Behçet's syndrome who have arthritis: a controlled and masked study. Ann Rheum Dis 60(11):1074–1076
54. Lin P, Liang G (2006) Behçet's disease: recommendation for clinical management of mucocutaneous lesions. J Clin Rheumatol 12:282–286
55. Jung JY, Kim DY, Bang D (2008) Leg ulcers in Behçet's disease. Br J Dermatol 158:172–203
56. Oh SH, Lee JH, Shin JU, Bang D (2008) Dermatological features in Behçet's disease-associated vena cava obstruction. Br J Dermatol 159:555–560
57. Golan G, Beeri R, Mevorach D (1994) Henoch–Schonlein purpura-like disease representing a flare of Behçet's disease. Br J Rheumatol 33:1198–1199
58. Park YW, Park JJ, Lee JB et al (2007) Development of Henoch–Schonlein purpura in a patient with Behçet's disease presenting with recurrent deep vein thrombosis. Clin Exp Rheumatol 25:S96–S98
59. Chen KR, Kawahara Y, Miyakawa S et al (1997) Cutaneous vasculitis in Behçet's disease: a clinical and histopathologic study of 20 patients. J Am Acad Dermatol 36:689–696

60. Bilic M, Mutasim DF (2001) Neutrophilic eccrine hidradenitis in a patient with Behçet's disease. Cutis 68:107–111
61. Nijsten TE, Meuleman L, Lambert J (2002) Chronic pruritic neutrophilic eccrine hidradenitis in a patient with Behçet's disease. Br J Dermatol 147:797–800
62. Mercader-Garcia P, Vilata-Corell JJ, Pardo-Sanchez J et al (2003) Neutrophilic eccrine hidradenitis in a patient with Behçet's disease. Acta Derm Venereol 83:395–396
63. Cantini F, Salvarani C, Niccoli L et al (1998) Behçet's disease with unusual cutaneous lesions. J Rheumatol 25:2469–2372
64. Korkmaz C, Aydinli A, Erol N et al (2001) Widespread nocardiosis in two patients with Behçet's disease. Clin Exp Rheumatol 19:459–462
65. King R, Crowson AN, Murray E et al (1995) Acral purpuric papulonodular lesions as a manifestation of Behçet's disease. Int J Dermatol 34:190–192
66. Aydin F, Senturk N, Yildiz L et al (2006) Behçet's disease with unusual cutaneous lesions. J Eur Acad Dermatol Venereol 20:106–107
67. Callen PR (2007) Sweet's syndrome-a comprehensive review of an acute febrile neutrophilic dermatosis. Orphanet J Rare Dis 2:34
68. Magro CM, Crowson AN (1995) Cutaneous manifestations of Behçet's disease. Int J Dermatol 34:159–165
69. Hui-li S, Zheng-ji H (1993) Study on cutaneous lesions in Behçet's disease and meanings of relative laboratory parameters. In: Godeau F, Weschler B (eds) Behçet's disease, Proceedings of the sixth international conference on Behçet's disease. Excerpta Medica, Amsterdam, p 325
70. Oguz A, Serdaroglu S, Tuzun Y, Erdogan N, Yazici H, Savaskan H (1992) Acute febrile neutrophilic dermatosis associated with Behçet's syndrome. Int J Dermatol 31:645–646
71. Azizlerli G, Ozarmagan G, Ovul C, Sarica R, Mustafa SO (1992) A new kind of skin lesion in Behçet's disease: extragenital ulcers. Acta Derm Venereol 72:286
72. Ozarmagan G, Saylan T, Azizlerli G, Ovul C, Aksungur VL (1991) Re-evaluation of the pathergy test in Behçet's disease. Acta Derm Venereol 71:75–76
73. Krause I, Molad Y, Mitrani M, Weinberger A (2000) Pathergy reaction in Behçet's disease: lack of correlation with mucocutaneous manifestations and systemic disease expression. Clin Exp Rheumatol 18:71–74
74. Cakir N, Yazici H, Chamberlain MA, Barnes CG, Yurdakul S, Atasoy S, Akcasu A, Iscimen A (1991) Response to intradermal injection of monosodium urate crystals in Behçet's syndrome. Ann Rheum Dis 50:634–636
75. Yazici H, Tüzün Y, Tanman AB, Yurdakul S, Serdaroglu S, Pazarli H, Müftüoglu A (1985) Male patients with Behçet's syndrome have stronger pathergy reactions. Clin Exp Rheumatol 3(2):137–141
76. Alpagut U, Ugurlucan M, Dayioglu E (2007) Major arterial involvement and review of Behçet's disease. Ann Vasc Surg 21(2):232–239
77. Tüzün H, Sayin A, Karaözbek Y, Erdağ A, Coskun H, Vural FS (1993) Peripheral aneurysms in Behçet's disease. Cardiovasc Surg 1(3):220–224
78. Tüzün H, Besirli K, Sayin A, Vural FS, Hamuryudan V, Hizli N, Yurdakul S, Yazici H (1997) Management of aneurysms in Behçet's syndrome: an analysis of 24 patients. Surgery 121(2):150–156
79. Yalcindag FN, Batioglu F (2008) Pathergy-like reaction following intravitreal triamcinolone acetonide injection in a patient with Behçet's disease. Ocul Immunol Inflamm 16(4):181–183
80. Choi IJ, Kim JS, Cha SD, Jung HC, Park JG, Song IS, Kim CY (2000) Long-term clinical course and prognostic factors in intestinal Behçet's disease. Dis Colon Rectum 43(5):692–700
81. Mat MC, Nazarbaghi M, Tüzün Y, Hamuryudan V, Hızlı N, Yurdakul S, Özyazgan Y, Yazici H (1998) Wound healing in Behçet's syndrome. Int J Dermatol 37:120–123
82. Ozarmagan G, Saylan T, Azizlerli G, Ovül C, Aksungur VL (1991) Re-evaluation of the pathergy test in Behçet's disease. Acta Derm Venereol 71(1):75–76
83. Dilsen N, Konice M, Aral O, Ocal L, Inanc M, Gül A (1993) Comparative study of the skin pathergy test with blunt and sharp needles in Behçet's disease: confirmed specificity but decreased sensitivity with sharp needles. Ann Rheum Dis 52:823–825

84. Fresko I, Yazici H, Bayramicli M, Yurdakul S, Mat C (1993) Effect of surgical cleaning of the skin on the pathergy phenomenon in Behçet's syndrome. Ann Rheum Dis 52:619–620
85. Fresko I, Ozsoy Y, Mat C, Melikoglu M, Tunc R, Yazici H (2000) The response to the intradermal injection to monosodium urate in Behçet's syndrome and its comparison to the pathergy test. Yonsei Med J 41(3):S25
86. Gul A, Esin S, Dilsen N, Konice M, Wigzell H, Biberfeld P (1995) Immunohistology of skin pathergy reaction in Behçet's disease. Br J Dermatol 132:901–907
87. Melikoglu M, Uysal S, Krueger JG, Kaplan G, Gogus F, Yazici H, Oliver S (2006) Characterization of the divergent wound-healing responses occurring in the pathergy reaction and normal healthy volunteers. J Immunol 177:6415–6421
88. Ben Ahmed M, Houman H, Miled M, Dellagi K, Louzir H (2004) Involvement of chemokines and Th1 cytokines in the pathogenesis of mucocutaneous lesions of Behçet's disease. Arthritis Rheum 50:2291–2295
89. Jorizzo JL, Solomon AR, Cavallo T (1985) Behçet's syndrome. Immunopathologic and histopathologic assessment of pathergy lesions is useful in diagnosis and follow-up. Arch Pathol Lab Med 109:747–751
90. Gilhar A, Winterstein G, Turani H, Landau J, Etzioni A (1989) Skin hyperreactivity response (pathergy) in Behçet's disease. J Am Acad Dermatol 21:547–552
91. Haim S, Sobel JD, Friedman-Birnbaum R, Lichtig C (1976) Histological and direct immunofluorescence study of cutaneous hyperreactivity in Behçet's disease. Br J Dermatol 95:631–636
92. Gilhar A, Haim S, Wolf V, Golan D (1983) Mast cells in Behçet's disease: ultrastructural and histamine content studies. J Dermatol 10:185–186
93. Budak-Alpdogan T, Demircay Z, Alpdogan O, Direskeneli H, Ergun T, Bayik M, Akoglu T (1997) Skin hyperreactivity of Behçet's patients (pathergy reaction) is also positive in interferon alpha-treated chronic myeloid leukaemia patients, indicating similarly altered neutrophil functions in both disorders. Ann Haematol 74:45–48
94. Tascilar K, Baran A, Melikoglu M, Gogus F, Hatemi G, Yazici H (2008) Effect of immunosuppressive treatment on skin pathergy reaction in Behçet's syndrome. Clin Exp Rheumatol 26(4):30
95. Melikoglu M, Fresko I, Mat C, Ozyazgan Y, Gogus F, Yurdakul S, Hamuryudan V, Yazici H (2005) Short-term trial of etanercept in Behçet's disease: a double blind, placebo controlled study. J Rheumatol 32:98–105
96. Jorizzo JL, Taylor RS, Schmalstieg FC, Solomon AR Jr, Daniels JC, Rudloff HE, Cavallo T (1985) Complex aphthosis: a forme fruste of Behçet's syndrome? J Am Acad Dermatol 13(1):80–84
97. Keogan MT (2009) Clinical immunology review series: an approach to the patient with recurrent orogenital ulceration, including Behçet's syndrome. Clin Exp Immunol 156(1):1–11
98. Rogers RS III (2009) Pseudo-Behçet's disease. Clin Exp Immunol 156(1):1–11
99. Hatemi I, Hatemi G, Celik AF, Melikoglu M, Arzuhal N, Mat C, Ozyazgan Y, Yazici H (2008) Frequency of pathergy phenomenon and other features of Behçet's syndrome among patients with inflammatory bowel disease. Clin Exp Rheumatol 26:S91–S95
100. Tunc R, Uluhan A, Melikoglu M, Ozyazgan Y, Ozdogan H, Yazici H (2001) A reassessment of the International Study Group criteria for the diagnosis (classification) of Behçet's syndrome. Clin Exp Rheumatol 19(5 Suppl 24):S45–S47
101. Jonsson R, Heyden G, Westberg NG, Nyberg G (1984) Oral mucosal lesions in systemic lupus erythematosus – a clinical, histopathological and immunopathological study. J Rheumatol 11(1):38–42
102. Fresko I, Yazici H, Isci H, Yurdakul S (1993) Genital ulceration in patients with systemic lupus erythematosus. Lupus 2(2):135
103. Gül A (2005) Behçet's disease as an autoinflammatory disorder. Curr Drug Targets Inflamm Allergy 4(1):81–83
104. Alpsoy E, Er H, Durusoy C, Yilmaz E (1999) The use of sucralfate suspension in the treatment of oral and genital ulceration of Behçet's disease: a randomized, placebo-controlled, double-blind study. Arch Dermatol 135:529–532

105. Mumcu G, Ergun T, Elbir Y et al (2005) Clinical and immunological effects of azithromycin in Behçet's disease. J Oral Pathol Med 34:13–16
106. Hamuryudan V, Yurdakul S, Serdaroglu S, Tuzun Y, Rosenkaimer F, Yazici H (1990) Topical alpha interferon in the treatment of oral ulcers in Behçet's syndrome: a preliminary report. Clin Exp Rheumatol 8:51–54
107. Ergun T, Gurbuz O, Yurdakul S, Hamuryudan V, Bekiroglu N, Yazici H (1997) Topical cyclosporine-A for treatment of oral ulcers of Behçet's syndrome. Int J Dermatol 36:720
108. Mat C, Tuzun T, Ozsoy Y, Erturk G, Mercan E, Fresko I, Baykal IE, Araman A,Yazici H (2000) Cromolyn gel 4%in the treatment of genital ulcers of Behçet's disease. In: Bang D, Lee ES, Lee S (eds) Proceeding of the International Conference on Behçet's disease, Seoul, p 907
109. Tasli L, Mat C, De Simone C, Yazici H (2006) Lactobacilli lozenges in the management of oral ulcers of Behçet's syndrome. Clin Exp Rheumatol 24:S83–S86

Chapter 5
Eye Disease in Behçet's Syndrome

Yılmaz Özyazgan and Bahram Bodaghi

Keywords Uveitis • Retinal vasculitis • Iridocyclitis • Optic disk edema • Hypopyon • Slit lamp • Vitreous haze • Synechia • Cystoid macular edema • Cataracts • Secondary glaucoma • Visual loss • Blindness • Corticosteroids • Azathioprine • Cyclosporine • Anti-TNF alpha agents • Interferon alpha

Ocular involvement is one of the principal manifestations of Behçet's syndrome (BS) and its main cause of morbidity. It has specific features that make it rather unique among the various forms of uveitis.

Epidemiology

The overall frequency of ocular involvement is around 50% among BS patients in general [1]. However, it might go up as high as 70% among males and the young and as low as 30% or less among the old and the female [2].

In a recent multicenter survey, BS was the most frequent diagnosis (32%) among uveitis patients who presented to ophthalmology clinics in different parts of Turkey [3]. This compares with ~25 and 6.2% in reports of similar surveys 18 years apart from Japan [4, 5] and 2.5% from Boston, USA [6]. These figures while obviously reflecting the differences in the parent disease frequency among these geographies also stand for the fact that BS is not very rare once one goes to subspecialty practices even in places like USA where the prevalence in the general population is quite low (also see Chaps. 1 and 3).

Studies based on hospital records show that ocular involvement commonly begins within the initial few years during the disease course [7, 8]. It usually starts

Y. Özyazgan (✉)
Department of Ophthalmology, Cerrahpasa Medical Faculty, University of Istanbul, Istanbul, Turkey
e-mail: ozyazgan@isbank.net.tr

Y. Yazıcı and H. Yazıcı (eds.), *Behçet's Syndrome*,
DOI 10.1007/978-1-4419-5641-5_5, © Springer Science+Business Media, LLC 2010

unilaterally, but in most patients the other eye also gets diseased in time. The eye disease is bilateral in around three-fourth to four-fifth of the patients [7, 8]. In the 20-year Cerrahpasa outcome survey, eye involvement was bilateral in 80% of the males and 64% of the females at the first visit. At the end of two decades, 87% of males and 71% of females had bilateral disease [7]. It is interesting to note that the prominent gender difference in more severe disease in BS is also apparent in this context, as well.

Ocular inflammation in patients with BS is most commonly a panuveitis and retinitis. Some patients do indeed present as isolated anterior uveitis [3, 8]. However, in many patients this progresses to a panuveitis with time. The duration of follow-up should be specified in reporting eye disease in BS.

Once the early phase is over, when the only symptoms can be slight impairment of vision associated with few floaters, the uveitis of BS is rather straightforward to recognize by the experienced ophthalmologist. In this line and in a formal factor analysis among a sizeable group of BS it was seen that the uveitis of BS had special differentiating features that allowed it to stand as a solo factor in a matrix of various other clinical findings [9]. There is nongranulomatous uveal inflammation that may be prominent in either the anterior or the posterior segments or more commonly in both. This is usually accompanied by occlusive retinal vasculitis.

The term uveitis, by definition, points out to those pathologies restricted to the uvea. However, in many other types of uveitis including that associated with BS, the retina is also involved whenever the inflammation involves the intermediate and the posterior poles [10].

Clinical Symptoms and Findings

In early disease, the only complaint may be a slight impairment of vision associated with few floaters. Some patients also complain of redness, pain in the globe, photophobia, and tearing.

These findings usually subside within the course of a few weeks. In advanced stages, the visual loss becomes permanent and acute flares are characterized by varying degrees of further visual loss, sometimes resulting in the ability to see only hand motion at a near distance.

A critical concept that underlies the various components of inflammatory changes that show periodicity is "activation." It plays a key role in the evaluation of different clinical presentations, clinical variations at long-term follow-up, and in the evaluation of prognosis.

The impossibility to predict the exact time when it will occur, its episodic nature, the nearly total disappearance of the nonpermanent inflammatory findings after each attack, and the potential damage it leads to renders its definition and recording crucially important.

BS patients with eye disease should be followed closely and patiently for prolonged periods, since many of the inflammatory findings may wax and wane and clinical findings may show dynamic changes. Short-term observations may be misleading and the specific signs and symptoms should be interpreted in the context of the big picture.

It is useful to classify the symptoms and findings as they relate to the anatomic localization in the eye while the permanent and nonpermanent findings should be carefully separated and recorded at each visit.

Anterior Chamber Findings Reflecting an Acute Attack

Inflammation which is limited to the anterior segment is commonly called nonspecific iridocyclitis. The normal physiological balance in the anterior segment is suddenly disrupted and pathological changes occur in the vascular permeability of the vessels in the iris.

The most characteristic finding is the presence of cells in the anterior chamber. Inflammatory cells which enter the anterior segment from the damaged vascular endothelium appear like floating dust particles in the light beam of the biomicroscope. Due to the temperature difference between the corneal apex and the iris-lens plain, inflammatory cells move freely in accord with the normal movement of the aqueous humor. When the globe is moved, the movement of cells in the anterior segment can be easily seen with the slit lamp.

Flare, another important sign of activation, is the exudation of protein from the inflamed iris vessels. Depending on its density, it gives a foggy appearance to the anterior segment and prevents the visualization of the iris details. Sometimes it becomes dense and is called a fibrin clot. Cells and flare may or may not coexist during activation in the anterior segment. When both cells and flare are present, their intensities may be different and should be graded separately [11]. Cells may disappear after a while, but the flare may persist longer, indicating persistent vascular injury.

Hypopyon, when present, is a pathognomonic sign of activation (Fig. 5.1). It is the collection of the fibrinous and a dense cellular infiltrate in the lower part of the anterior chamber. It forms due to gravity. It is mainly composed of polymorphonuclear leukocytes, inflammatory material, and tissue fragments. It is mobile and may change position with the movement of the head or a change in the posture of the patient. Although it might sometimes be seen with the naked eye or using a penlight, it is more easily visualized with the help of a slit lamp. Sometimes it may only be seen gonioscopically from the anterior chamber angle. Presence of hypopyon might point out to the severity of the inflammatory exacerbation. However, it disappears without leaving any sequelae. It is seen in around 6–12% of patients with ocular involvement either seen by the naked eye or more commonly by the biomicroscope/gonioscopy [8, 12–14]. It is generally thought that the frequency of hypopyon has decreased due to the use of steroids. The frequency of hypopyon would be higher if the patient is examined early during the onset of activation. Atypical hypopyon presenting without conjunctival hyperemia is called a white (cold) hypopyon.

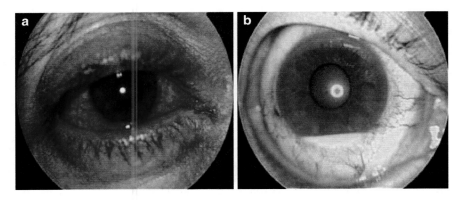

Fig. 5.1 Hypopyon ("hot" **a**/"cold" **b**)

This is usually seen during activations of patients under intense immunosuppressive treatment. Hypopyon of either kind is associated with a severe panuveitis in the majority of the instances.

Keratic precipitates result from the precipitation of inflammatory cells on the corneal endothelium. These cells are mainly polymorphonuclear leukocytes and lymphocytes. They are usually localized to the lower part of the cornea and persist for a long time.

Inflammatory cells can be localized behind the lens and anterior vitreous, similar to the cells in the anterior chamber. These usually point out to the involvement of the ciliary bodies and resemble opaque inflammatory debris. They persist for a long time and they are less mobile with the movements of the eye ball.

Other less frequent anterior segment findings are conjunctival aphthae, episcleritis, ciliary flush, and perilimbal circumferential ciliary injections [15, 16] (Fig. 5.2).

Anterior Chamber Findings Reflecting Permanent Damage

The pupillar margin and/or the posterior face of the iris may attach to the anterior face of the lens causing the organized adhesions called posterior synechia. When they are localized only to portions of the pupilla they are called partial synechia and when they surround 360° of the pupilla, they are called total or annular posterior synechia. When such synechia are present the pupillary margin becomes irreversibly irregular and stays in a fixed position (Fig. 5.3). With prolonged activation and inadequate treatment, fibrosis of the inflammatory material results in the formation of a cyclitic membrane covering the pupillary space and anterior part of the lens and the development of seclusio or occlusio pupillae. Less frequently, an anterior synechia may develop between the peripheral iris and the cornea by the same mechanism.

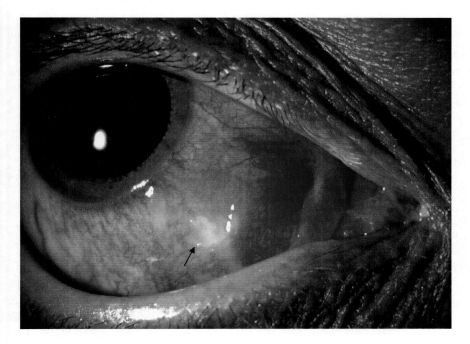

Fig. 5.2 Conjunctival ulcer

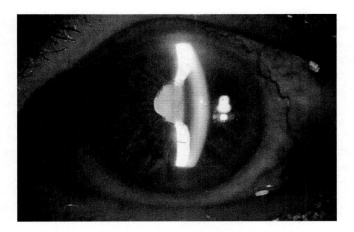

Fig. 5.3 Advanced anterior segment damage in a patient with Behçet's disease. Posterior synechia, peripheral anterior synechia, narrow anterior chamber, and complicated cataract can be seen

Seclusio or occlusio pupillae prevents the aqueous humor from passing through the pupillary space causing pupillary block glaucoma. Similarly, angle closure glaucoma develops as a result of peripheral anterior synechia. Secondary glaucoma develops in around 11% of BS patients with ocular involvement [17]. Neovascularizations in the iris which is an infrequent finding in BS may also cause a secondary glaucoma [18]. Inflammatory cells and debris plugging of the trabecular meshwork, trabeculitis, prolonged use of topical and systemic corticosteroids may also cause increased intraocular pressure and secondary glaucoma by preventing aqueous outflow.

The inflammatory mediators released during recurrent attacks in the anterior segment as well as the prolonged use of corticosteroids may cause changes in the lens metabolism resulting in cataract formation. Such cataracts are located mainly in the posterior subcapsular area. Mature and cortical cataract formation due to prolonged inflammatory activation and the use of therapeutic agents may also be seen.

Posterior Segment and Retinal Findings Reflecting an Acute Attack

Vitreal inflammatory signs in the form of haze or cells are the main inflammatory findings of posterior segment involvement pointing to blood–retinal barrier breakdown. The other findings relate directly to the retina.

Vitreous haze is due to protein leakage, arising from the ciliary bodies, choroid, or the retina. It is the most sensitive sign of an acute posterior segment inflammation. Density of the vitreous haze can be different in each flare and is used in grading its severity (Fig. 5.4). The grading is done by evaluating the details of the optic disk and retina, using a 20-diopter lens with indirect ophthalmoscopy or a 90-diopter lens with the slit lamp [4, 10].

Cells also may be seen in the vitreus during an acute attack. However, they are not as pathognomonic for the acute inflammation as they are in the anterior segment. On biomicroscopy, they seem to hang between vitreous fibrils in varying numbers. Although they can move when the globe moves, they do not move as freely as cells in the anterior segment. They usually persist for a long time in many different and non-descript shapes.

Retinal involvement is almost inevitable in patients with posterior segment involvement and the permanent damage in the retina causes more morbidity than damage in the uvea. Permanent loss of vision is directly related to the amount of retinal damage. Choroid, outer retinal layer, and retinal pigmented epithelium less frequently show signs of involvement.

The main retinal pathology is an occlusive vasculitis, which affects both the arterioles and veins in the posterior segment of the globe and accompanying inflammatory findings in the same area [19, 20]. Varying degrees of vitreous haze, retinal edema, deep or superficial hemorrhages, and inflammatory infiltrations in the retina may be seen during recurrent acute vasoocclusive attacks. As a sign of an acute attack diffuse retinal edema can be seen in BS patients, but it is not very frequent.

Cystoid macular edema (CME) is one of the deleterious findings that can be seen both during acute exacerbations and in silent periods (Fig. 5.5). CME is resistant

Fig. 5.4 Mild (**a**), moderate (**b**), and marked (**c**) activations in the posterior segment

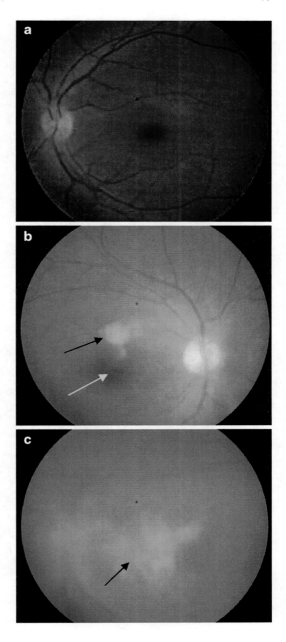

to treatment and resolves slowly causing visual impairment. Segmental and total vascular sheathing frequently occur during retinal involvement and persist for a long time.

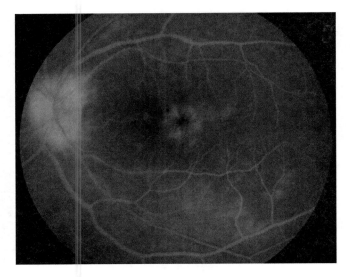

Fig. 5.5 Cystoid macular edema

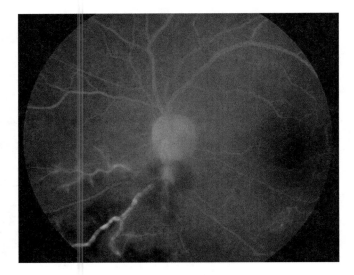

Fig. 5.6 Branch retinal vein occlusion

Branch retinal vein occlusion can occasionally be seen while central retinal vein occlusion is an uncommon finding (Fig. 5.6). Central retinal artery occlusion is also quite rare.

Hyperemia and edema of the optic disk and papillitis are among the other posterior findings frequently seen in BS during an attack and are usually observed along other findings of posterior segment involvement. Isolated papilledema is usually a manifestation of sagital sinus thrombosis [21]. However, there are also cases where isolated papilledema occurs in the absence of neurological involvement. These should be interpreted as a form of uveitis and should be treated as such until proven otherwise.

Posterior Chamber and Retinal Findings Reflecting Permanent Damage

Apart from the dysmorphic cells causing opacities remaining from an acute attack the homogenous collagenous structure of the vitreus is disrupted and fibrillation is seen on occasion. Posterior vitreal detachment is another consequence.

Multiple recurrent vasooclusive attacks may gradually lead to permanent atrophic changes in the retina. Parallel to the retinal damage, microvasculitis of the optic nerve vasculature can cause progressive optic atrophy. Neovascularization of the optic disk (Fig. 5.7) and retina may infrequently develop due to hypoxia resulting from vascular occlusion.

Recurrent activations, especially when localized to the posterior pole may cause damage in the whole posterior segment, primarily in the retina. Especially the macula and the optic disk are affected. This damage is proportionate to the number and severity of the attacks [10]. As the permanent damage in the macula and the optic nerve progresses, visual acuity decreases and may result in total loss of vision. Recurrent vasoocclusive attacks gradually lead to attenuated retinal vessels, retinal atrophy and fibrosis, degenerative changes in the macula, optic disk atrophy, variable degree of chorioretinal scars, retinal pigment epithelium alterations, and epiretinal membrane. Hemorrhage in the vitreous, vitreous contraction, and retinal detachment can rarely be seen [22].

Hypotonia, most often the end-stage complication of treatment resistant panuveitis results in phytysis bulbi, the shrunken and nonfunctional eye. It is the result of the total and irreversible atrophy and occlusive fibrosis of the ciliary body [23].

Fluorescein Angiography and Indocyanine Green Angiograpy

Fluorescein angiography (FFA) is a useful tool for evaluating the retina and the optic disk vasculature. It is mainly useful in making a management decision when there is vitrous haze but no active retinal inflammation detected by the biomicroscope. It also helps in differentiating associated vasculitis when there is optic disk edema. Atmaca and colleagues have shown that retinal vascular changes were present on FFA in 6.3% of the patients even in the absence of any temporary or permanent retinal damage, clinical signs of acute exacerbations and loss of vision [24]. The early phase of FFA shows diffuse vascular leakage during periods of activation and resolution in BS patients with posterior involvement. The later phase of FFA reveals leakage from the disk, capillary nonperfusion, collateral formation and

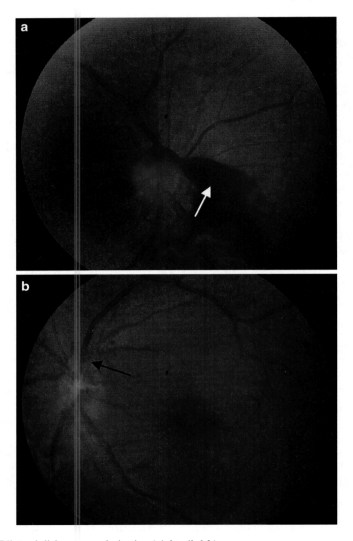

Fig. 5.7 Bilateral disk neovascularization (*right* **a**/*left* **b**)

neovascularization on the retina and the disk. When evaluating for CME, FFA is especially useful for detecting patelloid appearance and the ischemia in the macula, helping to confirm the diagnosis. Moreover, the additional use of optical coherence tomography (OCT) is very helpful in identifying lesions such as macular hole, epiretinal membrane formation, and degenerative changes in the retina. FFA can also be used in monitoring therapy.

Indocyanine green (ICG) angiography visualizes choroidal vascular changes in patients with posterior involvement and discloses several different types of angiographic images [25]. It may reveal hyper and/or hypofluorescent lesions, leakage of the choroidal vessels, and irregular filling defects of choroid [26]. These findings may correlate with disease duration [10].

Gedik and colleagues examined 49 eyes of 25 patients with BS during their activation phases, with FFA and ICG. They showed that there was only one patient (2%) who showed choroidal pathology on ICG angiography without detectable changes on FFA and suggested that findings on ICG angiography alone were not specific for BS [27] and that FFA was a more sensitive method for monitoring progression during therapy and follow-up.

Immunohistopathologic Evaluation

Histopathology of the ocular lesions in BS shows perivasculitis accompanied by tissue damage. There is usually no primary involvement in choroid and retinal pigmented epithelium [8]. Ocular tissues are infiltrated by CD 4+ T lymphocytes, B cells and plasma cells, forming a nongranulomatous inflammation [10]. Winter and Yukins have suggested that an obliterative vasculitis causes the pathological lesions [28]. Mullaney and Collum have reported necrotizing arteriolitis and phlebitis with thromboses in the eye of a patient with BS [29].

Necrotizing, neutrophilic obliterative perivasculitis, infiltration of veins, capillaries, and arteries with lymphocytic and mononuclear cells, and venous thrombosis are characteristic features of BS [12]. In the active stage, neutrophil infiltration is present in the anterior segment as hypopyon, in the corneal endothelium, iris, ciliary body, and the choroid, while perivascular infiltration with lymphocytes and plasma cells is also seen [30].

In more advanced stages, following recurrent attacks of activation, proliferation of collagen fibrils, choroidal thickness, cyclitic membrane formation, and eventually hypotonia and phytisis bulbi are observed [30]. Vasculitic process affects optic nerve vessels causing ischemia and as this progress complete and incomplete optic atrophy develops [22].

Retinal occlusive vasculitis, capillary nonperfusion, and development of capillary drop out leading to vascular remodeling and neovascularization may infrequently be observed in BS [31].

Clinical Course and Prognosis (See Also Chap. 17)

Depending on its extent retinal vasculitis causes varying degrees of visual loss. Especially, increased scar formation in the vascular arcade (the region around the macula made up of the vessels stemming out from the optic disk) and damage to the optic nerve results in irreversible visual loss.

The anatomical classification of the eye involvement as anterior, posterior or panuveitis as outlined above is important for therapeutic and prognostic purposes [10]. Inflammatory exacerbations localized to the anterior segment can generally be suppressed with topical treatment and the lesion may totally disappear without permanent damage. Nevertheless, in some patients who repeatedly have severe attacks restricted to the anterior segment, manageable complications such as secondary glaucoma and cataracts may develop due both to the inflammation itself and to the drugs used to suppress the inflammation. On the other hand, inflammation localized to the posterior segment always requires systemic treatment with corticosteroids and/or immunosuppressives. In posterior involvement or panuveitis the severity of the inflammation, the anatomical location, and the clinical course determines whether the treatment should be of short or long duration, or whether monotherapy or combination therapy is needed. Despite intensive medical interventions, progressive visual loss and even total blindness may develop in some cases due to irreversible damage in the optic disk and retina.

In a survey from North Africa where the frequency of ocular involvement was 80%, blindness was reported in a quarter of the patients [32]. In a study from Japan, visual acuity loss was significantly less in the period 1984–1993 than in 1974–1983. This was interpreted as resulting from better management [33]. In another study, Tugal-Tutkun et al. showed that male patients who had presented in 1990 had significantly lower risk of loss of vision compared to those who presented in 1980 [8]. This improvement in the prognosis of ocular involvement was also related to better treatment, including more aggressive and early use of immunosuppressives and to the use of combination therapy. Ocular involvement in BS mandates a close follow-up, detailed examinations and a more aggressive treatment plan.

Despite the noted improvement in the prognosis of eye disease, in general, there are some patients in whom the same agent(s) is able to control the eye disease in one eye and not the other. The patient course as outlined in Fig. 5.8 demonstrates this. We do not know why azathioprine, especially during its second term use in this patient was successful in one eye and not the other eye of this patient.

There is consensus that the main determinant of visual prognosis in any one patient is the number of ocular attacks during the disease course [10, 34] as is demonstrated in Fig. 5.9. On the other hand, the patient course outlined in Fig. 5.10 shows that the intensity of the attack is also important in some patients.

Disease Assessment

Visual acuity is usually the best indicator of disease burden in eye disease [10, 34]. Various other schemes like haze charts [35] or automated cell counters have also been proposed and are used mainly for research purposes [36] (see Chap. 18).

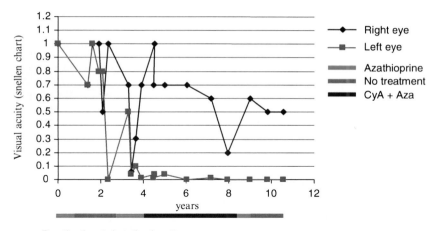

Fig. 5.8 Graph illustrating marked frequent eye activations observed during the clinical course of uveitis in a real patient. The patient had six attacks on the right and seven on the left during the follow-up. Although the patient received immunosuppressive treatment (single or combined), attacks continued to occur. At the end of 10 years of follow-up, the visual acuity was moderately preserved in the right eye but unfortunately, useful vision was lost in the left

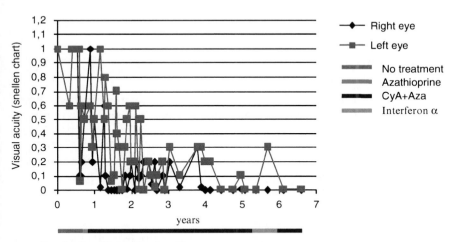

Fig. 5.9 Graph illustrating severe frequent activation in the right and left eye during the clinical course of uveitis in a real patient. The patient had 26 attacks in the right and 18 on the left during 7 years of follow-up. Mainly combined immunosuppressive treatment was given during most of the follow-up period. Despite intensive immunosuppressive treatment, frequent severe attacks continued to occur and the patient lost bilateral useful vision at the end of 7th year of follow-up

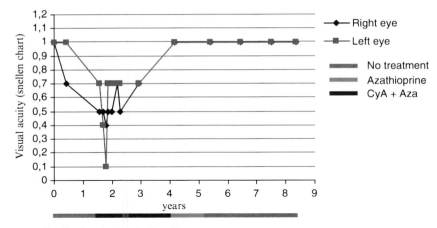

R activation 6; L activation 2

Fig. 5.10 Graph illustrating moderately frequent activations in the left eye and marked frequent activations in the right eye during the clinical course of uveitis in a real patient. The patient had six attacks on the right and two in the left during the follow-up. The sharp drop in the visual acuity of the left eye is due to the intensity rather than the number of activations. No systemic immuno-suppressive treatment was given during the first year. CyA+Aza were started on the second year and continued for 3 years until CyA was stopped. The treatment continued with Aza for 1 more year, then immunosuppressive treatment was stopped

Management

Ocular inflammation is perhaps the most dreaded feature of Behçet's syndrome. The disease course is unpredictable and challenging. The spectrum of outcomes range from spontaneous remission to acute visual loss or progressive blindness. Therefore, the aim of any therapeutic strategy in patients with ocular BS must be the strict control of ocular inflammation in order to prevent severe and sight-threatening relapses. Visual prognosis of BS has dramatically improved in the last two decades initially by first early use of conventional immunosuppressives, and biologic agents more recently. In the 70s, 73% of patient with ocular disease developed blindness within an average time of 3.5 years [37]. On the other hand, there was no decrease in mean visual acuity between the beginning and the end of the 2-year period among the azathioprine users in the azathioprine trial [38] and when these patients were reassessed at 8 years [39] blindness was present in 8/20 (40%) of the patients initially allocated to placebo and in 3/24 (13%) in those who initially received azathioprine. This improvement in visual outcome is probably still continuing with the current use of biologics but no hard data are yet at hand. (See also Chap. 19).

Systemic Therapy

Only a few randomized controlled clinical trials (RCTs) have been conducted in the field of uveitis in general, and the majority included series of patients with BS. One RCT has shown the efficacy of azathioprine over placebo in patients with eye involvement. In a series of 73 patients, the drug decreased occurrence of anterior attacks and preserved visual acuity when compared to placebo [39]. Interestingly, azathioprine also decreased the development of new eye disease among BS patients without eye involvement. Three RCTs have been published with different dosages of cyclosporine A showing efficacy [40–42]. Recently, European League Against Rheumatism (EULAR) recommendations for the management of BS became available [43]. They combine current evidence from clinical trials and the opinion of a multidisciplinary group of experts. The committee agreed on nine recommendations after two anonymous Delphi rounds. All nine recommendations were accepted with good levels of agreement. Two recommendations were established for ocular involvement as presented hereafter and should be taken into consideration in the face of patients with posterior uveitis related to BS.

1. Any patient with BS and inflammatory eye disease affecting the posterior segment should be on a treatment regime, which includes azathioprine and systemic corticosteroids.

    This is a major topic as mentioned previously. It will avoid dramatic visual loss or major ocular complications in most of the patients. Both drugs are widely available and systemic side effects remain well-known and limited allowing their large use worldwide. Duration of therapy is controversial but long-term regimens (at least 2 years) are usually required.
2. If the patient has severe eye disease defined as >2 lines of drop in visual acuity on a 10/10 scale and/or retinal disease, (retinal vasculitis or macular involvement), it is recommended that either cyclosporine A or infliximab be used in combination with azathioprine and corticosteroids; alternatively interferon alpha with or without corticosteroids could be used.

Cyclosporine A is frequently used in association with azathioprine for severe eye involvement and in cases resistant to azathioprine; however, there are no controlled data that support the use of this combination. High blood pressure and nephrotoxicity remain the major side effects. Moreover, the risk of developing neurological BS in patients treated with cyclosporine A remains to be determined. Also there is no consensus as to exactly when to introduce the biologics in treatment. The two major biologicals are TNF alpha blockers and interferon alpha 2a. Studies have been reported in the last decade in favor of either strategy with its advantages and limitations. Both have played a major role in the modern therapeutic management of the disease, especially in ocular disease.

TNF alpha blockers are the first major option, especially as a rescue therapy. Different reports have emphasized the rapid action of infliximab in severe cases of ocular BD resistant to conventional therapy. Clearance of vitreous haze and control of retinal involvement is efficiently and rapidly achieved with anti-TNF agents. Even though comparative data are lacking, it is probable that these drugs have the most rapid efficacy on intraocular inflammation, clearing up the vitreous haze in 24–72 h, decreasing retinal vasculitis in 2 weeks and retinal necrosis and hemorrhages in a few days or a few weeks. Therefore, they seem to be the drug of choice in severe and sight-threatening cases of ocular BS. A comprehensive review of the literature on the use of anti-TNF alpha agents has been recently published after discussion among experts [44].

More than 90% of the patients treated with anti-TNF alpha agents have received infliximab, mostly for eye disease. The first report in the literature was published by Sfikakis et al. in a series of three patients with major panuveitis despite aggressive immunosuppressors who received 5 mg/kg i.v. infusion of infliximab with an immediate efficacy within 24 h [45]. Three independent, open-label, self-controlled studies have confirmed these initial gratifying results [46–48]. Other retrospective studies have discussed the benefit of anti-TNF drugs in patients with ocular involvement [49–51].

Limited data suggest that adalimumab is also efficient for the same indication [52, 53]. However, results are less convincing with etanercept even though efficacy has been shown in extraocular manifestations of BS [54].

Safety issues include infections, demyelinating disease, malignancies, and congestive heart failure. It is highly important to exclude tuberculosis before anti-TNF alpha therapy [44]. Moreover, infliximab-induced formation of various autoantibodies, which appears to be clinically insignificant, commonly occurs but needs a close monitoring of patients. Due to its cost and potential side effects, anti-TNF alpha drugs are proposed in patients with severe posterior uveitis in order to control the sight-threatening episode with a later change for a more conventional molecule or interferon alpha. However, long-term infliximab may be proposed in severe resisting cases or in the face of intolerance to other drugs.

Interferon alpha is another interesting option. In the early 90s, IFN-alpha has shown encouraging results in the treatment of BS alone or combined with corticosteroid and/or immunosuppressives [55–59]. IFN-alpha 2b was initially proposed but IFN-alpha 2a seems more effective. Since 1996, Kotter et al. have extensively described the use of IFN-alpha 2a in patients with ocular BS [60–63]. Other groups have published retrospective open-label studies with encouraging results [64–66]. Initial treatment modalities, i.e. doses ranging from 3 to 9 million daily vs. thrice a week regimen, as well as duration of IFN-alpha 2a administration and corticosteroid therapy tapering vary widely among reported studies. One of the benefits of IFN therapy over other strategies is the possibility to rapidly taper corticosteroids without inducing a relapse.

Two major issues are important to consider when dealing with biologic agents such as IFN-alpha. Long-term efficacy seems now recognized and patients relapsing while under conventional immunosupressive therapy are generally controlled with IFN-alpha. However, rapid action in vision-threatening situations may require high-dose therapy which may be difficult to tolerate. Therefore, rescue therapy is more easily obtained with anti-TNF agents, which may be replaced by IFN-alpha for the long-term management. Lower dosage of IFN-alpha is then sufficient to control the disease, giving a better tolerance. Recent reports have shown for the first time that prolonged remission may be obtained after long-term therapy with IFN-alpha [67]. It is too early to discuss a curative effect of IFN-alpha therapy in patients with BS and further international randomized studies are needed.

Another biologic agent has been proposed in patients with uveitis. The safety and efficacy of daclizumab has been investigated by Buggage et al. in a randomized, double-masked, placebo-controlled clinical trial including 17 patients. In this small study, there was no suggestion that daclizumab was beneficial when compared to placebo [68].

Papilledema may be due to dural sinus thrombosis in the absence of uveitis. Rapid visual field defect or blindness may occur in the absence of an aggressive anti-inflammatory treatment, which must be initiated rapidly.

Local Therapy

Patients with isolated anterior uveitis usually require high-dose topical corticosteroids and cycloplegic agents. A series of three subconjunctival injections of corticosteroids may be proposed in severe cases of anterior uveitis with hypopyon. Topical corticosteroids will be tapered progressively based on clinical findings and sometimes on findings on laser flare photometry. It is important to emphasize that secondary glaucoma and cataract may occur during long-term topical therapy.

Intravitreal injections of triamcinolone have been proposed in patients with severe and intractable posterior uveitis with immediate macular threat or those with recalcitrant macular edema [69–73]. However this remains a rare procedure with a short-lived effect, needing further systemic anti-inflammatory and immunosuppressive management. Furthermore, monitoring is important as side effects such as secondary glaucoma, cataract endophthalmitis, or CMV retinitis may occur [74].

More recently, the use of anti-VEGF (Vascular Endothelial Growth Factor) agents has been advocated in patients with macular edema or neovascularisation due to diffuse retinal ischemia [75, 76]. Efficacy on macular edema is shorter than what was observed with triamcinolone. Even though this drug does not have the same side effects of corticosteroids, it must still be used with caution and in appropriate situations.

Argon laser photocoagulation may be indicated in patients with severe retinal ischemia in order to avoid retinal neovascularisation and further intravitreal hemorrhages or neovascular glaucoma inducing severe pain in a blind eye. Retinal vein occlusions are associated with a high risk of neovascularization. FFA is previously performed to identify with accuracy the extent of retinal ischemia. Laser procedure is applied under topical anesthesia during one or multiple sequences. However, the physician must keep in mind that neovascularisation is also due to intraocular inflammation. Therefore, a systemic therapy must always be initiated as a first step followed by laser photocoagulation if necessary.

Surgical Procedures

Peripheral Iridectomy

Secondary glaucoma due to posterior seclusion may require a peripheral iridectomy in order to decrease intraocular pressure and avoid further visual field defects or blindness. Nd: YAG laser iridotomy may also be performed with a subsequent risk of failure or complication [77]. In other cases of uncontrolled secondary glaucoma not related to a pupillary block, deep sclerectomy of trabeculectomy with per-operative use of mitomycine C may be proposed [78]. Long-term postoperative success remains inconsistant, highlighting the absolute necessity of the control of intraocular inflammation and the initiation of immunosuppressive medications or immunomodulators in order to avoid the occurrence of steroid-induced glaucoma.

Cataract Surgery

Recently, the success of cataract extractions has significantly improved. Phacoemulsification is now a routine procedure despite difficulties related to previous episodes of uveitis [79, 80]. Long-term postoperative results are encouraging. However, the optimal outcome depends on the strict control of ocular inflammation during at least 3 months prior to surgery. A special anti-inflammatory protocol is proposed in all cases before and a few weeks after surgery. The use of intraocular lenses is now proposed in almost all patients. Hydrophobic acrylic lenses are one of the best options in inflammatory eyes. Postoperative visual recovery depends on the degree of preoperative retinal damage.

Vitrectomy

Pars plana vitrectomy may be necessary in case of intravitreal hemorrhage without spontaneous resolution. Vitreous removal will disclose areas of retinal ischemia and neovessels requiring endo ocular laser photocoagulation. Posterior segment surgery may also be required in cases of retinal detachment.

References

1. Sakane T, Takeno M, Suzuki N, Inaba G (1999) Behçet's disease. N Engl J Med 341: 1284–1291
2. Yazici H, Tüzün Y, Pazarli H et al (1984) Influence of age of onset and patient's sex on the prevalence and severity of manifestations of Behçet's syndrome. Ann Rheum Dis 43:783–789
3. Kazokoglu H, Onal S, Tugal-Tutkun I et al (2008) Demographic and clinical features of uveitis in tertiary centers in Turkey. Ophthalmic Epidemiol 15:285–293

4. Mishima S, Masuda K, Izawa Y et al (1979) Behçet's diesae in Japan: ophthalmologic aspects. Tr Am Ophthalmol Soc 76:225–279
5. Goto H, Mochizuki M, Yamaki K et al (2007) Epidemiological survey of intraocular inflammation in Japan. Jpn J Ophthalmol 51:41–44
6. Rodriguez A, Calonge M, Pedroza-Serez M et al (1996) Referral patterns of uveitis in a tertiary eye care center. Arch Ophthalmol 114:593–599
7. Kural-Seyahi E, Fresko I, Seyahi N et al (2003) The long-term mortality and morbidity of Behçet's syndrome: a 2-decade outcome survey of 387 patients followed at a dedicated center. Medicine 82:60–76
8. Tugal-Tutkun I, Onal S, Altan Yaycıoglu R et al (2004) Uveitis in Behçet's disease: an analysis of 880 patients. Am J Ophthalmol 138:373–380
9. Tunc R, Keyman E, Melikoglu M, Fresko I, Yazici H (2002) Target organ associations in Turkish patients with Behçet's disease: a cross sectional study with exploratory factor analysis. J Rheumatol 29:2393–2396
10. Nussenblatt RB, Whitcup SM, Paletsine AG (2004) Behçet's disease. In: Nussenblatt RB, Whitcup SM, Paletsine AG (eds) Uveitis: fundamentals and clinical practice. Mosby, Philadelphia, pp 350–371
11. Jabs DA, Nussenblatt RB, Rosenbaum JT (2005) Standardization of uveitis nomenclature for reporting clinical data. Results of the First International Workshop. Am J Ophthalmol 140:509–516
12. George RK, Chan CC, Whitcup SM et al (1997) Ocular immunopathology of Behçet's disease. Surv Ophthalmol 42:157–162
13. Ramsay A, Lightman S (2001) Hypopyon uveitis. Surv Ophthalmol 46:1–18
14. Pazarlı H, Ozyazgan Y, Aktunc T (1989) Clinical observations on hypopyon attacks of Behçet's disease in Turkey. In: Seventh international conference on Behçet's disease (abstracts), Rochester, MN, 14–15 Sept
15. Tugal-Tutkun I, Urgancioglu M, Foster CS (1995) Immunopathologic study of the conjunctiva in patients with Behçet's disease. Ophthalmology 102:1660–1668
16. Zamir E, Bodaghi B, Tugal-Tutkun I et al (2003) Conjunctival ulcers in Behçet's disease. Ophthalmology 110:1137–1141
17. Elgin U, Berker N, Batman A (2004) Incidence of secondary glaucoma in Behçet's disease. J Glaucoma 13:441–444
18. Yalvaç IS, Sungur G, Turhan E et al (2004) Trabeculectomy with mitomycin-C in uveitic glaucoma associated with Behçet's disease. J Glaucoma 13:450–453
19. Baer JC, Raizman MB, Foster CS (1990) Ocular Behçet's disease in the United States: clinical presentation and visual outcome in 29 patients. In: Masahiko U, Shigeaki O, Koki A (eds) Proceedings of the 5th international symposium on the immunology and immunopathology of the eye, Tokyo. Elsevier Science, New York, p 383
20. Ehrlich GE (1997) Vasculitis in Behçet's disease. Int Rev Immunol 14:81–88
21. Akman-Demir G, Serdaroglu P, Tasci B (1999) Clinical patterns of neurological involvement in Behçet's disease: evaluation of 200 patients. The Neuro-Behçet's Study Group. Brain 122:2171–2182
22. Foster CS, Vitale AT (2002) Adamantiades-Behçet's disease. In: Foster CS, Vitale AT (eds) Diagnosis and treatment of uveitis. W.B. Saunders Company, Philadelphia, pp 632–652
23. Kacmaz RO, Kempen JH, Newcomb C et al, Systemic Immunosuppressive Therapy for Eye Diseases Cohort Study Group (2008) Ocular inflammation in Behçet's disease: incidence of ocular complications and of loss of visual acuity. Am J Ophthalmol 146:828–836
24. Atmaca LS (1989) Fundus changes associated with Behçet's disease. Graefes Arch Clin Exp Ophthalmol 227:340–344
25. Bozzoni-Pantaleoni F, Gharbiya M, Pirraglia MP et al (2001) Indocyanine gren angiographic findings in Behçet's disease. Retina 21:230–236
26. Atmaca LS, Sönmez PA (2003) Fluorescein and indocyanine green angiography findings in Behçet's disease. Br J Ophthalmol 87:1466–1468
27. Gedik S, Akova YA, Yılmaz G et al (2005) Indocyanine green and fundus fluorescein angiographic findings in patients with active ocular Behçet's disease. Ocul Immunol Inflamm 13:51–58

28. Winter FC, Yukins RE (1966) The ocular pathology of Behçet's disease. Am J Ophthmol 62:257–262
29. Mullaney J, Collum LM (1985) Ocular vasculitis in Behçet's disease: a pathological and immunohistochemical study. Int Ophthalmol 7:183–191
30. Hegab S, Al-Mutawa S (2000) Immunopathogenesis of Behçet's diseae. Clin Immunol 96:174–186
31. Atmaca LS, Batioglu F, Idil A (1996) Retinal and disc neovascularization in Behçet's disease and efficacy of laser photocoagulation. Graefes Arch Clin Exp Ophthalmol 234:94–99
32. El Belhadji M, Hamdani M, Laouissi N et al (1997) L'attente ophthalmologique dans la maladie d Behçet: a propos de 520 cas. J Fr Ophthalmol 20:592–598
33. Ando K, Fujino Y, Hijikata K et al (1999) Epidemiological features and viusal prognosis of visual prognosis of Behçet's disease. Jpn J Ophthalmol 43:312–317
34. Sakamoto M, Akazawa K, Nishioka Y et al (1995) Prognostic factors of vision in patients with Behçet's disease. Ophthalmology 102:317–321
35. Nussenblatt RB, Palestine AG, Chan CC et al (1985) Standardization of vitreal inflammatory activity in intermediate and posteror uveitis. Ophthalmology 92:467–471
36. Tugal-Tutkun I, Cingu K, Kir N, Yeniad B, Urgancioglu M, Gul A (2008) Use of laser flare-cell photometry to quantify intraocular inflammation in patients with Behçet's uveitis. Graefes Arch Clin Exp Ophthalmol 246:1169–1177
37. Mamo JG (1970) The rate of visual loss in Behçet's disease. Arch Ophthalmol 84:451–452
38. Yazici H, Pazarli H, Barnes CG et al (1990) A controlled trial of azathioprine in Behçet's syndrome. N Engl J Med 322:281–285
39. Hamuryudan V, Ozyazgan Y, Hizli N et al (1997) Azathioprine in Behçet's syndrome: effects on long-term prognosis. Arthritis Rheum 40:769–774
40. BenEzra D, Cohen E, Chajek T et al (1988) Evaluation of conventional therapy versus cyclosporine A in Behçet's syndrome. Transplant Proc 20(3 Suppl 4):136–143
41. Masuda K, Nakajima A, Urayama A, Nakae K, Kogure M, Inaba G (1989) Double-masked trial of cyclosporin versus colchicine and long-term open study of cyclosporin in Behçet's disease. Lancet 1:1093–1096
42. Ozyazgan Y, Yurdakul S, Yazici H et al (1992) Low dose cyclosporin A versus pulsed cyclophosphamide in Behçet's syndrome: a single masked trial. Br J Ophthalmol 76:241–243
43. Hatemi G, Silman A, Bang D et al (2008) Management of Behçet's disease: a systematic literature review for the EULAR evidence based recommendations for the management of Behçet's disease. Ann Rheum Dis 68:1528–1534
44. Sfikakis PP, Markomichelakis N, Alpsoy E et al (2007) Anti-TNF therapy in the management of Behçet's disease – review and basis for recommendations. Rheumatology (Oxford) 46:736–741
45. Sfikakis PP, Theodossiadis PG, Katsiari CG, Kaklamanis P, Markomichelakis NN (2001) Effect of infliximab on sight-threatening panuveitis in Behçet's disease. Lancet 358:295–296
46. Tugal-Tutkun I, Mudun A, Urgancioglu M et al (2005) Efficacy of infliximab in the treatment of uveitis that is resistant to treatment with the combination of azathioprine, cyclosporine, and corticosteroids in Behçet's disease: an open-label trial. Arthritis Rheum 52:2478–2484
47. Sfikakis PP, Kaklamanis PH, Elezoglou A et al (2004) Infliximab for recurrent, sight-threatening ocular inflammation in Adamantiades-Behçet's disease. Ann Intern Med 140:404–406
48. Ohno S, Nakamura S, Hori S et al (2004) Efficacy, safety, and pharmacokinetics of multiple administration of infliximab in Behçet's disease with refractory uveoretinitis. J Rheumatol 31:1362–1368
49. Tabbara KF, Al-Hemidan AI (2008) Infliximab effects compared to conventional therapy in the management of retinal vasculitis in Behçet's disease. Am J Ophthalmol 146:845.e1–850.e1
50. Bodaghi B, Bui Quoc E, Wechsler B et al (2005) Therapeutic use of infliximab in sight threatening uveitis: retrospective analysis of efficacy, safety, and limiting factors. Ann Rheum Dis 64:962–964
51. Niccoli L, Nannini C, Benucci M et al (2007) Long-term efficacy of infliximab in refractory posterior uveitis of Behçet's disease: a 24-month follow-up study. Rheumatology (Oxford) 46:1161–1164

52. Mushtaq B, Saeed T, Situnayake RD, Murray PI (2007) Adalimumab for sight-threatening uveitis in Behçet's disease. Eye 21:824–825
53. van Laar JA, Missotten T, van Daele PL, Jamnitski A, Baarsma GS, van Hagen PM (2007) Adalimumab: a new modality for Behçet's disease? Ann Rheum Dis 66:565–566
54. Melikoglu M, Fresko I, Mat C et al (2005) Short-term trial of etanercept in Behçet's disease: a double blind, placebo controlled study. J Rheumatol 32:98–105
55. Durand JM, Soubeyrand J (1994) Interferon-alpha 2b for refractory ocular Behçet's disease. Lancet 344:333
56. Feron EJ, Rothova A, van Hagen PM, Baarsma GS, Suttorp-Schulten MS (1994) Interferon-alpha 2b for refractory ocular Behçet's disease. Lancet 343:1428
57. Pivetti-Pezzi P, Accorinti M, Pirraglia MP, Priori R, Valesini G (1997) Interferon alpha for ocular Behçet's disease. Acta Ophthalmol Scand 75:720–722
58. Sánchez Román J, Pulido Aguilera MC, Castillo Palma MJ et al (1996) [The use of interferon alfa-2r in the treatment of autoimmune uveitis (primary or associated with Behçet's disease)]. Rev Clin Esp 196:293–298
59. Kötter I, Eckstein AK, Stübiger N, Zierhut M (1998) Treatment of ocular symptoms of Behçet's disease with interferon alpha 2a: a pilot study. Br J Ophthalmol 82:488–494
60. Kotter I, Deuter C, Stubiger N, Zierhut M (2005) Interferon-a (IFN-a) application versus tumor necrosis factor-a antagonism for ocular Behçet's disease: focusing more on IFN. J Rheumatol 32:1633
61. Kötter I, Vonthein R, Zierhut M et al (2004) Differential efficacy of human recombinant interferon-alpha2a on ocular and extraocular manifestations of Behçet's disease: results of an open 4-center trial. Semin Arthritis Rheum 33:311–319
62. Kötter I, Zierhut M, Eckstein A et al (2003) Human recombinant interferon-alpha2a (rhIFN alpha2a) for the treatment of Behçet's disease with sight-threatening retinal vasculitis. Adv Exp Med Biol 528:521–523
63. Kötter I, Zierhut M, Eckstein AK et al (2003) Human recombinant interferon alfa-2a for the treatment of Behçet's disease with sight threatening posterior or panuveitis. Br J Ophthalmol 87:423–431
64. Bodaghi B, Gendron G, Wechsler B et al (2007) Efficacy of interferon alpha in the treatment of refractory and sight threatening uveitis: a retrospective monocentric study of 45 patients. Br J Ophthalmol 91:335–339
65. Krause L, Turnbull JR, Torun N, Pleyer U, Zouboulis CC, Foerster MH (2003) Interferon alfa-2a in the treatment of ocular Adamantiades-Behçet's disease. Adv Exp Med Biol 528:511–519
66. Tugal-Tutkun I, Güney-Tefekli E, Urgancioglu M (2006) Results of interferon-alfa therapy in patients with Behçet's uveitis. Graefes Arch Clin Exp Ophthalmol 244:1692–1695
67. Gueudry J, Wechsler B, Terrada C et al (2008) Long-term efficacy and safety of low-dose interferon alpha2a therapy in severe uveitis associated with Behçet's disease. Am J Ophthalmol 146:837.e1–844.e1
68. Buggage RR, Levy-Clarke G, Sen HN et al (2007) A double-masked, randomized study to investigate the safety and efficacy of daclizumab to treat the ocular complications related to Behçet's disease. Ocul Immunol Inflamm 15:63–70
69. Atmaca LS, Yalcindag FN, Ozdemir O (2007) Intravitreal triamcinolone acetonide in the management of cystoid macular edema in Behçet's disease. Graefes Arch Clin Exp Ophthalmol 245:451–456
70. Karacorlu M, Mudun B, Ozdemir H, Karacorlu SA, Burumcek E (2004) Intravitreal triamcinolone acetonide for the treatment of cystoid macular edema secondary to Behçet's disease. Am J Ophthalmol 138:289–291
71. Ohguro N, Yamanaka E, Otori Y, Saishin Y, Tano Y (2006) Repeated intravitreal triamcinolone injections in Behçet's disease that is resistant to conventional therapy: one-year results. Am J Ophthalmol 141:218–220
72. Oueghlani E, Pavesio CE (2008) Intravitreal triamcinolone injection for unresponsive cystoid macular oedema in probable Behçet's disease as an additional therapy. Klin Monatsbl Augenheilkd 225:497–499

73. Tuncer S, Yilmaz S, Urgancioglu M, Tugal-Tutkun I (2007) Results of intravitreal triamcinolone acetonide (IVTA) injection for the treatment of panuveitis attacks in patients with Behçet's disease. J Ocul Pharmacol Ther 23:395–401

74. Saidel MA, Berreen J, Margolis TP (2005) Cytomegalovirus retinitis after intravitreous triamcinolone in an immunocompetent patient. Am J Ophthalmol 140:1141–1143

75. Mirshahi A, Namavari A, Djalilian A, Moharamzad Y, Chams H (2009) Intravitreal bevacizumab (Avastin) for the treatment of cystoid macular edema in Behçet's disease. Ocul Immunol Inflamm 17:59–64

76. Erdurman FC, Durukan AH, Mumcuoglu T, Hürmeric V (2009) Intravitreal bevacizumab treatment of macular edema due to optic disc vasculitis. Ocul Immunol Inflamm 17:56–58

77. Elgin U, Berker N, Batman A, Soykan E (2007) Nd:YAG laser iridotomy in the management of secondary glaucoma associated with Behçet's disease. Eur J Ophthalmol 17:191–195

78. Elgin U, Berker N, Batman A, Soykan E (2007) Trabeculectomy with mitomycin C in econdary glaucoma associated with Behçet's disease. J Glaucoma 16:68–72

79. Berker N, Soykan E, Elgin U, Ozkan SS (2004) Phacoemulsification cataract extraction and intraocular lens implantation in patients with Behçet's disease. Ophthalmic Surg Lasers Imaging 35:215–218

80. Kadayifcilar S, Gedik S, Eldem B, Irkec M (2002) Cataract surgery in patients with Behçet's disease. J Cataract Refract Surg 28:316–320

Chapter 6
Behçet's Syndrome and the Nervous System

Aksel Siva and Shunsei Hirohata

Keywords Behçet's disease • Neurologic involvement • Classification • Differential diagnosis • Therapy

Introduction

Patients with Behçet's syndrome (BS) may present with different neurological problems which are either direct or indirect consequences of the systemic disease (Table 6.1) [1–3]. It is common to name the former, with documented involvement of the nervous system as a part of the systemic disease, as "neuro-Behçet's syndrome" (NBS). The most common form of neurological complication seen in BS is parenchymal-central nervous system (CNS) involvement, which is believed to be due to inflammatory small vessel disease and may present as acute disease or may have a chronic progressive form. The second common form is the cerebral venous sinus thrombosis (CVST), in which CNS-parenchymal involvement is unlikely. This pattern had led some authors to name this form of presentation as vasculo-Behçet's [4, 5]. However, as in both parenchymal CNS involvement and CVST, in varying degrees, vascular involvement is part of the picture. Therefore, we choose to name these patterns as intra-axial-NBS and extra-axial-NBS, respectively. Headache is the most common neurological symptom seen in patients with NBS, but occurs commonly in patients with BS in general, as well, and may be due to different causes and therefore deserves to be discussed separately.

The neuro-psycho-Behçet variant in which an organic psychotic syndrome is prominent is a rare form of NBS [6]. Peripheral nervous system involvement is also extremely rare, and it may be either directly related to BS or may occur as a consequence of treatments given for systemic manifestations of the disease, such as

A. Siva (✉)
Department of Neurology, Clinical Neuroimmunology Unit, Cerrahpaşa School of Medicine, University of Istanbul, Istanbul, Turkey
e-mail: asiva@tnn.net

Y. Yazıcı and H. Yazıcı (eds.), *Behçet's Syndrome*,
DOI 10.1007/978-1-4419-5641-5_6, © Springer Science+Business Media, LLC 2010

Table 6.1 The neurological spectrum of Behçet's syndrome*

Primary neurological involvement (neurological involvement directly related to BS)
Cerebral venous sinus thrombosis (extra-axial NBS)
Central nervous system involvement (intra-axial NBS)
Acute intra-axial NBS
Chronic progressive intra-axial NBS
Neuro-Psycho-Behçet's Syndrome
Peripheral nervous system involvement
Subclinical NBS
Headache (migraine-like, nonstructural)
Secondary neurological involvement (neurological involvement indirectly related to BS)
Neurologic complications secondary to systemic involvement of BS (i.e., cerebral emboli from cardiac complications of BS, increased intracranial pressure secondary to superior vena cava syndrome)
Neurologic complications related to BS treatments (i.e., CNS neurotoxicity with cyclosporine; peripheral neuropathy secondary to thalidomide or colchicine)
Coincidental – unrelated (non-BS) neurological involvement
Primary headaches and any other coincidental neurological problem

*Modified from refs. [1–3]

BS Behçet's syndrome, *NBS* neuro-Behçet's syndrome, *CNS* central nervous system

colchicine or thalidomide. Other neurologic complications secondary to systemic involvement of BS or related to BS treatments are considered as indirect consequences of the syndrome (Table 6.1).

In recent years an increasing number of reports had pointed to cases, who demonstrated silent clinical signs, or neurophysiological, or neuroimaging findings without any corresponding neurological symptom. This pattern is considered as subclinical neurologic disease and its long-term implications is not currently known [1].

Diagnosis of NBS

The diagnosis of NBS is accomplished mainly by clinical means. It should be noted, however, that it is uncommon for NBS to arise in the absence of systemic features of Behçet's disease. It is therefore recommended that the satisfaction of the international diagnostic criteria for Behçet's disease is a prerequisite for diagnosis [7]. Therefore, although there is not a definite validated diagnostic criteria for NBS, in a patient who fulfills the International Diagnostic Criteria for Behçet's Disease, it seems reasonable to consider the diagnosis of NBS, when neurological symptoms develop which cannot be otherwise explained by any other known systemic or neurological disease or drugs used. To confirm the diagnosis of NBS in such a patient, objective abnormalities should be detected either on neurological examination, and/or with neuroimaging studies (MRI disclosing findings suggestive of NBS) and/or abnormal cerebrospinal fluid (CSF) findings consistent with NBS [1].

Epidemiology of NBS

The prevalence of NBS in BS is around 5% in nonselected large series [8–10]. However, in a prospective study with two decades of follow-up the frequency of neurological involvement was 13.0% among the males and 5.6% among the females [11]. The mean age of onset for BS is around 26–27, and NBS develops after a mean of 5 years. However, when CVST is the main neurologic problem, ages of onset for both BS and the NBS are much earlier [10, 12]. Neurological involvement in BS occurs more commonly in men, with a male-to-female ratio of up to 4:1, whereas the sex ratio in BS, in general, is almost equal [1]. Such a significant male predominance has also been noted in other vascular complications of BS [11].

Extra-axial NBS

CVST is seen in 10–20% of NBS patients with neurologic involvement [8, 10, 13–15]. Thrombosis of the venous sinuses may cause increased intracranial pressure with severe headache, papilledema, motor ocular cranial nerve (sixth nerve) palsies, and mental changes, but in some patients the only manifestation may be a moderate headache [8, 10, 13–15]. CVST in BS evolves relatively slowly in most cases, but acute onset with seizures and focal neurologic signs have also been reported [4]. Superior sagittal sinus is most frequently involved with a substantial number of these patients also having lateral sinus thrombosis. Intracranial hypertension with initially normal neuroimaging with subsequent finding of CVST has been reported where patients might have CVT that couldn't be visualized due to technical problems such as being beyond the resolution of the imaging techniques or as the CVT developing very insidiously – being still partially patent early in the disease.

The onset of CVST in patients with BS tends to occur earlier than the clinical onset of parenchymal CNS involvement and this difference is significant mainly among the male patients [4, 12, 16]. Focal venous hemorrhagic cerebral infarction commonly seen in patients with CVST due to other causes is uncommon in BS, and the occurrence of CVST together with primary CNS involvement in the same patient is also rare [10, 14, 15]. CVST in BS is strongly associated with systemic major vessel disease, such as thrombosis of major veins, and systemic arterial disease, such as pulmonary aneurysms, whereas such an association isn't the case in patients with intra-axial NBS [12, 14, 16]. BS patients with CVST have a better neurological prognosis than the patients with intra-axial NBS, as recurrence and neurologic deficits are less likely to occur. However, due to an increased association with major systemic vessel disease they may have a higher overall morbidity and mortality, and therefore a diagnosis of CVST in a patient with BS may not be always associated with a favorable outcome [1]. All these observations support the notion that the two major forms of neurological disease (*intra- and extra-axial NBS*) in BS might have different pathogenic mechanisms [10, 14, 15].

Intra-axial NBS

Parenchymal involvement in BS may present with symptoms and signs consistent with focal or multifocal CNS dysfunction with or without headache. The most common presentations are pyramidal weakness, brainstem and cerebellar signs, and cognitive/behavioral changes [1]. The onset of a subacute brainstem syndrome in a young man, especially of Mediterranean, Middle-Eastern, or Oriental origin, with cranial nerve findings, dysarthria, corticospinal tract signs and a mild confusion with severe headache should promptly raise the probability of "NBS." Such a patient needs to be interviewed for the presence of systemic findings of BS. In the case of BS, it will be very likely to obtain a past or present history of recurrent oral aphthous ulcers and some other systemic manifestations of the disease. Emotional lability, seizures, a self limited or progressive myelopathy, may be seen but are less common, whereas isolated optic neuritis, aseptic meningitis, and extrapyramidal syndromes are rare presentations [1, 13, 17]. Patients with intra-axial NBS may remain with a single neurologic attack or initially have a relapsing-remitting course, with some of them developing a secondary progression later, while a few will have a progressive CNS dysfunction from the onset [1–3]. The latter progressive manifestation may be referred to chronic progressive NBS, which is discussed below.

Classification of Intra-axial NBS

Intra-axial NBS can be classified into acute NBS and chronic progressive NBS forms [2, 3]. Thus, acute NBS is characterized by an acute CNS syndrome, which responds well to corticosteroids and is usually self-limiting [2]. As already mentioned, a significant number of patients with acute NBS will remain with a single attack, while roughly a third will continue to have further attacks [8–10]. By contrast, chronic progressive NBS is characterized by intractable, slowly progressive neuro-behavioral changes and ataxia, along with persistent marked elevation of CSF IL-6 (usually more than 20 pg/ml) [2]. These patients with a chronic progressive form are also considered to have intra-axial NBS with a primary or secondary progressive course with gradual neurologic deterioration leading to significant disability [8–10].

Arterial-NBS

Arterial involvement resulting in CNS vascular disease is rare in BS, but an increasing number of cases with bilateral internal carotid artery occlusion, vertebral artery dissection or thrombosis, aneurysms, intracranial arteritis, and intra-axial small arterial occlusions are being reported [16–22]. These observations suggest that arterial involvement may be a subgroup of NBS [1], but whether this subdivision has any pathognomonic or other meaning is currently not known. Intracranial hemorrhages may occur but are extremely rare, most occurring within ischemic lesions [23, 24].

Headache in BS

Headache can occur as the presenting symptom of NBS either due to CNS involvement or CVST. It can also be seen in association with ocular inflammation. Headache is the most common neurological symptom seen in patients with BS. It usually is not associated with intracranial disease [1, 25]. In several studies on headache in BS, the most common type of headache was reported to be migraine [26–29]. When BS patients with headache are studied in detail, it will be found that some report a bilateral, frontal, moderate paroxysmal migraine-like pain, which is not a true idiopathic migraine, since it generally starts after the onset of BS and commonly accompanies the exacerbations of systemic findings of the disease, such as oral ulcerations or skin lesions, though this is not always the rule [25]. It may be explained by a vascular headache triggered by the immunomediated disease activity in susceptible individuals. Finally, coexiting primary headaches such as migraine and tension type headaches in patients with BS also are seen.

Neuro-Psycho-Behçet's Syndrome

Some patients with BS may develop a neuro-behavioral syndrome, which consists of euphoria, loss of insight/disinhibition, indifference to their disease, psychomotor agitation or retardation, with paranoid attitudes and obsessive concerns not associated with glucocorticosteroid or any other drug use, we name as "neuro-psycho-Behçet's Syndrome" [6]. This form of presentation has been suggested to be closely associated with the chronic progressive subgroup of intra-axial NBS [30].

Cognitive Changes Observed in Patients with NBS

Memory impairment was found to be the major cognitive function problem in patients with NBS with delayed recall being the most severely affected memory process, seen in all patients either in the verbal and/or visual modalities [31].

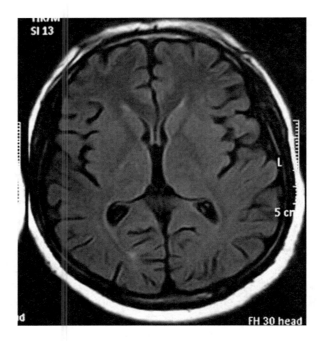

Fig. 6.1 An MRI image showing moderately enlarged third ventricle and mild sulcal enlargement in a patient with neuro-psycho-Behçet's Syndrome, who had mild cognitive deficits and behavioral changes

An impairment in the process of acquisition and storage; attention deficit and deficits of executive functions of frontal system were the other cognitive functions involved in the declining order. Neuropsychological status deteriorated insidiously, regardless of the neurological attacks during the follow-up period in most of the patients. The presence of cognitive decline was not directly related to detectable lesions on neuroimaging at early stages of the disease. However, an enlargement of the third ventricle and atrophy of the posterior fossa structures were observed in the late stages of the disease and this was correlated with memory loss (Fig. 6.1). This form of presentation might be also closely associated with the chronic progressive subgroup of intra-axial NBS [30].

Neuromuscular Disease in BS

Peripheral nervous system (PNS) involvement with clinical manifestations is rare in BS. Reported PNS involvement includes mononeuritis multiplex, a distal sensory motor neuropathy, an axonal sensory neuropathy and isolated muscle involvement with focal or generalized myositis [5, 10, 13, 33–36]. However, electroneuromyographic studies may disclose a subclinical neuropathy in patients who do not report symptoms suggestive of neuropathy [5, 36]. Besides, it should be kept in mind, that the neuropathy may develop secondary to a various drugs used in the treatment of BS, such as thalidomide or colchicine [7], or may also be coincidental.

Subclinical NBS

The incidental finding of neurological signs in patients with BS without neurological symptoms was reported in some series, with a minority of these patients developing mild neurological attacks later [8, 37]. In another study looking at silent neurological involvement in BS, the authors also concluded that this group of patients represented a milder form of the disease, since the mortality and disability rate was found to be significantly low when followed prospectively [38].

Brainstem auditory and somatosensory evoked potentials, and transcranial magnetic stimulation were studied in patients with intra-axial NBS in several studies and showed a wide range of abnormalities, mainly due to the involvement the basal parts of the brainstem and corticospinal tracts [1, 13]. The demonstration of subclinical involvement by detection of abnormal responses in examined areas without corresponding clinical symptoms and signs in some of these patients is noteworthy in providing information for the extent of the CNS involvement. In another study, subclinical involvement was investigated by using P300 (event related potential = P300) in Behçet's patients without neurological manifestations [39]. The findings suggested that the delayed P300 measures and motor response time may reflect subclinical neurologic involvement.

Electroneuromyographic studies, as already mentioned have also shown a subclinical neuropathy in some patients who did not report symptoms suggestive of a neuropathy. Similarly clinically silent muscle involvement was reported in patients without overt muscle involvement, by electron microscopy [32]. Autonomic nervous system involvement was also reported in asymptomatic patients with BS [40]. On the other hand, subclinical CNS involvement was also detected by single photon emission computed tomography studies in some patients without prominent neurological problems [41–43].

The detection of abnormalities in neurophysiological studies, as well as by neuroimaging in asymptomatic patients further suggests that the subgroup of patients with subclinical CNS and PNS involvement may not be so uncommon [44]. However, the clinical and prognostic value of detecting abnormalities in such diagnostic studies in this subgroup of patients is still not clear.

Neuropathology of NBS

The neuropathology of intra-axial NBS in the acute phase lesions is characterized by infiltration of mononuclear cells around small vessels, consisting of T lymphocytes and monocytes, but very few B lymphocytes, with most neurons undergoing apoptosis [45]. Of note, neither fibrinoid necrosis nor infiltration of inflammatory cells in the vessel walls was noted, indicating that NBS is not strictly a cerebral vasculitis, but rather a perivasculitis [45–47]. However, fibrinoid necrosis was also reported to be observed in a few studies [48, 49]. In chronic progressive lesions of NBS, similar histopathological changes were noted in pons, cerebellum, medulla, internal capsule, and midbrain, although the degree of mononuclear cell infiltration was modest. There were also scattered foci of neurons undergoing apoptosis with formation of a few binucleated neurons [45]. It is suggested that soluble factors produced by infiltrating cells, including IL-6, might play a role in the induction of apoptosis of neurons in NBS. The most prominent feature of NBS at long-term remission for as long as 15 years, was atrophy of basal pons with formation of cystic or moth-eaten lesions, consisting of isomorphic gliosis with viable neurons although being in remission is not necessarily a prerequisite for these observations [45]. There were still scattered foci of perivascular cuffing of T lymphocytes and monocytes, emphasizing the common features throughout the course of NBS.

The most frequent CNS sites involved in NBS are the brainstem-diencephalic and pontobulbar regions. Koçer et al. suggested that the anatomic variability of venous structural arrangements at different levels of the CNS might explain this predilection [23]. On the other hand, arterial involvement resulting in CNS vascular disease is rare in BS [1]. Of note, the demonstration of the preservation of viable neurons within the parenchymal lesions with isomorphic gliosis in a patient with a long course of NBS renders unlikely the possibility that such lesions result from ischemia secondary to vasculitic involvement of arteries at least in some patients [45]. Rather, these findings suggest that a continuum of relapsing-remitting small attacks with perivascular cuffing of mononuclear cells might be taking place during the long disease course.

Neuroimmunology of NBS

CSF analysis findings, when available, usually show abnormalities including leuko-cytosis and an increase in protein concentration in most patients with intra-axial NBS [8–10]. More importantly, it has been shown that the concentration of IL-6 is mark-edly elevated in CSF from patients with acute NBS and chronic progressive NBS, correlating with the disease activity [2, 50]. Thus, CSF IL-6 was decreased when the disease activity was successfully suppressed [51]. Previous studies also demonstrated that proinflammatory cytokines, including IL-6, play important role in the neuron damage [52–54]. Accordingly, there has been a growing appreciation of the destructive potential of elevated levels of IL-6 in the CNS. IL-6 has been found to cause neuronal degeneration and cell death also in various other disorders [55]. It is therefore most likely that high amounts of proinflammatory cytokines, especially IL-6, might be important in the induction of neuronal apoptosis in NBS.

In another study in which serum and CSF levels of cytokines and chemokines were studied in NBS, multiple sclerosis, and other inflammatory and noninflammatory neurological diseases, the authors pointed to the importance of chemokine effects in NBS CSF, and that this pattern resembled nonspecific inflammation compared to autoimmune disorders such as MS [56].

Diagnostic Studies in NBS

Neuroimaging

In BS patients with neurological problems consistent with intra-axial-NBS, cranial magnetic resonance imaging (MRI) is usually quite diagnostic. The lesions are generally located within the brainstem, extending to the diencephalon and/or basal ganglia (Figs. 6.2a–d and 6.3a–c). They are less often at the periventricular and subcortical white matter [23]. However, the pattern of parenchymal lesions can also be suggestive of a small vessel vasculitis, reminding us that the pathologlical changes in CNS involvement is not always typical in NBS. As discussed above a definite vasculitis is not observed in most cases. Brainstem lesions with extension into the diencephalic and basal ganglia region in the acute phase of the disease may disclose mass effect due to vasogenic edema and therefore may resemble tumors. A number of tumefactive lesions confused with primary or metastatic tumors have been reported but only a few were located elsewhere from the brainstem and deep hemispheric structures, such as the frontoparietal lobe, temporal lobe, or cerebellum in the cerebrum [13, 57]. Spinal cord involvement is not common, but when seen the major site to be involved is the cervical cord, with a myelitis-like lesion continuing more than two segments sometimes mimicking neuromyelitis optica (NMO), with the lesion extending to the brainstem. Gadolinium enhancement of the lesions, subsequent resolution of these lesions, and thoracic cord involvement have also been reported.

The probability of detecting a significant finding in the cerebral arteriography is low. As in most cases with CNS parenchymal disease, the vascular involvement is most likely to be prominent in the postcapillary venules. Therefore cerebral arteriography is not a priority in NBS, as well as in cases with extra-cerebral vascular involvement. It should be kept in mind that more than a neutrophilic infiltration with arterial injury may occur at the site of arteriographic puncture in patients with BS. Recently a fatal rebleeding during the arterial injection of the contrast medium was reported in a Behçet patient with a basilar artery aneurysm [58]. Since patients with BS have vascular inflammatory changes that may increase the rebleeding tendency of the aneurysm, the authors suggested that once an intracranial aneurysm is suspected or detected by noninvasive studies, further investigation of the aneurysm may be done by multi-slice computed tomography, which is known to be a sensitive diagnostic tool [58].

MR-venography (MRV) is the preferred imaging modality to diagnose or confirm CVST in BS, and T1&T2-weighted images also may disclose the venous sinus thrombosis (Fig. 6.4).

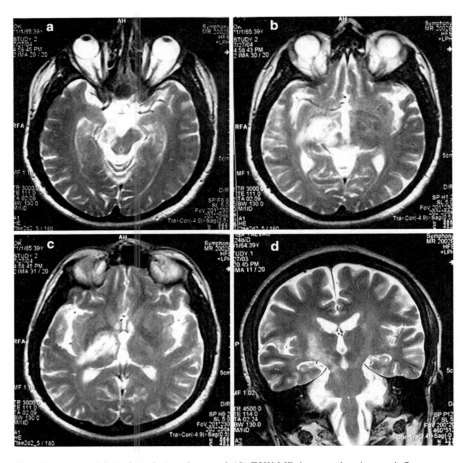

Fig. 6.2 a–d: Axial (**a, b** and **c**) and coronal (**d**) T2W-MR images showing an inflammatory lesion in the right meso-diencephalic region extending toward the basal ganglia in a patient with neuro-Behçet's Syndrome

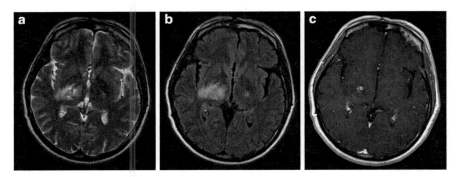

Fig. 6.3 a–c: Axial cranial T2 (**a**) and Flair (**b**) images showing an active-contrast enhancing lesion (T1 Gadolinium image, **c**) in the right deep hemispheric structures extending from the brainstem to the basal ganglia, posterior internal capsule and thalami of a male patient with intra-axial neuro-Behçet's Syndrome

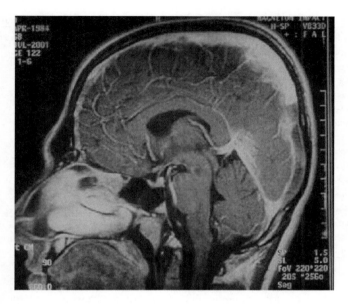

Fig. 6.4 A T2-weighted image showing thrombosis of the posterior part of the superior sagital sinus thrombosis in a patient with extra-axial neuro-Behçet's syndrome

Cerebrospinal Fluid

During the acute stage, CSF examination usually shows inflammatory changes in most cases of intra-axial NBS with increased number of cells (up to a few hundred cells per ml) and modestly elevated protein levels [13]. Besides, as already mentioned markedly elevated concentrations of IL-6 in the CSF of patients with both acute and chronic progressive NBS in relation to disease activity can be found [2]. Oligoclonal bands may be seen but this will be an infrequent finding, seen in about less than 20% of cases. CSF in patients with CVST may be under increased pressure, but the cellular and chemical composition is usually normal.

Differential Diagnosis

Differential Diagnosis of Intra-axial (Parenchymal) NBS

Patients with NBS are young and frequently present with a subacute brainstem syndrome or hemiparesis, as well as with other various neurological manifestations. Hence, the possibility of BS is often included in the differential diagnosis of multiple sclerosis and in the stroke of the young adult [17] (Table 6.2).

Table 6.2 The differential diagnosis of intra-axial (CNS) neuro-Behçet's syndrome

Neurologic diseases
Multiple sclerosis
Stroke in young adults
Primary CNS vasculitis
Primary CNS lymphoma
Brainstem glioma
Systemic diseases with neurologic involvement
Connective tissue diseases and systemic vasculitides with CNS involvement
Neuro-sarcoidosis
CNS-tuberculosis
Vogt–Koyanagi–Harada syndrome
Reiter syndrome
Eales' disease
Cogan's syndrome
Susac syndrome
Sweet syndrome

Optic neuritis, sensory symptoms, and spinal cord involvement, which are common in MS, are rarely seen in NBS. However, sometimes the clinical presentation of NBS may be confused with MS, but the MRI findings are clearly different. MS has more discrete and smaller brainstem lesions in contrast to the large extensive lesions of NBS. The supratentorial, periventricular ovoid lesions and corpus callosum involvement are more prominent in MS compared to the small, bi-hemispheric, and subcortical lesions of NBS [1, 17]. Spinal cord involvement is unlikely to extend more than two vertebral segments in MS, whereas more extensive lesions are reported in NBS, similar to NMO. The CSF also reveals different patterns, with a more prominent pleocytosis and low rate of positivity for oligoclonal bands in CNS-NBS (Table 6.3).

An acute stroke-like onset is not common in NBS, and MRI lesions within the classical arterial territories are also not expected. The absence of systemic symptoms and signs will serve to differentiate the primary CNS vasculitis from NBS, and the difference in some of the systemic symptoms and signs, as well as the MRI findings and specific blood tests from the secondary CNS vasculitides.

Sarcoidosis can be confused with BS due to uveitis, arthritis, and CNS involvement, but the absence of oral and genital ulcers, and the presence of peripheral lymphadenopathy, and bilateral hilar lymph nodes on chest X-ray, as well as the presence of noncaseating granulomatous lesions in biopsy specimens in sarcoidosis help in the differential diagnosis.

Tuberculosis may resemble BS because of its multisystem involvement and for its potential to affect the nervous system. Hilar lymphadenopathy and pulmonary cavities are not expected in BS, and the mucocutaneus manifestations of BS are unusual for tuberculosis. Furthermore the cellular and biochemical constituent of CSF and the MRI findings are likely to be different brainstem or hemispheric tumors and primary CNS lymphoma may be included in the differential diagnosis

Table 6.3 The differential diagnosis of multiple sclerosis and intra-axial (CNS) neuro-Behçet's syndrome

	Multiple sclerosis	CNS-neuro-Behçet's syndrome
Gender	Female > male	Male > female
Symptoms at onset		
Common	ON; sensory; spinal cord; brainstem/INO; motor; cerebellar	Headache; motor; cerebellar; brainstem
Uncommon	Headache; brainstem	ON; sensory; spinal cord; brainstem/INO
MRI		
PV&SC lesions	(+++)	(±)
Brainstem lesions	Small, discrete, extension (−)	Large, diffuse, extension (+)
Spinal cord lesions	(++)	(±)
CSF		
Inflammatory changes	(±)	(++)
OCB (+)	>90%	<20%

From ref. [17]

CNS central nervous system, *MRI* magnetic resonance imaging, *CSF* cerebrospinal fluid, *OCB* oligoclonal bands, *ON* optic neuritis, *BS* brainstem, *IN* internuclear ophtalmoplegia, *PV* Periventricular, *SC* subcortical

of NBS in patients who present with space occupying lesions on their MRIs, but the presence of systemic findings and the resolution of the MRI lesion following high-dose steroids that will remain without expanding and/or enhancing on follow-up imaging studies will help to distinguish NBS from brain neoplasia.

Due to the presence of eye disease and some other systemic manifestations rare diseases such as Vogt–Koyanagi–Harada syndrome, Reiter syndrome, Eales' disease, Cogan's syndrome, and Susac syndrome are other considerations in the differential diagnosis of BS. All may present with nervous system manifestations and therefore are included in the differential diagnosis of NBS, too. However, a complete ophthalmologic examination will reveal the true nature of eye involvement in each of these syndromes, which will have differences from the eye involvement seen in BS [17].

"Neuro-Sweet disease" (NSD) is the rare CNS involvement that is seen with Sweet disease (SD), which is an idiopathic multisystem inflammatory disorder characterized by peculiar erythematous skin lesions and fever that resembles BS. It may be difficult to differentiate it from BS, but the ocular signs seen in Sweet's disease are episcleritis and conjunctivitis rather than uveitis. HLA-Cw1 and B54 association has been reported for SD compared with the high frequency of HLA-B51 in BS [59, 60]. In NSD any region of the CNS can be involved without site predilection, resulting in a variety of neurologic symptoms. The neurologic events may be recurrent but the prognosis is benign, as the disease isn't a true vasculitis [59, 60].

Gastrointestinal symptoms in BS may mimic Crohn's disease or chronic ulcerative colitis. Eye disease is rare and genital ulcers are absent in inflammatory bowel diseases.

The diagnosis can be confirmed by intestinal biopsy. Whipple's disease with its gastro-intestinal and various nervous system symptoms may also resemble BS.

Prognosis

Neurological involvement in BS is an important cause of morbidity. Approximately 50% of NBS patients are moderate-to-severely disabled after 10 years of disease [10]. Onset with cerebellar symptoms and a progressive course were found to be unfavor-able factors, while onset with headache, a diagnosis of CVST, and disease course limited to a single episode were favorable [1]. An elevated protein level and pleocy-tosis in the CSF were also reported to be associated with a poorer prognosis [8].

Treatment

Neurological involvement in BS is heterogeneous and it is difficult to predict its course, prognosis, and assess response to treatment. Therefore, it is not possible to reach a conclusion on the efficacy of any treatment unless properly designed studies are carried for each form of NBS. However, this is difficult to accomplish, as num-bers of new NBS cases seen yearly are limited even in large centers. Currently, we have no first-rate evidence for the efficacy of any treatment for any form of NBS. Empirical impressions currently create the guidelines for management.

Intra-axial NBS: Acute Episodes

Glucocorticoids are used to treat acute CNS involvement, but the effect is short-lived and they do not prevent further attacks or progression. Acute attacks of intra-axial NBS are treated with either oral prednisolone (1 mg/kg for up to 4 weeks, or until improve-ment is observed) or with high-dose intravenous methyl prednisolone (IVMP-1 g/day) for 5–7 days. Both forms of treatment should be followed with an oral tapering dose of glucocorticoids over 2–3 months in order to prevent early relapses [61, 62].

Intra-axial NBS: Long-term Treatments

Colchicine, azathioprine, cyclosporine-A, cyclophosphamide, methotrexate, chloram-bucil, immunomodulatory agents such as interferon-α and thalidomide have been shown to be effective in treating some of the systemic manifestations of BS; however, none of these agents have been shown to be beneficial in NBS in a properly designed study [30, 61–63]. Cyclosporine was reported to cause neurotoxicity or to accelerate the development of CNS symptoms and therefore its use in NBS is not recommended [64–66]. The common clinical practice is to add an immunosuppresant drug, such as azathioprine or monthly pulse cyclophosphamide to glucocorticoids in progressive NBS cases, but the efficacy of such a combination has not been proven. Although limited to a small case series in an open study with long-term follow-up of 4 years, low dose methotrexate (5–15 mg/weekly) was reported to have some beneficial effect in patients with chronic progressive NBS and the beneficial effect was reported to be correlated with the decreased CSF IL-6 concentrations [67].

Successful treatment of neurologic manifestations of BS with monoclonal anti-TNF alpha antibody (infliximab) in a few patients has been recently reported [68–73]. The occurrence of neuro-relapses after stopping infliximab, formation of neutralizing antibodies, and the probability of increased CNS auto-immunity with monoclonal anti-TNF alpha antibody treatment should be kept in mind. Mycophenolate mofetil and tacrolimus are other immunosupressant/immunomodulator agents that were used to treat ocular inflammation and significant systemic manifestations in patients with BS, but there is no information regarding the potential effect of all these drugs in preventing CNS involvement or new neurologic attacks. Data on the use of intravenous immunoglobulin and plasma exchange in NBS is also limited and unclear.

Cerebral aneurysms are rare in BS, but when small unruptured aneurysms are detected medical therapy with steroids with or without cytotoxic agents may be tried. As an alternative to surgery, endovascular treatment is another option in the management of Behçet's disease-associated intracranial aneurysms [21].

Treatment of CVST in NBS

There is no consensus on the treatment of CVST in NBS. Some authors use a combination of anticoagulation with glucocorticoids [4, 14, 61], while others administer glucocorticoids alone [15]. As BS patients with CVST are more likely to have also systemic large vessel disease including pulmonary and peripheral artery aneurysms, anticoagulation should be considered only after such possibilities are ruled out to avoid the possibility of fatal bleeding [74]. However, in a recently reported large series of patients with CVST (extra-axial NBS), who were treated successfully with anticoagulation no serious side effects were observed [14], recurrence of CVST is uncommon after the initial episode.

EULAR (European League Against Rheumatism) Recommendations for the Treatment of NBS

According to the recently published EULAR recommendations for the treatment of Behçet's Disease, there are no controlled data to guide the management of CNS involvement in BD. For parenchymal involvement agents to be tried may include corticosteroids, interferon-α, azathioprine, cyclophosphamide, methotrexate and TNF-α antagonists. For dural sinus thrombosis corticosteroids are recommended. Cyclosporine A should not be used in BD patients with central nervous system involvement unless necessary for intraocular inflammation [74].

References

1. Siva A, Altıntas A, Saip S (2004) Behçet's syndrome and the nervous system. Curr Opin Neurol 17:347–357
2. Hirohata S, Isshi K, Oguchi H, Ohse T, Haraoka H, Takeuchi A, Hashimoto T (1997) Cerebrospinal fluid interleukin-6 in progressive Neuro-Behçet's syndrome. Clin Immunol Immunopathol 82:12–17
3. Kawai M, Hirohata S (2000) Cerebrospinal fluid beta(2)-microglobulin in neuro-Behçet's syndrome. J Neurol Sci 179:132–139
4. Wechsler B, Vidailhet M, Bousser MG et al (1992) Cerebral venous sinus thrombosis in Behçet's disease: long term follow-up of 25 cases. Neurology 42:614–618
5. Serdaroglu P (1998) Behçet's disease and the nervous system. J Neurol 245:197–205
6. Siva A, Özdogan H, Yazici H et al (1986) Headache, neuro-psychiatric and computerized tomography findings in Behçet's syndrome. In: Lehner T, Barnes CG (eds) Recent advances in Behçet's disease. Royal Society of Medicine Service, London, pp 247–254
7. International Study Group for Behçet's Disease (1990) Criteria for diagnosis of Behçet's disease. Lancet 335:1078–1080
8. Akman-Demir G, Serdaroglu P, Tasci B, The Neuro-Behçet Study Group (1999) Clinical patterns of neurological involvement in Behçet's disease: evaluation of 200 patients. Brain 122:2171–2182
9. Kidd D, Steuer A, Denman AM, Rudge P (1999) Neurological complications in Behçet's syndrome. Brain 122:2183–2194
10. Siva A, Kantarci OH, Saip S et al (2001) Behçet's disease: diagnostic and prognostic aspects of neurological involvement. J Neurol 248:95–103
11. Kural-Seyahi E, Fresko I, Seyahi N et al (2003) The long-term mortality and morbidity of Behçet's syndrome: a 2-decade outcome survey of 387 patients followed at a dedicated center. Medicine (Baltimore) 82:60
12. Tunc R, Saib S, Siva A, Yazici H (2004) Cerebral venous thrombosis is associated with major vessel disease in Behçet's syndrome. Ann Rheum Dis 63:1693–1694
13. Al-Araji A, Kidd DP (2009) Neuro-Behçet's disease: epidemiology, clinicalcharacteristics, and management. Lancet Neurol 8:192–204
14. Saadoun D, Wechsler B, Resche-Rigon M et al (2009) Cerebral venous thrombosis in Behçet's disease. Arthritis Rheum (Arthritis Care Res) 61:518–526
15. Yesilot N, Bahar S, Yilmazer S et al (2009) Cerebral venous thrombosis in Behçet's disease compared to those associated with other etiologies. J Neurol 256(7):1134–1142
16. Houman MH, Hamzaoui-B'Chir S, Ben Ghorbel I et al (2002) Neurologic manifestations of Behçet's disease: analysis of a series of 27 patients. Rev Med Interne 23:592–606
17. Siva A, Saip S (2009) The spectrum of nervous system involvement in Behçet's syndrome and its differential diagnosis. J Neurol 256:513–529
18. Bahar S, Coban O, Gürvit H et al (1993) Spontaneus dissection of the extracranial vertebral artery with spinal subarachnoid hemorrhage in a patient with Behçet's disease. Neuroradiology 35:352–354
19. Krespi Y, Akman-Demir G, Poyraz M et al (2001) Cerebral vasculitis and ischaemic stroke in Behçet's disease: report of one case and review of the literature. Eur J Neurol 8(6):719–722
20. Sagduyu A, Sirin H, Oksel F et al (2002) An unusual case of Behçet's disease presenting with bilateral internal carotid artery occlusion. J Neurol Neurosurg Psychiatry 73:343

21. Kizilkilic O, Albayram S et al (2003) Endovascular treatment of Behçet's disease-associated intracranial aneurysms: report of two cases and review of the literature. Neuroradiology 45:328–334
22. Aktas EG, Kaplan M, Ozveren MF (2008) Basilar artery aneurysm associated with Behçet's Disease: a case report. Turk Neurosurg 18:35–38
23. Kocer N, Islak C, Siva A et al (1999) CNS involvement in Neuro-Behçet's syndrome: an MR study. AJNR 20:1015–1024
24. Kikuchi S, Niino M, Shinpo K et al (2002) Intracranial hemorrhage in neuro-Behçet's syndrome. Intern Med 41:692–695
25. Saip S, Siva A, Altıntas A et al (2005) Headache in Behçet's syndrome. Headache 45:911–919
26. Monastero R, Mannino M, Lopez G et al (2002) Prevalence of headache in patients with Behçet's disease without overt neurological involvement. Cephalalgia 23:105–108
27. Aykutlu E, Baykan B, Akman-Demir G et al (2006) Headache in Behçet's disease. Cephalalgia 26:180–186
28. Kidd D (2006) The prevalence of headache in Behçet's syndrome. Rheumatology 45:621–623
29. Haghighi AB, Aflaki E, Ketabchi L (2008) The prevalence and characteristics of different types of headache in patients with Behçet's disease, a casecontrol study. Headache 48:424–429
30. Hirohata S (2007) Potential new therapeutic options for involvement of central nervous system in Behçet's disease (neuro-Behçet's syndrome). Curr Rheumatol Rev 3:297–303
31. Oktem-Tanor O, Baykan-Kurt B, Gurvit IH et al (1999) Neuropsychological follow-up of 12 patients with neuro-Behçet's disease. J Neurol 246:113–119
32. Serdaroglu P (1989) Neuromuscular manifestations in the course of Behçet's disease. Acta Myologica 2:41–45
33. Namer IJ, Karabudak R, Zileli T et al (1987) Peripheral nervous system involvement in Behçet's disease. Eur Neurol 26:235–240
34. Lannuzel A, Lamaury I, Charpentier D, Caparros-Lefebvre D (2002) Neurological manifestations of Behçet's disease in a Caribbean population: clinical and imaging findings. J Neurol 249:410–418
35. Sarui H, Maruyama T, Ito I et al (2002) Necrotising myositis in Behçet's disease: characteristic features on magnetic resonance imaging and a review of the literature. Ann Rheum Dis 61:751–752
36. Atasoy HT, Tunc TO, Unal AE et al (2007) Peripheral nervous system involvement in patients with Behçet's disease. Neurologist 13:225–230
37. Al-Araji A, Sharquie K, Al-Rawi Z (2003) Prevalence and patterns of neurological involvement in Behçet's disease: a prospective study from Iraq. J Neurol Neurosurg Psychiatry 74:608–613
38. Yesilot N, Shehu M, Oktem-Tanor O et al (2006) Silent neurological involvement in Behçet's disease. Clin Exp Rheumatol 24:S65–S70
39. Kececi H, Akyol M (2001) P300 in Behçet's patients without neurological manifestations. Can J Neurol Sci 28:66–69
40. Karatas GK, Onder M, Meray J (2002) Autonomic nervous system involvement in Behçet's disease. Rheumatol Int 22:155–159
41. Huang WS, Chiu PY, Kao A, Tsai CH, Lee CC (2002) Decreased cerebral blood flow in neuro-Behçet's syndrome with neuropsychiatricmanifestations and normal magnetic resonance imaging – a preliminary report. J Neuroimaging 12:355–359
42. Nobili F, Cutolo M, Sulli A et al (2002) Brain functional involvement by perfusion SPECT in systemic sclerosis and Behçet's disease. Ann NY Acad Sci 966:409–414
43. Cengiz N, Sahin M, Onar M (2004) Correlation of clinical, MRI and Tc-99m HMPAO SPECT findings in neuro-Behçet's disease. Cengiz N, Sahin M, Onar M. Correlation of clinical, MRI and Tc-99 m HMPAO SPECT findings in neuro-Behçet's disease. Acta Neurol Belg 104:100–105
44. Tunc T, Ortapamuk H, Naldoken S et al (2006) Subclinical neurological involvement in Behçet's disease. Neurol India 54:408–411

45. Hirohata S (2008) Histopathology of central nervous system lesions in Behçet's disease. J Neurol Sci 267:41–47
46. Hadfield MG, Aydin F, Lippman HR et al (1996) Neuro-Behçet's disease. Clin Neuropathol 15:249–255
47. Arai Y, Kohno S, Takahashi Y et al (2006) Autopsy case of neuro-Behçet's disease with multifocal neutrophilic perivascular inflammation. Neuropathology 26:579–585
48. Kawakita H, Nishimura M, Satoh Y, Shibata N (1967) Neurological aspects of Behçet's disease: a case report and clinico-pathological review of the literature in Japan. J Neurol Sci 5:417–438
49. Scardamaglia L, Desmond PM, Gonzales MF et al (2001) Behçet's disease with cerebral vasculitis. Int Med J 31:560–561
50. Akman-Demir G, Tuzun E, Icoz S et al (2008) Interleukin-6 in neuro-Behçet's disease: association with disease subsets and long-term outcome. Cytokine 44:373–376
51. Hirohata S, Suda H, Hashimoto T (1998) Low-dose weekly methotrexate for progressive neuropsychiatric manifestations in Behçet's disease. J Neurol Sci 159:181–185
52. Kessler JA, Ludlam WH, Freidin MM et al (1993) Cytokine-induced programmed death of cultured sympathetic neurons. Neuron 11:1123–1132
53. Heyser CJ, Masliah E, Samimi A et al (1997) Progressive decline in avoidance learning paralleled by inflammatory neurodegeneration in transgenic mice expressing interleukin 6 in the brain. Proc Natl Acad Sci USA 94:1500–1505
54. Gruol DL, Nelson TE (2005) Purkinje neuron physiology is altered by the inflammatory factor interlukin-6. Cerebellum 4:198–205
55. Gadient RA, Otten UH (1997) Interleukin-6 (IL-6)-a molecule with both beneficial and destructive potentials. Prog Neurobiol 52:379–390
56. Saruhan-Direskeneli G, Yentur SP, Akman-Demir G et al (2003) Cytokines and chemokines in neuro-Behçet's disease compared to multiple sclerosis and other neurological diseases. J Neuroimmunol 145:127–134
57. Matsuo K, Yamada K, Nakajima K, Nakagawa M (2005) Neuro-Behçet's disease mimicking brain tumor. Am J Neuroradiol 26:650–653
58. Aktas EG, Kaplan M, Ozveren MF (2008) Basilar artery aneurysm associated with Behçet's disease: a case report. Turk Neurosurg 18:35–38
59. Hisanaga K, Iwasaki Y, Itoyama Y (2005) Neuro-Sweet disease: clinical manifestations and criteria for diagnosis. Neurology 64:1756–1761
60. Hisanaga K (2007) Neuro-neutrophilic disease: neuro-Behçet's disease and neuro-Sweet disease. Intern Med 46:153–154
61. Siva A, Fresko I (2000) Behçet's disease. Curr Treat Options Neurol 2:435–448
62. Kantarci O, Siva A (2006) Behçet's disease: diagnosis and management (Chapter 96). In: Noseworthy J (ed) Neurological therapeutics principles and practice, 2nd edn. Informa Healthcare, New York, pp 1196–1206
63. Sakane T, Takeno M, Suzuki N, Inaba G (1999) Behçet's disease. N Engl J Med 341:1284–1291
64. Kotake S, Higashi K, Yoshikawa K et al (1999) Central nervous system symptoms in patients with Behçet's disease receiving cyclosporine therapy. Ophthalmology 106:586
65. Mitsui Y, Mitsui M, Urakami R et al (2005) Behçet's disease presenting with neurological complications immediately after conversion from conventional cyclosporin A to microemulsion formulation. Intern Med 44:149–152
66. Kotter I, Gunaydin I, Batra M et al (2006) CNS involvement occurs more frequently in patients with Behçet's disease under cyclosporin A than under other medications results of a retrospective analysis of 117 cases. Clin Rheumatol 25:482–486
67. Kikuchi H, Aramaki K, Hirohata S (2003) Low dose MTX for progressive neuro-Behçet's disease. A follow-up study for 4 years. Adv Exp Med Biol 528:575–578
68. Licata G, Pinto A, Tuttolomondo A et al (2003) Anti-tumor necrosis factor alpha monoclonal antibody therapy for recalcitrant cerebral vasculitis in a patient with Behçet's syndrome. Ann Rheum Dis 62:280–281
69. Ribi C, Sztajzel R, Delavelle J, ChizzoliniC J (2005) Efficacy of TNF a blockade in cyclophosphamide resistant neuro-Behçet's disease. Neurol Neurosurg Psychiatry 76:1733–1735

70. Sarwar H, McGrath H Jr, Espinoza LR (2005) Successful treatment of long-standing neuro-Behçet's disease with infliximab in patients with refractory disease. J Rheumatol 32:181–183
71. Fujikawa K, Aratake K, Kawakami A et al (2007) Successful treatment of refractory neuro-Behçet's disease with infliximab: a case report to show its efficacy by magnetic resonance imaging, transcranial magnetic stimulation and cytokine profile. Ann Rheum Dis 66:136–137
72. Piptone N, Olivieri I, Padula A et al (2008) Infl iximab for the treatment of neuro-Behçet's disease: a case series and review of the literature. Arthritis Rheum 59:285–290
73. Kikuchi H, Aramaki K, Hirohata S (2008) Effect of infliximab in progressive Neuro-Behçet's syndrome. J Neurol Sci 272:99–105
74. Hatemi G, Silman A, Bang D et al (2008) EULAR recommendations for the management of Behçet's disease. Ann Rheum Dis 67:1656–1662

Chapter 7
Vascular Disease in Behçet's Syndrome

Vedat Hamuryudan and Melike Melikoğlu

Keywords Aneurysm • Deep vein thrombosis • Intracardiac thrombosis • Pulmonary artery aneurysm • Thromboembolism • Thrombophlebitis • Thrombosis • Vascular disease • Vasculitis • Vena cava

Arterial Involvement

Behçet's syndrome (BS) may affect practically any artery regardless of the size leading to the formation of aneurysms or occlusions [1–3]. Aneurysms are usually more common than occlusions but the reverse has also been reported [4, 5]. Arterial involvement makes up 15% of all vascular complications of BS [6–8]. Its frequency has been around 5% in most reports [7, 9, 10] but higher figures reaching 18% have been also published [6, 11]. Like the more severe manifestations of BS, arterial involvement mostly occurs in men. In a two decade outcome survey on 387 BS patients (262 being men) four men (1.5%) but no woman had arterial involvement at their initial visits [12]. However, at the end of the survey, 20 men (7.6%) and one woman (0.8%) had developed arterial involvement. In this survey a median of 7 years had elapsed between the onset of the disease and arterial involvement, which was consistent with other reports about the late development of this complication [3, 7, 12]. An important feature of arterial involvement is its coexistence with venous thrombosis [6, 13]. This association is highest when the pulmonary arteries are involved [14]. Like all manifestations of BS arterial involvement can be recurrent [15–17]. Aneurysms at different sites may develop either simultaneously or within variable intervals. Aneurysms and arterial occlusions may also be detected in the same patient [18].

V. Hamuryudan (✉)
Division of Rheumatology, Department of Medicine, Cerrahpasa Medical Faculty, University of Istanbul, Istanbul, Turkey
e-mail: vhamuryudan@yahoo.com

Y. Yazıcı and H. Yazıcı (eds.), *Behçet's Syndrome*,
DOI 10.1007/978-1-4419-5641-5_7, © Springer Science+Business Media, LLC 2010

Clinical Picture

Systemic symptoms like fever and fatigue may be seen during the early stages of arterial involvement. Symptoms of active BS along with elevated acute phase responses may be present.

Arterial occlusions may be asymptomatic or may cause ischemic symptoms depending on the site of involvement and adequacy of the collateral circulation. Loss of pulses, intermittent claudication or even gangrene of the extremities [19, 20], hemiplegia [21], and acute myocardial infarction, both due to coronary artery occlusion [22, 23] and intestinal infarction due to mesenteric artery thrombosis [24] have been reported.

The most common sites for aneurysm formation are abdominal aorta, pulmonary arteries, femoral, popliteal, and carotid arteries [3, 6, 7, 9–11]. In contrast to Takayasu's arteritis, thoracic aorta is rarely affected in BS [25–27]. Involvement of the coronary arteries and cerebral arteries is also not frequent [28–30].

Peripheral artery aneurysms are manifested as painful, hyperemic, pulsatile masses, which enable their early recognition [31] (Fig. 7.1). They usually do not cause distal ischemia but carry the risk of rupture or leakage [32]. They are mostly saccular, punched-out pseudoaneurysms with or without thrombosis [4].

In contrast to peripheral artery aneurysms, abdominal aortic aneurysms are often diagnosed in the later stages since their nonspecific symptoms like back or flank pain, abdominal discomfort and constipation are often interpreted as being related to other causes [32]. These aneurysms carry the risk of rupture resulting in medical emergencies or death [33, 34]. They are false aneurysms originating from the punched-out defects on the posterior or lateral wall of the aorta (Fig. 7.2). The aneurysmal sac usually lies in the retroperitoneal area between the aorta and verte-

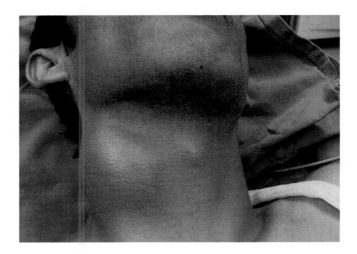

Fig. 7.1 Carotid artery aneurysm (Photo courtesy Dr. Hasan Tüzün)

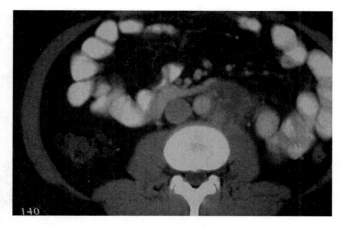

Fig. 7.2   Abdominal aortic aneurysm at computerized tomography

bral column and may erode the vertebral body or even cause hydronephrosis [32]. The aorta is usually surrounded by a thick fibrotic tissue and enlarged lymph glands. During attacks additional punched-out defects can develop on the posterior wall of the aorta. A pulsatile abdominal mass on physical examination is of paramount importance for the diagnosis. On the other hand physical examination is often unrewarding because of the posterior localization of the aneurysm and the surrounding fibrotic tissue [32].

Pathology

In the early stages, an acute inflammation characterized by intense infiltration of neutrophils and lymphoplasmocytic cells is seen in the media and adventitia with few cells in the intima. There is also an intense infiltration of inflammatory cells in the vasa vasorum with severe medial destruction and loss of elastic and muscle fibers [32, 35, 36] (Fig. 7.3). This picture is different from Takayasu's arteritis, which characteristically shows granulomatous inflammation, severe disruption of the elastic lamina, and marked thickening of all three layers of the arteries [27]. In BS the infiltrating lymphocytes in the media are predominantly CD3+ T cells and expression of IL-1 and TNF-β are seen in neutrophils, lymphocytes, and endothelial cells in the vasa vasorum [36]. Chronic stages are characterized by the destruction of the media, fibrous thickening of the intima as well as adventitial and periadventitial fibrosis [32]. These changes are also different from atherosclerotic changes which include intimal hyperplasia, medial degeneration and calcification [36]. Occlusion of the vaso vasorum speeds the transmural necrosis which results in the perforation of the vessel wall leading to pseudoaneurysm formation [37].

Fig. 7.3 Removed iliac artery with
destroyed aneurysm wall (Photo
courtesy Dr. Hasan Tüzün)

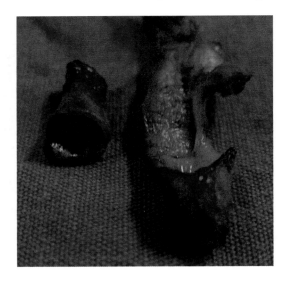

Radiology

Arterial puncture carries the risk of aneurysm formation at the insertion site [9]. Therefore conventional angiography should be avoided unless endovascular interventions are planned. The preferred methods for the detection of arterial involvement are contrast-enhanced CT angiography and MR angiography [38]. The development of multidetector CT has enabled reconstructions of three-dimensional, high resolution images within a short time. This intervention also allows the assessment of the vessel wall and can show the mural thrombus. The experience with PET scanning is limited [39].

Management

Peripheral arterial aneurysms of BS only rarely regress under medical treatment and should be managed surgically [40]. Immunosuppressive therapy should be initiated ideally before surgery to decrease recurrences and postoperative complications [41, 42]. Surgery is complicated by the formation of aneurysms at the anastomosis site and graft thrombosis [43–45] (Fig. 7.4). Occlusions necessitate arterial by-pass surgery [46]. Aneurysms of BS should be operated with synthetic grafts since venous grafts increase the risk of new aneurysm formation [32, 41]. Peripheral aneurysms can be managed with ligation when the collateral circulation is adequate [32, 47]. In recent years, endovascular replacement of stent grafts

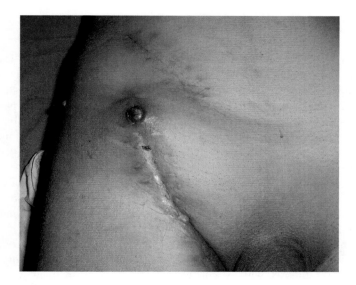

Fig. 7.4 New aneurysm formation at the operation site (Photo courtesy Dr. Hasan Tüzün)

has emerged as an alternative to surgery but long-term results of this intervention are not known [48, 49].

Pulmonary Artery Involvement

BS may involve the entire pulmonary artery tree leading to the formation of pulmonary artery aneurysms (PAA) or pulmonary artery occlusions [50–52]. Pulmonary artery occlusions usually accompany PAA and cause perfusion defects [53, 54]. PAA commonly develop in large and medium-sized pulmonary arteries and constitute the leading cause of mortality in BS [12, 53, 54]. In a literature review, 89% of the 201 patients with PAA were men [53]. We had observed PAA in 3.8% of the 262 male patients but in none of the 125 female patients during our 20-year survey [12].

Patients develop PAA at a significantly younger age as compared to other types of arterial involvement. In a retrospective study, the mean age of 91 patients was 31 years when they had developed PAA whereas it was 39 years among the 69 patients developing other types of arterial involvement [55]. The mean disease duration until the emergence of PAA is around 5 years [56]. However, it should be mentioned that the development of PAA can, on occasion, precede the onset of BS [50, 55]. There are also reports of young men, not with the usual characteristics of BS developing PAA along with venous thrombosis [57, 58]. This clinical picture was described in 1959 and is referred to as the Hughes–Stovin syndrome [59]. The clinical and histologic similarities of Hughes–Stovin syndrome suggest that it is most probably an incomplete form of BS [60].

Clinical Picture

Hemoptysis is the most frequent and usually the presenting symptom of PAA [50]. It occurs with the rupture of the aneurysm into an eroded bronchi and may be abundant and life threatening. Chest pain, cough, dyspnea are other symptoms and occur in varying frequencies. Patients with PAA also often have systemic symptoms like fever and fatigue and may have active manifestations of BS. Occasionally, infiltrations in the lung parenchyma and nodular lesions can precede the development of PAA [61]. A case of bronchiolitis organizing pneumonia, a nonspecific pathologic response to lung injury, has been also reported in a BS patient with PAA [62].

PAA are often multiple and bilateral (Fig. 7.5). A radiologic study using serial CT scans demonstrated 46 PAA in 13 BS patients ranging between two and seven aneurysms per patient [63]. Eleven (24%) of these aneurysms had developed in the main pulmonary arteries, 25 (54%) in the lobar arteries and 10 (22%) were located on segmental branches. Fifteen (33%) aneurysms were partially or totally thrombosed.

PAA show a strong association with vascular involvement elsewhere in the body [50]. Venous thrombosis, while occurring in <25% of all BS patients, was present in 81% of our patients with PAA [56]. Thrombosis of the vena cava (15%), intracardiac thrombus formation (12%), and peripheral artery aneurysms (15%) were other vascular lesions accompanying PAA [50, 56, 64]. However, despite the widespread thrombosis thromboembolism is uncommon in BS most probably because the thrombus in the diseased veins is tightly adhered to the endothelium with its entire body [65] (Fig. 7.6).

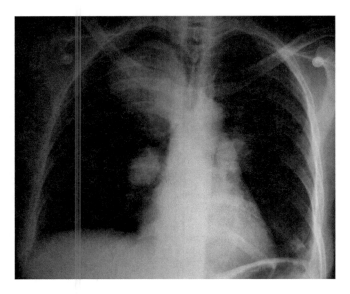

Fig. 7.5 Chest radiograph showing multiple pulmonary artery aneurysms

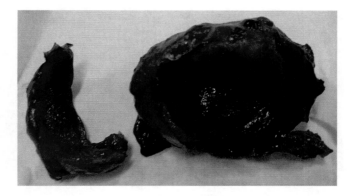

Fig. 7.6 Macroscopic appearance of the thrombus in BS (Photo courtesy Dr. Hasan Tüzün)

Radiology

Plain chest radiographs are useful initially in the symptomatic patient and during the follow-up [66, 67]. On chest radiographs, PAA usually appear as round, hilar, or peripheral opacities. Spiral CT scan of the lungs is usually sufficient for the diagnosis of PAA and for monitoring the response of the patients to treatment (Fig. 7.7). The regression or even complete disappearance of PAA under medical treatment has been shown in serial CT scans [63]. On the other hand, a retrospective study suggests that the probability of routine CT screening for detecting PAA in patients with no pulmonary or vascular symptoms is very low [68].

Conventional pulmonary angiography carries the risk of inducing the formation of aneurysms or thrombosis at the puncture site and therefore should be done only when there are plans for endovascular interventions. Intravenous digital subtraction angiography appears to be safe but may not show the thrombosed aneurysms [54]. Multislice CT provides multiplanar, high definition images of the pulmonary vasculature as well as the lung parenchyma [69]. MR angiography may be another alternative in showing thrombosed and nonthrombosed pulmonary aneurysms [67, 70, 71]. Limited experience suggests that FDG-PET/CT may have some value in showing the inflammatory activity in pulmonary arteries [72].

Differential Diagnosis

Hemoptysis in an adult, especially when the diagnosis of BS has not been established may lead to the misdiagnosis of pulmonary tuberculosis [14]. Here, we should remember that tuberculosis is especially more common in geographies where BS is endemic. The more abundant nature of hemoptysis in PAA and hilar

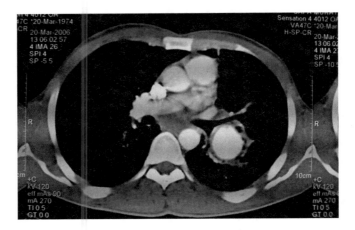

Fig. 7.7 Pulmonary artery aneurysm CT image

opacities in the chest X-ray may be helpful in differentiating the two. However, it should be kept in mind that pulmonary tuberculosis and PAA can also coexist in the same patient [56].

The frequent presence of venous thrombosis in patients with PAA may also lead to the misdiagnosis of pulmonary thromboembolism. Since in BS thrombi are common within pulmonary arteries, ventilation-perfusion scintigraphies may show perfusion defects suggesting thromboembolism, which apart from delaying the diagnosis of PAA, may lead to grave consequences if anticoagulants are initiated [14, 50]. In situ thrombi of the small pulmonary vessels frequently accompany PAA [53]. These can be seen as nodules or cavitating nodules on chest radiographs or CT scans during follow-up [73]. Since these patients will be usually on immunosuppressives these images often necessitate investigations to rule out infection. Thrombi in the pulmonary vessels may also lead to the development of pulmonary artery hypertension [74].

Pathology

Pathological changes are seen in the vasa vasorum of the pulmonary arteries [75]. A dense inflammatory infiltration consisting mainly of mononuclear cells can be seen in and around the vessel wall along with neovascularization of the vasa vasorum. These changes lead to ischemia of the affected arteries resulting in the loss of elastic fibers, muscle cells, and transmural necrosis, ending finally with the formation of aneurysms [76]. PAA are usually true aneurysms surrounded by dense adventitial fibrosis which prevents their early rupture. On the other hand, thrombotic occlusions and recanalizations along with focal hemorrhages and infarct areas may lead to the disruption of the vessel wall and to the formation of pseudoaneurysms. Thus, side by side presence of a true and a pseudoaneurysm is not rare in BS [75].

Management

PAA constitute the leading cause of mortality in BS [77]. Prompt diagnosis and prompt initiation of immunosuppressive treatment are very important in achieving a better outcome. Fifteen years ago we had reported a 50% mortality among 24 BS patients within 1 year following the diagnosis of PAA [14]. However, 10 years later we reported a better outcome for 26 patients who had been diagnosed as having PAA after our initial report [56]. The 1-year mortality in the latter group was 15% and the 5-year survival rate was 62%. The clinical characteristics of both groups were similar and there was no major change in the treatment. The only difference explaining the improved outcome was the significantly earlier diagnosis and treatment of PAA in the latter group.

There are no formal data on the management of PAA, which currently consists of monthly boluses of cyclophosphamide along with high dose corticosteroids [56, 78]. In our center, we treat our patients initially with three boluses of 1 g methylprednisolone followed by 1 mg/kg/day prednisolone and monthly boluses of 1 gm cyclophosphamide. The dose of prednisolone is tapered down according to the clinical response and discontinued if possible within 1 year. Monthly cyclophosphamide boluses are given for 1 year and the dose intervals are extended to every second month thereafter. This treatment is usually continued for 2 years and then is either stopped or maintained with azathioprine according to the patient response. In case of recurrence the treatment is initiated again. There are isolated reports on the beneficial effects of infliximab [79] or autologous hematopoietic stem cell transplantation [80].

Because the aneurysms are usually multiple the results of surgery are often not satisfactory [14, 81]. Endovascular embolization may be an alternative to surgery in emergencies [82, 83]. However the presence of the widespread thrombosis in these patients may preclude this potentially life-saving intervention. The development of an air cavity at the site of the aneurysm sac following embolization treatment has been also reported [84] (Fig. 7.8).

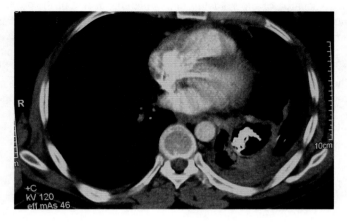

Fig. 7.8 Formation of air cavity following embolization treatment

Venous Thrombosis

Deep vein thrombosis (DVT) is the most frequent vascular manifestation of BS. The prevalence of vascular involvement in BS ranges from 15 to 50% and approximately 85% of this involvement is on the venous side [7, 8, 10, 12, 55]. DVT can take place in any localization in the venous system, but most commonly in deep veins of the legs. Superior and inferior vena cava, cerebral venous sinuses, and hepatic veins are other sites of involvement [7, 8, 10, 12, 55].

Risk for DVT in BD is significantly higher in men (40%) than in women (5%) [7, 8, 10, 12, 85]. Age of onset of venous involvement is significantly lower than that is true for aortic and peripheral arterial involvement [12, 55]. A case-controlled study of 73 Behçet's patients found a 14-fold increased risk of venous thrombosis compared to controls [86].

The majority of the vascular events occur within 5 years of disease onset [7, 10, 12, 55]. However, in 7–30% of the patients, it may occur before or shortly before the clinical diagnosis of BS [10, 55]. There is still some discussion whether vascular manifestation should be incorporated into ISG criteria set [87, 88]. Vascular involvement, at both venous and arterial sites has considerable specificity, but low sensitivity and hence has not been included in this criteria set [89].

In retrospective surveys, 13–35% of patients with vascular involvement had multiple types of vascular events [10, 55]. As many as 90% of the patients with pulmonary or systemic arterial involvement develop venous thrombosis during the disease course [14, 55, 56]. Grouping of vascular manifestations has been shown to be one of the symptom clusters and gives rise to the concept of a vasculo-Behçet's disease [90, 91]. This clustering is important to determine accurate risk assessment for potentially mortal vascular complication in patients with BS. In a retrospective survey of 882 BS patients with vascular involvement, the risk for recurrent episode of vascular involvement was found as 23% after 2 years and 38% after 5 years [55]. Among the potential predictive factors, only being male was a significant risk factor for the recurrence. Risk association of superficial thrombophlebitis, as one of the prominent skin manifestation, with vascular involvement has not been formally studied but retrospective surveys indicate its frequent coexistence with major vessel involvement [7, 8, 92]. The precise molecular and cellular mechanisms underlying the thrombotic risk of BS remain unknown. There is an occlusive inflammatory thrombus formation, strictly adherent to inflamed vessel wall, which is typically not complicated with thromboembolism [35–37]. The current evidence suggests that the pathogenesis of thrombosis in BS is probably not due to a hypercoagulable state but rather to vascular damage induced by inflammation or intrinsic endothelial dysfunction which by itself may serve as a source of thrombogenic stimuli [93–95].

Deep Vein Thrombosis of Lower Extremities

DVT of the legs make up 70% of all vascular manifestations and the first vascular events in 78% of the patients [55]. In a retrospective radiologic evaluation the most

Fig. 7.9 Deep vein thrombosis in leg

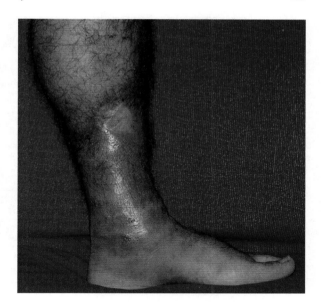

commonly involved sites were popliteal and superficial femoral veins, followed by tributary veins of the calves, common femoral, external iliac, and common iliac veins [4]. In 59% of the patients the involvement was bilateral.

Long-term morbidity due to a postthrombotic syndrome is not rare and can be substantial. On the other hand, the exact incidence and risk factors for it to develop have not been fully evaluated. Besides the pain, swelling, and stasis dermatitis, the chronic nonhealing leg ulceration can be debilitating (Fig. 7.9). A small patient series focused on leg ulcers in BD suggested that stasis ulceration should be differentiated from vasculitic lesions and pyoderma gangrenosum [96].

Vena Caval Thrombosis

BD should be included in the differential diagnosis of vena caval thrombosis, especially in young males [97–99]. Superior vena caval (SVC) and inferior vena caval (IVC) thrombosis make up 9 and 4% of major vessel manifestations of BS, respectively [8, 55]. In many patients, caval thrombosis is associated with vascular events at various other sites [97–99].

SVC thrombosis in BS usually results in characteristic signs and symptoms of SVC syndrome. These patients have swelling and cyanosis of the face, neck and upper extremities, and prominent venous collaterals in the area drained by the SVC. It usually has a benign course with efficient collateral circulation. It might rarely be complicated with pleural effusion, chylothorax, and mediastinal fibrosis [100]. Contrast-enhanced CT scan or MR angiography as noninvasive radiological interventions are the preferred imaging methods to diagnose SVC thrombosis [66].

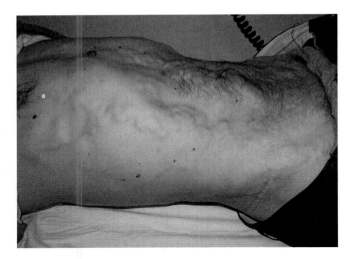

Fig. 7.10 Venous collaterals of inferior vena cava thrombosis

IVC in BS has a chronic, progressive course. It is potentially disabling and is characterized by leg swelling, pain, skin induration, intractable venous leg ulcers, and venous collaterals (Fig. 7.10). Striking feature of IVC is its frequent association with thromboses of the hepatic and deep veins of legs [98, 101–103].

Budd–Chiari Syndrome

While the Budd–Chiari syndrome is a rare vascular manifestation of BS (1.5–3.2%), BS has been reported as one of the leading causes of the Budd–Chiari syndrome in regions where BS is endemic [101] Among all the venous thrombotic manifestation of BS, hepatic vein thrombosis is the most lethal complication with 50% of mortality rate within a year [101]. It has been reported that the hepatic vein thrombosis is frequently associated with IVC occlusion, which determines the survival [101–103]. Similarly, in a recent retrospective survey from Turkey, 12 of 22 patients with Budd–Chiari syndrome had inferior vena cava thrombosis at initial presentation and 19 of them had vena caval disease in their disease course [55]. Splenomegaly is not common in BS and should raise the possibility of portal vein thrombosis [103].

Cerebral Venous Thrombosis (Also See Chap. 6)

Cerebral venous thrombosis (CVT) is a major type of vascular neurologic manifestation of BS. It accounts for 17–30% of central nervous system involvement [104, 105]. Males are more frequently affected than females [104–107].

Fig. 7.11 Cerebral MRI image of superior sagital sinus thrombosis

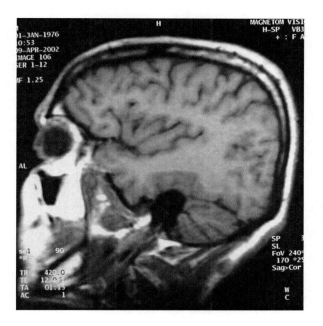

Characteristically, CVT presents with the symptoms and signs of isolated intracranial hypertension [105–107]. Headache is the most common presenting symptom followed by papilledema (62%), fever (28%), nausea/vomiting (18%), focal deficits (12%), seizure (8%), and confusion (6%) [106]. Cerebral MRI seems to be safe and reliable alternative radiologic method to conventional angiography in the diagnosis [108], although comparative studies are lacking (Fig. 7.11). Cerebrospinal fluid examination was usually normal except for an increased pressure found in 60% of the patients [106]. The patient series with CVT and isolated intracranial hypertension indicated that BD was a leading inflammatory disorder underlying CVT and should be considered in the differential diagnosis [109]. It has been reported that CVT in BS differs in certain aspects from those of CVT associated with other disorders [107]. The occlusion of cerebral veins leading to localized brain edema, so-called venous infarction was significantly less in BD patients with CVT than those of non-BS patients. Subacute mode of onset, younger age, and male predominance were the other distinguishing features of CVT associated with BS [107].

CVT in BS is strongly associated with peripheral major vessel disease [92, 106] and occurs earlier in the disease course than the parenchymal type of central nervous system disease [92]. A analysis of 64 consecutive patients from a single center revealed that parenchymal central nervous system involvement was significantly less in BS patients with CVT compared to BS patients without CVT, 4.7 and 28.7%, respectively [106].

In contrast to parenchymal central nervous system involvement, the prognosis of CVT is usually favorable [105–107]. A retrospective long-term follow-up study revealed that approximately 90% of the patients had good response to the treatment within 1 month [106]. However, 35% of the patients might develop certain types of the sequelae; severe visual loss due to optic atrophy being the most frequent [106]. Risk for such complications was associated with the presence of papilledema and prothrombotic risk factors. The presence of peripheral venous thrombosis and prothrombotic risk factors, on the other hand, related to increased risk for the recurrence [106].

Cardiac Involvement (See Also Chap. 8)

Intracardiac Thrombosis

Intracardiac thrombosis is a rare complication of BS (Fig. 7.12). In an attempt to clarify the clinical and pathologic correlates of intracardiac thrombus in BS, 24 published cases were reviewed in 2000 [64]. The patients were mostly reported from the Mediterranean basin and the Middle East. There was a clear predominance of young males. It was the initial manifestation of the disease in half of the patients. Fever, hemoptysis, dyspnea, and cough were the most common presenting symptoms. Thrombosis was usually located at the right side of the heart. Heart valves were rarely affected. Pathological findings showed an organizing thrombus formation containing mononuclear inflammatory cell infiltrates with or without involvement

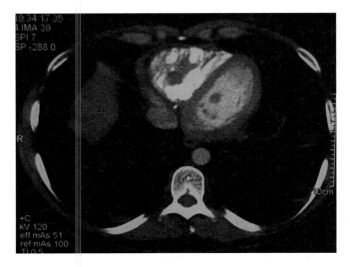

Fig. 7.12 CT image of right ventricular intracardiac thrombi

of underlying cardiac tissue. In 50% of the patients, intracardiac thrombosis was associated with large arterial involvement, notably PAA. DVT was observed in 56% of the patients. It has been reported that BS patients with intracardiac thrombus had a high frequency of pulmonary embolism (56–67%) [110]. Although the right-sided thrombosis might explain the increased risk for pulmonary emboli, it is difficult to rule out a coexisting in situ pulmonary artery vasculitis [111].

References

1. Lie JT (1992) Vascular involvement in Behçet's disease: arterial and venous and vessels of all sizes. J Rheumatol 19:341–343
2. Calamia KT, Schirmer M, Melikoglu M (2004) Major vessel involvement in Behçet's disease. Curr Opin Rheumatol 17:1–8
3. Hamza M (1987) Large artery involvement in Behçet's disease. J Rheumatol 14:554–559
4. Ko GY, Byun JY, Choi BG, Cho SH (2000) The vascular manifestations of Behçet's disease: angiographic and CT findings. Br J Rheumatol 73:1270–1274
5. Tohme A, Aoun N, El-Rassi B, Ghayad E (2003) Vascular manifestations in Behçet's disease. Joint Bone Spine 70:384–389
6. Duzgun N, Ates A, Aydintug OT, Demir O, Olmez U (2006) Characteristics of vascular involvement in Behçet's disease. Scand J Rheumatol 35:65–68
7. Koc Y, Güllü I, Akpek G et al (1992) Vascular involvement in Behçet's disease. J Rheumatol 19:402–410
8. Kuzu MA, Ozaslan C, Koksoy C, Gürler A, Tüzüner A (1994) Vascular involvement in Behçet's disease: 8 year audit. World J Surg 18:948–953
9. Le Thi Huong D, Wechsler B, Papo T et al (1995) Arterial lesions in Behçet's disease. A study in 25 patients. J Rheumatol 22:2103–2113
10. Sarica-Kucukoglu R, Akdag-Kose A, Kayabali M et al (2006) Vascular involvement in Behçet's disease: a retrospective analysis of 2319 cases. Int J Dermatol 45:919–921
11. Al-Dalaan AN, Al Balaa SR, K El Ramahi et al (1994) Behçet's disease in Saudi Arabia. J Rheumatol 21:658–661
12. Kural-Seyahi E, Fresko I, Seyahi N et al (2003) The long term mortality and morbidity of Behçet's syndrome. A 2 decade outcome survey of 387 patients followed at a dedicated center. Medicine (Baltimore) 82:60–76
13. Ceyran H, Akcali Y, Kahraman C (2003) Surgical treatment of vasculo-Behçet's disease. A review of patients with concomitant multiple aneurysms and venous lesions. Vasa 32:149–153
14. Hamuryudan V, Yurdakul S, Moral F et al (1994) Pulmonary arterial aneurysms in Behçet's syndrome: a report of 24 cases. Br J Rheumatol 33:48–51
15. Sherif A, Stewart P, Mendes DM (1992) The repetitive vascular catastrophes of Behçet's disease: a case report with review of the literature. Ann Vasc Surg 6:85–89
16. Planer D, Leibowitz D, Elitzur Y, Korach A, Hiller N, Chajek-Shaul T (2007) Chronicle of a death foretold: a case of catastrophic vascular Behçet's disease. Clin Rheumatol 26:457–459
17. Jayachandran NV, Rajasekhar L, Chandrasekhara PK, Kanchinadham S, Narsimulu G (2008) Multiple peripheral arterial and aortic aneurysms in Behçet's syndrome: a case report. Clin Rheumatol 27:265–267
18. Wechsler B, Le Thi Huong Du LT, De Gennes C et al (1989) Arterial manifestations of Behçet's disease. 12 cases. Rev Med Interne 10:303–311
19. Cooper AM, Naughton MN, Williams BD (1994) Chronic arterial occlusion associated with Behçet's disease. Br J Rheumatol 33:170–172
20. Gera C, Jose W, Malhotra N, Malhotra V, Dhanoa J (2008) Radial artery occlusion, a rare presentation of Behçet's disease. J Assoc Physicians India 56:643–644

21. Sagduyu A, Sirin H, Oksel F, Turk T, Ozenc D (2002) An unusual case of Behçet's disease presenting with bilateral internal carotid artery occlusion. J Neurol Neurosurg Psychiatry 73:343

22. Calguneri M, Aydemir K, Ozturk MA, Haznedaroglu IC, Kiraz S, Ertenli I (2006) Myocardial infarction and deep venous thrombosis in a young patient with Behçet's disease. Clin Appl Thromb Hemost 12:105–109

23. Atzeni F, Sarzi-Puttini P, Doria A, Boiardi L, Pipitone N, Salvarani C (2005) Behçet's disease and cardiovascular involvement. Lupus 14:723–726

24. Bayraktar Y, Soylu AR, Balkanci F, Gedikoglu G, Cakmakci M, Sayek I (1998) Arterial thrombosis leading to intestinal infarction in a patient with Behçet's disease associated with protein C deficiency. Am J Gastroenterol 93:2556–2558

25. Suzuki K, Kazui T, Yamashita K, Terada H, Washiyama N, Suzuki T (2005) Emergency operation for distal aortic arch aneurysm in Behçet's disease. Jpn J Thorac Cardiovasc Surg 53:389–392

26. Marzban M, Mandegar MH, Karimi A et al (2008) Cardiac and great vessel involvement in Behçet's disease. J Card Surg 23:765–768

27. Hoffman GS (2003) Large vessel vasculitis. Unresolved issues. Arthritis Rheum 48:2406–2414

28. Kaku Y, Hamada JI, Kuroda JI, Kai Y, Morioka M, Kuratsu JI (2007) Multiple peripheral middle cerebral artery aneurysms associated with Behçet's disease. Acta Neurochir (Wien) 149:823–827

29. Nakasu S, Kaneko M, Matsuda M (2001) Cerebral aneurysms associated with Behçet's disease: a case report. J Neurol Neurosurg Psychiatry 70:682–684

30. Tezcan H, Yavuz S, Fak AS, Aker U, Direskeneli H (2002) Coronary stent implantation in Behçet's disease. Clin Exp Rheumatol 20:704–706

31. Cakir O, Eren N, Ülkü R, Nazaroglu H (2002) Bilateral subclavian arterial aneurysm and ruptured abdominal aorta pseudoaneurysm in Behçet's disease. Ann Vasc Surg 16:516–520

32. Tuzun H, Besirli K, Sayin A et al (1997) Management of aneurysms in Behçet's syndrome: an analysis of 24 patients. Surgery 121:150–156

33. Erentug V, Bozbuga N, Omeroglu SN et al (2003) Rupture of abdominal aortic aneurysms in Behçet's disease. Ann Vasc Surg 17:682–685

34. Iscan ZH, Vural KM, Bayazit M (2005) Compelling nature of arterial manifestations in Behçet's disease. J Vasc Surg 41:53–58

35. Lakhanpal S, Tani K, Lie JT et al (1985) Pathologic features of Behçet's syndrome: a review of Japanese autopsy registry data. Hum Pathol 16:790–795

36. Kobayashi M, Ito M, Nakagawa A et al (2000) Neutrophil and endothelial cell activation in the vasa vasorum in vasculo-Behçet's disease. Histopathology 36:362–371

37. Matsumoto T, Uekusa T, Fukuda Y (1991) Vasculo-Behçet's disease. A pathologic study of eight cases. Hum Pathol 22:45–51

38. Cho YK, Lee W, Choi SI, Jae HJ, Chung JW, Park JH (2008) Cardiovascular Behçet's disease: the variable findings of rare complications with CT angiography and conventional angiography and its interventional management. J Comput Assist Tomogr 32:679–689

39. Wenger M, Baltaci M, Klein-Weigel P et al (2003) 18-FDG-positron emission tomography for diagnosis of large vessel arteritis in Behçet's disease. Adv Exp Med Biol 528:435–436

40. Yekeler E, Tunaci A, Tunaci M, Kamali S, Gul A, Acunas B (2005) Successful medical treatment of abdominal aortic aneurysms in a patient with Behçet's disease: imaging findings. Australas Radiol 49:182–184

41. Alpagut U, Ugurlucan M, Dayioglu E (2007) Major arterial involvement and review of Behçet's disease. Ann Vasc Surg 21:232–239

42. Park MC, Hong BK, Kwon HM, Hong YS (2007) Surgical outcomes and risk factors for postoperative complications in patients with Behçet's disease. Clin Rheumatol 26:1475–1480

43. Robenshtok E, Krause I (2004) Arterial involvement in Behçet's disease: the search for new treatment strategies. Isr Med Assoc J 6:162–163

44. Kalko Y, Basaran M, Aydin U, Kafa U, Basaranoglu G, Yasar T (2005) The surgical treatment of arterial aneurysms in Behçet's disease: a report of 16 cases. J Vasc Surg 42:673–677

45. Hosaka A, Miyata T, Shigematsu H et al (2005) Long term outcome after surgical treatment of arterial lesions in Behçet's disease. J Vasc Surg 42:116–121
46. Ozeren M, Mavioglu I, Dogan OV, Yucel E (2000) Reoperation results of arterial involvement in Behçet's disease. Eur J Vasc Endovasc Surg 20:512–519
47. Goz M, Cakir O, Eren MN (2007) Huge popliteal aneurysms in Behçet's syndrome: is ligation an alternative treatment? Vascular 15:46–48
48. Vasseur MA, Haulon S, Beregi JP, Le Tourneau T, Prat A, Warembourgh H (1998) Endovascular treatment of abdominal aneurysmal aortitis in Behçet's disease. J Vasc Surg 27:974–976
49. Nitecki SS, Ofer A, Karram T, Schwartz H, Engel A, Hoffman A (2004) Abdominal aortic aneurysm in Behçet's disease: new treatment options for an old and challenging problem. Isr Med Assoc J 6:152–155
50. Uzun O, Akpolat T, Erkan L (2005) Pulmonary vasculitis in Behçet's disease: a cumulative analysis. Chest 127:2243–2253
51. Erkan F, Gul A, Tasali E (2001) Pulmonary manifestations of Behçet's disease. Thorax 56:572–578
52. Efthimiou J, Johnston C, Spiro SG, Turner-Warwick M (1986) Pulmonary disease in Behçet's syndrome. Q J Med 58:259–280
53. Uzun O, Erkan L, Akpolat I, Findik S, Atici AG, Akpolat T (2008) Pulmonary involvement in Behçet's disease. Respiration 75:310–321
54. Numan F, Islak C, Berkmen T, Tuzun H, Cokyüksel O (1994) Behçet's disease: pulmonary arterial involvement in 15 cases. Radiology 192:465–468
55. Melikoglu M, Ugurlu S, Tascilar K et al (2008) Large vessel involvement in Behçet's syndrome: a retrospective survey. Ann Rheum Dis 67(Suppl II):67
56. Hamuryudan V, Er T, Seyahi E et al (2004) Pulmonary artery aneurysms in Behçet's syndrome. Am J Med 117:867–870
57. Charlton RW, Du Plessis LA (1961) Multiple pulmonary artery aneurysm. Thorax 16:364–371
58. Kopp W, Green RA (1962) Pulmonary artery aneurysms with recurrent thrombophlebitis. The Hughes–Stovin syndrome. Ann Intern Med 56:105–114
59. Hughes JP, Stovin PG (1959) Segmental pulmonary artery aneurysms with peripheral venous thrombosis. Br J Dis Chest 53:19–27
60. Erkan D, Yazici Y, Sanders A, Trost D, Yazici H (2004) Is Hughes–Stovin syndrome Behçet's disease? Clin Exp Rheumatol 22(4 Suppl 34):s64–s68
61. Cosan F, Artim-Esen B, Cagatay Y, Kamali S, Tunaci A, Gul A (2008) Parenchymal inflammatory infiltrations preceding pulmonary artery aneurysm in Behçet's disease. Clin Exp Rheumatol 26 (Suppl 50):s19
62. Gul A, Yilmazbayhan D, Buyukbabani N et al (1999) Organizing pneumonia associated with pulmonary artery aneurysm in Behçet's disease. Rheumatology (Oxford) 38:1285–1289
63. Tunaci M, Özkorkmaz B, Tunaci A, Gul A, Engin G, Acunas B (1999) CT findings of pulmonary artery aneurysms during treatment for Behçet's disease. Am J Roentgenol 172:729–733
64. Mogulkoc N, Burgess MI, Bishop PW (2000) Intracardiac thrombosis in Behçet's disease a systematic review. Chest 118:479–487
65. Leiba M, Sidi Y, Gur A et al (2001) Behçet's disease and thrombophilia. Ann Rheum Dis 60:1081–1085
66. Tunaci A, Berkmen YM, Gokmen E (1995) Thoracic involvement in Behçet's disease: pathologic, clinical and imaging features. Am J Roentgenol 164:51–56
67. Hiller N, Lieberman S, Chajek-Shaul T, Bar-Ziv J, Shaham D (2004) Thoracic manifestations of Behçet's disease at CT. Radiographics 24:801–808
68. Cosan F, Artim-Esen B, Cagatay Y, Tunaci Y, Gul A (2008) Pulmonary artery aneurysm screening in patients with Behçet's disease. Clin Exp Rheumatol 26(4 Suppl 50):s19
69. Emad Y, Abdel-Razek N, Gheita T, El-Wakd M, El Gohary T, Samadoni A (2007) Multislice CT pulmonary findings in Behçet's disease (report of 16 cases). Clin Rheumatol 26:879–884
70. Celenk C, Celenk P, Akan H et al (1999) Pulmonary artery aneurysms due to Behçet's disease: MR imaging and digital subtraction angiography findings. Am J Roentgenol 172:844–845

71. Akpolat T, Danaci M, Belet U, Erkan ML, Akar H (2000) MR imaging and MR angiography in vascular Behçet's disease. Magn Reson Imaging 18:1089–1096

72. Denecke T, Staeck O, Amthauer H, Hanninen EL (2007) PET/CT visualizes inflammatory activity of pulmonary artery aneurysms in Behçet's disease. Eur J Nucl Med Mol Imaging 34:970

73. Seyahi E, Melikoglu M, Akman C et al (2006) Pulmonary vascular involvement (PVI) in Behçet's syndrome (BS). Clin Exp Rheumatol 24(Suppl 42):s22

74. Santana AN, Antunes T, Barros JM, Kairalla RA, Carvalho CR, Barbas CS (2008) Pulmonary involvement in Behçet's disease: a positive single-center experience with the use of immunosuppressive therapy. J Bras Pneumol 34:362–366

75. Hamuryudan V, Oz B, Tuzun H, Yazici H (2004) The menacing pulmonary artery aneurysms in Behçet's syndrome. Clin Exp Rheumatol 22(4 Suppl 34):s1–s3

76. Takahama M, Yamamoto R, Nakajima R, Tada H (2009) Successful surgical treatment of pulmonary artery aneurysm in Behçet's syndrome. Interact Cardiovasc Thorac Surg 8:390–392

77. Yazici H, Esen F (2008) Mortality in Behçet's syndrome. Clin Exp Rheumatol 26(Suppl 51):s138–s140

78. Hatemi G, Silman A, Bang D et al (2008) EULAR recommendations for the management of Behçet's disease. Ann Rheum Dis 67:1656–1662

79. Baki K, Villiger PM, Jenni D, Meyer T, Beer JH (2006) Behçet's disease with life threatening hemoptoe and pulmonary aneurysms: complete remission after infliximab treatment. Ann Rheum Dis 65:1531–1532

80. Daikeler T, Kotter I, Bocelli-Tyndall C et al (2007) Haematopoietic stem cell transplantation for vasculitis including Behçet's disease and polychondritis: a retrospective analysis of patients recorded in the European Bone Marrow Transplantation and European League Against Rheumatism databases and a review of the literature. Ann Rheum Dis 66:202–207

81. De Montpreville VT, Macchiarani P, Dartevelle PG, Dulmet EM (1996) Large bilateral pulmonary artery aneurysms in Behçet's disease: rupture of the contralateral lesion after aneurysmorraphy. Respiration 63:49–51

82. Cantasdemir M, Kantarci F, Mihmanli I et al (2002) Emergency endovascular management of pulmonary artery aneurysms in Behçet's disease: report of two cases and review of the literature. Cardiovasc Intervent Radiol 25:533–537

83. Pelage JP, El Hajjam M, Lagrange C et al (2005) Pulmonary artery interventions: an overview. Radiographics 25:1653–1667

84. Cil BE, Turkbey B, Canyigit M, Kumbasar OO, Celik G, Demirkazik FB (2006) Transformation of a ruptured giant pulmonary artery aneurysm into an air cavity following transcatheter embolization in a Behçet's patient. Cardiovasc Intervent Radiol 29:1514–1515

85. Tursen U, Gurler A, Boyvat A (2003) Evaluation of clinical findings according to sex in 2313 Turkish patients with Behçet's disease. Int J Dermatol 42:346–351

86. Ames PR, Steuer A, Pap A, Denman AM (2001) Thrombosis in Behçet's disease: a retrospective survey from a single UK centre. Rheumatology (Oxford) 40:652–655

87. Silman A, Gul A (2000) Is there a place for large vessel disease in the diagnostic criteria of Behçet's disease? J Rheumatol 27:2050–2051

88. Schirmer M, Calamia KT, O'Duffy JD (1999) Is there a place for large vessel disease in the diagnostic criteria of Behçet's disease? J Rheumatol 26:2511–2512

89. International Study Group for Behçet's Disease (1990) Criteria for diagnosis of Behçet's disease. Lancet 335:1078–1080

90. Tunc R, Keyman E, Melikoglu M, Fresko I, Yazici H (2002) Target organ associations in Turkish patients with Behçet's disease: a cross sectional study by exploratory factor analysis. J Rheumatol 29:2393–2396

91. Krause I, Leibovici L, Guedj D, Molad Y, Uziel Y, Weinberger A (1999) Disease patterns of patients with Behçet's disease demonstrated by factor analysis. Clin Exp Rheumatol 17:347–350

92. Tunc R, Saip S, Siva A, Yazici H (2004) Cerebral venous thrombosis is associated with major vessel disease in Behçet's syndrome. Ann Rheum Dis 63:1693–1694

93. Espinosa G, Font J, Tàssies D, Vidaller A, Deulofeu R, López-Soto A, Cervera R, Ordinas A, Ingelmo M, Reverter JC (2002) Vascular involvement in Behçet's disease: relation with thrombophilic factors, coagulation activation, and thrombomodulin. Am J Med 112: 37–43

94. Leiba M, Seligsohn U, Sidi Y, Harats D, Sela BA, Griffin JH, Livneh A, Rosenberg N, Gelernter I, Gur H, Ehrenfeld M (2004) Thrombophilic factors are not the leading cause of thrombosis in Behçet's disease. Ann Rheum Dis 63:1445–1449

95. Chambers JC, Haskard DO, Kooner JS (2001) Vascular endothelial function and oxidative stress mechanisms in patients with Behçet's syndrome. J Am Coll Cardiol 37:517–520

96. Jung JY, Kim DY, Bang D (2008) Leg ulcers in Behçet's disease. Br J Dermatol 158:178–179

97. Kansu E, Ozer FL, Akalin E, Güler Y, Zileli T, Tanman E, Kaplaman E, Muftuoglu E (1972) Behçet's syndrome with obstruction of the venae cavae. A report of seven cases. Q J Med 41:151–168

98. Houman H, Lamloum M, Ben Ghorbel I, Khiari-Ben Salah I, Miled M (1999) Vena cava thrombosis in Behçet's disease. Analysis of a series of 10 cases. Ann Med Interne (Paris) 150:587–590

99. Oh SH, Lee JH, Shin JU, Bang D (2008) Dermatological features in Behçet's disease-associated vena cava obstruction. Br J Dermatol 159:555–560

100. Benjilali L, Harmouche H, Alaoui-Bennesser H, Mezalek ZT, Adnaoui M, Aouni M, Maaouni A (2008) Chylothorax and chylopericardium in a young man with Behçet's disease. Joint Bone Spine 75:743–745

101. Bayraktar Y, Balkanci F, Bayraktar M, Calguneri M (1997) Budd–Chiari syndrome: a common complication of Behçet's disease. Am J Gastroenterol 92:858–862

102. Bismuth E, Hadengue A, Hammel P, Benhamou JP (1990) Hepatic vein thrombosis in Behçet's disease. Hepatology 11:969–974

103. Bayraktar Y, Balkanci F, Kansu E, Dundar S, Uzunalimoglu B, Kayhan B, Telatar H, Gurakar A, Van Thiel DH (1995) Cavernous transformation of the portal vein: a common manifestation of Behçet's disease. Am J Gastroenterol 90:1476–1479

104. Akman-Demir G, Serdaroglu P, Tasci B (1999) Clinical patterns of neurological involvement in Behçet's disease: evaluation of 200 patients. The Neuro-Behçet's Study Group. Brain 122:2171–2182

105. Wechsler B, Vidailhet M, Piette JC, Bousser MG, Dell Isola B, Blétry O, Godeau P (1992) Cerebral venous thrombosis in Behçet's disease: clinical study and long-term follow-up of 25 cases. Neurology 42:614–618

106. Saadoun D, Wechsler B, Resche-Rigon M, Trad S, Le Thi Huong D, Sbai A, Dormont D, Amoura Z, Cacoub P, Piette JC (2009) Cerebral venous thrombosis in Behçet's disease. Arthritis Rheum 61:518–526

107. Yesilot N, Bahar S, Yilmazer S, Mutlu M, Kurtuncu M, Tuncay R, Coban O, Akman-Demir G (2009) Cerebral venous thrombosis in Behçet's disease compared to those associated with other etiologies. J Neurol 256:1134–1142

108. Wechsler B, Dell'Isola B, Vidailhet M, Dormont D, Piette JC, Blétry O, Godeau P (1993) MRI in 31 patients with Behçet's disease and neurological involvement: prospective study with clinical correlation. J Neurol Neurosurg Psychiatry 56:793–798

109. Biousse V, Ameri A, Bousser MG (1999) Isolated intracranial hypertension as the only sign of cerebral venous thrombosis. Neurology 53:1537–1542

110. Kajiya T, Anan R, Kameko M, Mizukami N, Minagoe S, Hamasaki S, Maruyama I, Sakata R, Tei C (2007) Intracardiac thrombus, superior vena cava syndrome, and pulmonary embolism in a patient with Behçet's disease: a case report and literature review. Heart Vessels 22:278–283

111. Hamuryudan V, Seyahi E, Yazici H (2008) Comment on "Cardiac Behçet's disease presenting as aortic valvulitis/aortitis or right heart inflammatory mass: a clinicopathologic study of 12 cases". Am J Surg Pathol 32:1914–1915

Chapter 8
Endothelial Dysfunction and Atherosclerosis in Behçet's Syndrome

Emire Seyahi, İzzet Fresko, and Hasan Yazıcı

Keywords Endothelial dysfunction • Arterial stiffness • Atherosclerosis • Intima-media thickness • Atherosclerotic plaque • Cardiac disease • Cardiovascular disease • Behçet's syndrome

Endothelium

Endothelium is a monolayer of cells located between the blood and the underlying tissues [1–7]. It plays an important role in the regulation of vascular tone, thrombosis, vascular inflammation, and smooth muscle cell proliferation [1–7]. A healthy endothelium balances the effects of relaxing and contracting factors, anticoagulant and procoagulant mediators or growth-inducing and inhibiting factors [1–7]. Relaxing factors produced and secreted by endothelial cells are endothelium-derived relaxing factors (EDRFs) of which nitric oxide (NO) is the major one, endothelium-derived hyperpolarizing factors (EDHFs) and prostacycline [1–7]. Besides being a potent relaxing factor, NO also inhibits arterial thrombosis and leukocyte adhesion [1–7]. It is synthesized in response to the shear stress caused by the blood flow over the endothelium and in response to biochemical stimuli like bradykinin or acetylcholine release [1–7]. Vasoconstricting factors include endothelin, tromboxane A_2, and angiotensin II.

E. Seyahi (✉)
Department of Medicine, Division of Rheumatology,
Cerrahpasa Medical Faculty,
University of Istanbul, Istanbul, Turkey
e-mail: eseyahi@yahoo.com

Y. Yazıcı and H. Yazıcı (eds.), *Behçet's Syndrome*,
DOI 10.1007/978-1-4419-5641-5_8, © Springer Science+Business Media, LLC 2010

Endothelial Cell Dysfunction:
What Is It and How Is It Measured?

Endothelial cell dysfunction (ECD) is characterized by reduced vasodilation which is by itself also a prothrombotic and proinflammatory state. ECD can be assessed by measuring endothelium-dependant vasodilatation with various tests [1–8]. Tests are based mainly on the stimulation of endothelial NO release. This could be achieved either by infusion of vasoactive substances like acetylcholine or by causing transient ischemia [8]. Endothelium-dependant vasodilation is often compared to the endothelium-independent vasodilatation which occurs after nitroglycerine administration. Flow-mediated dilatation (FMD) of the brachial artery by ultrasound has emerged as the widely used technique for assessing ECD [8, 9]. It is noninvasive, reproducible, fast, and safe [8, 9]. In this technique, the diameter of the brachial artery is measured with ultrasound first at rest. Then a pneumatic cuff is inflated for 5 min over the forearm to cause arterial occlusion. A second measurement is done 1 min after cuff deflation during reactive hyperemia [8, 9]. The change in arterial diameter divided by the baseline diameter gives the FMD.

The measurement of arterial stiffness can be considered as an alternative approach to assess ECD [10]. Arterial stiffness is recognized as an important predictor of atherosclerosis and cardiovascular disease [11]. Pulse wave analysis and pulse wave velocity (PWV) are two methods that assess arterial stiffness [10]. In the former, an augmentation index is derived from peripheral and/or central artery wave form analyses [10]. In the latter, arterial wave propagation velocity is measured. In the simplest way to measure PWV, arterial pulse wave is recorded at radial and femoral artery and the time delay along with distance traveled between two recording points are measured [10].

Endothelial Cell Dysfunction in Various Diseases

Impaired endothelial function has been found in essential hypertension, diabetes, coronary heart disease, congestive heart failure, and chronic renal failure [1–9, 12]. It has been shown in the earliest stages of atherosclerosis [9, 13, 14] and has been associated with each of the known atherosclerotic risk factors including aging, male gender, obesity, menopause, several forms of dyslipidemia, hyperhomocystinemia, and smoking [1–9, 12–14]. Interestingly, it has been shown that treatment or reduction of these risk factors result in improvement of endothelial dysfunction [1–9].

Endothelial dysfunction has been identified also in both acute and chronic inflammation [15–29]. Periodontitis, HIV infection, various acute nonspecific infections or even a mild temporary inflammatory reaction generated by Salmonella typhi vaccine could impair endothelial function [16–20]. Longitudinal studies have shown that intensive periodontal therapy results in improvement in endothelial function [17]. Rheumatoid arthritis (RA) and systemic lupus erythematosus (SLE) are chronic inflammatory diseases having extensive evidence of vascular inflammation and endothelial dysfunction [15, 21, 22]. Furthermore, ECD is a well-known feature of several types of vasculitis including ANCA-associated systemic vasculitis, polyarteritis nodosa, Kawasaki disease, Takayasu arteritis, and giant cell arteritis [15, 23, 24]. Similarly, suppression of inflammation with anti-TNF treatment or immunosuppressives has been demonstrated to improve ECD in patients with RA or systemic vasculitis [25–29].

Endothelial Cell Dysfunction in Behçet's Syndrome

Endothelial function and arterial stiffness have been investigated in a number of studies as shown in Table 8.1 [30–37]. The presence of ECD in patients with Behçet's syndrome (BS) was first reported by Chambers et al. in a controlled study [30]. Endothelial function, tested by FMD, was significantly impaired and rapidly improved with vitamin C treatment suggesting that ECD could be mediated by increased oxidative stress. FMD was independent of atherosclerotic risk factors such as age, gender, blood pressure, and lipid levels [30]. This study raised the question whether brachial artery FMD test might recognize patients with BS who have increased susceptibility to vascular complications [30]. Subsequent studies investigating FMD using the same method addressed whether impaired endothelial function is related to vascular or any particular organ involvement within BS [31–37]. While almost all confirmed the presence of ECD in BS, FMD in association with vascular involvement has been shown in only one [33]. One other study found reduced FMD levels among patients with eye disease [32]. Another demonstrated that endothelial function was more impaired in patients with active disease compared to those in the inactive state [37]. Recently, Protogerou et al. studied the effect of corticosteroid treatment on endothelial function by measuring FMD in 87 patients with BS [38]. Patients with active disease who were treated with corticosteroids were found to have higher FMD values compared to those who were not [38]. In contrast, among patients with inactive disease, those who were receiving corticosteroids had impaired endothelial function compared to those who were not. In addition, a 7 day follow-up of 11 patients demonstrated that endothelial functions significantly improved after corticosteroid treatment [38]. Authors suggested that corticosteroids may have dual effects on endothelial function [38].

Most of the studies that looked at arterial elastic properties found evidence for increased arterial resistance [39–44]. Alan et al. measured carotid artery end systolic and diastolic diameters using USG and showed that arterial distensibility was decreased in BS patients [39]. Ikonomidis et al. performed echocardiography of the aortic root and simultaneously measured brachial artery pressure to assess aortic functions [40]. They found that aortic diameters were increased, whereas aortic distensibility and strain were significantly decreased in patients compared to the controls [40]. The same investigators later evaluated aortic distensibility and arterial wave reflections by pulse wave analysis. They utilized applanation tonometry of the radial

Table 8.1 Studies investigating endothelial cell dysfunction by flow-mediated dilatation (FMD) in Behçet's syndrome

References	n	Age	FMD (%)	P value	Comment
[30]	BS: 9 M/10 F	40±2	0.7±0.9	0.001	Endothelial dysfunction was rapidly improved with vitamin C
	HC: 10 M/11 F	41±2	5.7±0.9		
[31]	BS: 12 M/36 F	39±11	3.9±3.8	0.01	FMD was not correlated with disease activity and with the presence or absence of vascular disease
	HC: 18 (sex matched)	Matched	6.6±2.7		
[32]	BS: 20 M/16 F	36±8	1.4±3.0	<0.001	FMD was correlated independently with homocysteine levels
	HC: 20 M/10 F	35±8	4.4±3.4		
[33]	BS: 41 M/9 F	39±9	10.41±3.85	<0.001	Reduction in FMD was more prominent among those with vascular involvement
	HC: 37 M/9 F	36±9	14.41±3.39		
[34]	BS: 40 M/25 F	38±9	11.4±6.3	0.001	FMD was similar between those with and without vascular involvement
	HC: 18 M/12 F	41±8	20.4±9.1		
[35]	BS (vascular): 8 M/7 F	38±12	16.3±6.8	0.608	FMD did not differ between BS patients with and without vascular involvement
	BS (nonvascular): 16 M/12 F	35±10	16.5±9.1		
	HC: 19 M/16 F	38±8	18.5±8.0		
[36]	BS: 24 M/4 F	31±7	15.7±2.4	0.001	FMD was impaired among BS patients with only mucocutaneous involvement
	HC: 24 M/5 F	30±6	21.4±6.4		

BS Behçet's syndrome, *HC* healthy controls

artery in a group of BS patients and controls with similar atherosclerotic risk factors [41]. The study confirmed once again the presence of arterial stiffness in BS. Both studies suggested that aortic stiffness could contribute to LV diastolic dysfunction [40, 41].

The same authors showed in a subsequent study that patients with active disease have decreased pressure wave reflections [42]. This finding was independent of the atherosclerotic risk factors and aortic function [42]. The same group also looked at the effect of corticosteroid therapy on arterial stiffness in a cross-sectional study [43]. They found that arterial stiffness was somewhat diminished in patients who were treated with steroids compared to those who were not, implying again that control of inflammation improves ECD [43]. Contrary to these findings, Kurum et al. measured PWV in a relatively small number of patients and controls and could not find an increase [44].

Atherosclerosis in Behçet's Syndrome

Atherosclerosis is strongly associated with chronic inflammatory diseases such as RA and SLE [45–48]. Inflammation itself plays a pivotal role in the development of atherosclerosis [49–51]. There are also studies showing evidence for subclinical atherosclerosis in vasculitides such as Takayasu arteritis [52], and in various forms of systemic necrotizing vasculitis [53, 54]. We discuss here data on the prevalence of cardiovascular diseases and atherosclerosis in BS.

Cardiovascular Diseases and Its Associated Mortality

There is no evidence that clinical cardiovascular disease or its associated mortality is increased in BS. We had observed 42 deaths (11%) among a cohort of 387 BS patients during a follow-up of 20 years [55]. Standardized mortality ratios (SMRs) were specifically increased among young males and the causes of death were due to mainly BS or its associated morbidities (30/42; 71%), such as large vessel disease (17/42; 40%), neurological involvement (5/42; 12%), amyloidosis with chronic renal disease (4/42; 10%). There were also neoplasms (4/42; 10%). However, cardiovascular complications such as ischemic heart disease (IHD) or congestive heart failure were the main cause of death in only five patients (12%). Furthermore, the majority of deaths occurred during the early years of the disease and the SMRs tended to decrease with time [55]. An increase in the mortality rate late in the course indicating mainly atherosclerotic cardiovascular disease mortality as reported for SLE was not observed [56]. More recently by the help of a questionnaire, we assessed the prevalence of angina and past history of IHD in 225 (141 M/84 F) patients with BS (mean age: 52 ± 8) and 117 (74 M/43 F) apparently healthy controls (mean age: 50 ± 5) [57]. Patients with BS were more likely to be older and hypertensive and less likely to smoke while the rest of the atherosclerotic risk factors were similar between patients and controls. The prevalence of angina and history of IHD were found to be similar between patients and controls even after adjustment for risk factors [57]. Furthermore, in an uncontrolled survey we found a relatively low number of patients with elevated coronary artery calcification [58]. With electron beam computed tomography we studied 24 males with BS and extensive and long-standing major vessel disease. The mean age was 37.8 ± 4.5; the majority were smokers (21/24; 88%), 42% (10/24) had hyperlipidemia and one had diabetes. Even under this worst case conditions only 3/24 (12.5%) had elevated coronary artery calcification scores. Considering historical evidence it was rather evident that one would expect considerably more coronary artery calcification if SLE patients with similar long standing and severe disease had been studied [59, 60].

Cardiac Involvement and Cardiac Functions in BS

Cardiac involvement due to BS is rare [55, 61–65] and has mainly been mentioned in sporadic case reports [66–77]. It appears in the form of valvular heart disease, endomyocardial involvement or coronary artery vasculitis. Valvular heart disease mostly involves aortic valve with or without aortitis and is relatively frequent in the Far East [77]. Endomyocardial involvement manifests itself as endomyocardial fibrosis or mural thrombi in the right heart [74–77]. Histopathologic examinations of valvular, aortic, and endomyocardial lesions show mixed acute and chronic inflammation at various stages and fibrosis [77]. Importantly, atherosclerotic changes are absent. Coronary artery vasculitis in the form of aneurysms or occlusion may lead to myocardial infarction or rupture of the aneurysm [66–73]. Characteristically, patients in these case reports have been young and lesions in the coronary angiographies were compatible with vasculitis rather than atherosclerotic plaques [66–73]. Furthermore, a review of 170 (122 M/48 F) autopsies of patients with BS, revealed that cardiomegaly was the most common cardiac abnormality observed ($n = 12$), followed by coronary arteritis or thrombosis ($n = 6$), endocarditis ($n = 4$), pericardial effusion ($n = 4$), myocardial fibrosis ($n = 2$), and aortic valve disease [78]. While arterial changes suggestive of vasculitis such as aneurysms, thrombosis, arteritis, and stenosis have been observed in 50 (29%) cases, atherosclerotic arterial lesions have been present in only 7 (4%) [78].

We and others had previously studied cardiac functions in patients with BS by echocardiography and found no significant differences when compared to those observed among healthy controls [37, 79–81].

On the other hand, there are reports of left ventricular diastolic dysfunction in patients with BS suggesting myocardial small vessel disease as an early sign of cardiac involvement [40, 41, 82–84]. Myocardial thallium scintigraphy studies showing increased frequency of silent myocardial ischemia with intact coronary arteries by angiography coupled by work showing low coronary flow reserve again suggest disturbances in the microcirculatory system due to vasculitis rather than coronary atherosclerosis [85–87].

Subclinical Atherosclerosis

A number of studies assessed subclinical atherosclerosis in BS using carotid artery ultrasonography [31, 33, 35, 39, 88–91]. As shown in Table 8.2, results are somewhat conflicting with respect to intima-media thickness (IMT) and the presence of atherosclerotic plaques. In a recent study, we evaluated the presence of carotid and femoral artery atherosclerosis in a sizeable group ($n=239$) with BS both with severe ($n=167$) and mild disease ($n=72$) along with controls such as patients with RA ($n=100$), ankylosing spondylitis (AS) ($n=74$), and healthy controls ($n=156$) [92]. We found that subclinical atherosclerosis occurred with similar frequency in patients with BS, AS, and healthy controls, in both males and females. Moreover, frequency of atherosclerotic plaques and IMT of carotid and femoral artery were similar between patients with intensive organ involvement and mild disease. In this large study population, only male patients with RA were found to have significantly increased frequency of carotid artery plaques after adjustment for age and other atherosclerotic risk factors [92]. Similar to our results, three studies found no statistically significant increase in carotid-IMT (C-IMT) among BS patients when compared to healthy controls [31, 35, 90]. In five others, BS patients were found to have increased C-IMT [33, 39, 88, 89, 91] while an increased prevalence of carotid artery plaques were noted in two studies [88, 89]. In one of these two, the frequency of patients with carotid artery plaques was found to be significantly higher among patients with BS, than in healthy controls, but significantly lower than that found among patients with SLE [88].

Evidence for increased frequency of carotid artery plaques (positive in two of nine studies) and increased IMT (present in five of nine studies) are not so strong [31, 33, 35, 39, 88–92]. In this setting, we have to remind ourselves that the presence of carotid artery plaques rather than increased IMT is a more reliable predictor of atherosclerosis. The role of IMT as a marker of atherosclerosis is questioned [93–97]. It has been also reported that carotid IMT could be reduced with intensive anti-TNF treatment in patients with RA, suggesting a close and perhaps reversible association between IMT and inflammation as seen in endothelial dysfunction [98, 99].

Lipid Abnormalities in BS

We and others could not find significant difference in serum lipid concentrations between BS patients and healthy controls [57, 92]. However, there are studies in which increased levels of cholesterol or triglycerides were described [100, 101]. Increased lipid peroxidation [101–106], serum lipoprotein [107–110] and anti-oxLDL antibody levels were also reported [111]. Lipid peroxidation and lipoprotein levels were found to be increased in the active compared to that found in the inactive disease periods [102, 103, 105, 109]. Observed increases in lipid and lipoproteins levels, susceptibility of LDL to oxidation, auto-antibodies against oxLDL may indicate a tendency toward atherosclerosis. Whether these changes are secondary to inflammation or whether they are true precursors of atherosclerosis are open to debate.

Table 8.2 Studies investigating carotid artery atherosclerosis in BS

References	n	Age	C-IMT (mm±sd)		P value	C-Plaques		P value	Comment
[31]	BS: 12 M/36 F HC: 18 (sex matched)	39±11 Matched	0.59±0.11 0.55±0.09		NS	Not investigated		–	C-IMT was not correlated with disease activity and vascular disease
[33]	BS: 41 M/9 F HC: 37 M/9 F	39±9 36±9	0.69±0.15 0.55±0.14		0.001	Not investigated		–	Higher IMT in vascular involvement
[35]	BS (vascular): 8 M/7 F BS (nonvascular): 16 M/12 F HC: 19 M/16 F	38±12 35±10 38±8	0.52±0.14 0.51±0.09 0.46±0.09		NS	Not investigated		–	IMT did not differ between those patients with vascular involvement and those without.
[39]	BS: 19 M/21 F HC: 25 M/15 F	39±8 40±9	0.81±0.12 0.59±0.12		<0.05	4/40 2/40		NS	Higher IMT in vascular involvement;
[88]	BS: 68 M/46 F SLE: 6 M/40 F HC: 46 M/31 F	38±9 41±10 37±8	0.55±0.14 0.66±0.24 0.48±0.09		<0.01	5/114 8/46 0/77		0.08 0.0002	Subgroups of BS were not different. C-IMT was only correlated with age.
[89]	BS: 21 M/13 F HC: 21 M/13 F	35±9 35±9	0.81±0.17 0.54±0.13		<0.001	6/34 0/34		<0.05	No correlation of IMT with disease activity or other risk factors.
[90]	BS: 20 M/21 F HC: 26 M/27 F	38±8 37±7	0.52±0.09 0.52±0.06		NS	0/41 0/53		–	IMT was similar between patients and controls.
[91]	BS: 24 M/16 F HC: 13 M/7 F	39±9 40±5	0.71±0.22 0.59±0.09		<0.01	1/40 0/20		–	Carotid IMT in the patients with eye disease was higher than those without.
[92]	BS: 162 M/77 F RA: 24 M/76 F AS: 58 M/16 F HC: 83 M/73 F	41±7 45±7[a] 39±7 39±7	**Males** 0.73±0.09 0.81±0.20 0.69±0.10 0.71±0.10	**Females** 0.68±0.09 0.70±0.12 0.66±0.07 0.65±0.06	Males: 0.000[a] Females: 0.023[a]	**Males** 31/162 11/24 9/58 10/83	**Females** 14/77 16/76 1/16 5/73	Males: 0.002[a] Females: 0.055	

BS Behçet's syndrome, *C-IMT* carotid artery intima-media thickness, *HC* healthy controls, *RA* rheumatoid arthritis, *AS* ankylosing spondylitis, *NS* not significant

[a]Only patients with RA were significantly different

Why Is Atherosclerosis Not Overtly Accelerated in BS?

The presence of endothelial dysfunction, arterial stiffness, and lipid peroxidation abnormalities are all in favor of atherosclerosis. However, data from clinical studies together with weak evidence for carotid atherosclerosis are against this contention and suggest that atherosclerosis is not accelerated in BS. There may be several reasons including (a) the episodic nature of the inflammation with usually modest elevations of inflammatory indices [112]; (b) the general tendency for the disease activity to decrease with the passage of time in many patients [55]; (c) the more disease burden on the venous, rather than the arterial side and finally (d) perhaps the fact that BS is not a true to form autoimmune disease [113].

References

1. Vogel RA (2001) Measurement of endothelial function by brachial artery flow-mediated vasodilation. Am J Cardiol 88(2):31E–34E
2. Poredos P (2001) Endothelial dysfunction in the pathogenesis of atherosclerosis. Clin Appl Thromb Hemost 7:276–280
3. Bijl M (2003) Endothelial activation, endothelial dysfunction and premature atherosclerosis in systemic autoimmune diseases. Neth J Med 61:273–277
4. Endemann DH, Schiffrin EL (2004) Endothelial dysfunction. J Am Soc Nephrol 15:1983–1992
5. Kasprzak JD, Kłosińska M, Drozdz J (2006) Clinical aspects of assessment of endothelial function. Pharmacol Rep 58(Suppl):33–40
6. Giannotti G, Landmesser U (2007) Endothelial dysfunction as an early sign of atherosclerosis. Herz 32:568–572
7. Al-Qaisi M, Kharbanda RK, Mittal TK, Donald AE (2008) Measurement of endothelial function and its clinical utility for cardiovascular risk. Vasc Health Risk Manag 4:647–652
8. Deanfield JE, Halcox JP, Rabelink TJ (2007) Endothelial function and dysfunction: testing and clinical relevance. Circulation 115:1285–1295
9. Celermajer DS, Sorensen KE, Gooch VM et al (1992) Non-invasive detection of endothelial dysfunction in children and adults at risk of atherosclerosis. Lancet 340:1111–1115
10. Oliver JJ, Webb DJ (2003) Noninvasive assessment of arterial stiffness and risk of atherosclerotic events. Arterioscler Thromb Vasc Biol 23:554–566
11. Duprez DA, Cohn JN (2007) Arterial stiffness as a risk factor for coronary atherosclerosis. Curr Atheroscler Rep 9:139–144
12. Ganz P, Vita JA (2003) Testing endothelial vasomotor function: nitric oxide, a multipotent molecule. Circulation 108:2049–2053
13. Gokce N, Keaney JF Jr, Hunter LM et al (2002) Risk stratification for postoperative cardiovascular events via noninvasive assessment of endothelial function: a prospective study. Circulation 105:1567–1572
14. Neunteufl T, Katzenschlager R, Hassan A et al (1997) Systemic endothelial dysfunction is related to the extent and severity of coronary artery disease. Atherosclerosis 129:111–118
15. Bacon PA (2005) Endothelial cell dysfunction in systemic vasculitis: new developments and therapeutic prospects. Curr Opin Rheumatol 17:49–55
16. Amar S, Gokce N, Morgan S, Loukideli M, Van Dyke TE, Vita JA (2003) Periodontal disease is associated with brachial artery endothelial dysfunction and systemic inflammation. Arterioscler Thromb Vasc Biol 23:1245–1249

17. Tonetti MS, D'Aiuto F, Nibali L et al (2007) Treatment of periodontitis and endothelial function. N Engl J Med 356:911–920
18. Hingorani AD, Cross J, Kharbanda RK et al (2000) Acute systemic inflammation impairs endothelium-dependent dilatation in humans. Circulation 102:994–999
19. Charakida M, Donald AE, Green H et al (2005) Early structural and functional changes of the vasculature in HIV-infected children: impact of disease and antiretroviral therapy. Circulation 112:103–109
20. Charakida M, Donald AE, Terese M et al (2005) ALSPAC (Avon Longitudinal Study of Parents and Children) Study Team. Endothelial dysfunction in childhood infection. Circulation 111:1660–1665
21. Piper MK, Raza K, Nuttall SL et al (2007) Impaired endothelial function in systemic lupus erythematosus. Lupus 16:84–88
22. Gonzalez-Gay MA, Gonzalez-Juanatey C, Vazquez-Rodriguez TR, Martin J, Llorca J (2008) Endothelial dysfunction, carotid intima-media thickness, and accelerated atherosclerosis in rheumatoid arthritis. Semin Arthritis Rheum 38:67–70
23. Filer AD, Gardner-Medwin JM, Thambyrajah J et al (2003) Diffuse endothelial dysfunction is common to ANCA associated systemic vasculitis and polyarteritis nodosa. Ann Rheum Dis 62:162–167
24. Booth AD, Wallace S, McEniery CM et al (2004) Inflammation and arterial stiffness in systemic vasculitis: a model of vascular inflammation. Arthritis Rheum 50:581–588
25. Gonzalez-Juanatey C, Llorca J, Vazquez-Rodriguez TR, Diaz-Varela N, Garcia-Quiroga H, Gonzalez-Gay MA (2008) Short-term improvement of endothelial function in rituximab-treated rheumatoid arthritis patients refractory to tumor necrosis factor alpha blocker therapy. Arthritis Rheum 59:1821–1824
26. Gonzalez-Juanatey C, Llorca J, Garcia-Porrua C, Sanchez-Andrade A, Martín J, Gonzalez-Gay MA (2006) Steroid therapy improves endothelial function in patients with biopsy-proven giant cell arteritis. J Rheumatol 33:74–78
27. Booth AD, Jayne DR, Kharbanda RK et al (2004) Infliximab improves endothelial dysfunction in systemic vasculitis: a model of vascular inflammation. Circulation 109(14):1718–1723
28. Raza K, Carruthers DM, Stevens R, Filer AD, Townend JN, Bacon PA (2006) Infliximab leads to a rapid but transient improvement in endothelial function in patients with primary systemic vasculitis. Ann Rheum Dis 65:946–948
29. Raza K, Thambyrajah J, Townend JN et al (2000) Suppression of inflammation in primary systemic vasculitis restores vascular endothelial function: lessons for atherosclerotic disease? Circulation 102:1470–1472
30. Chambers JC, Haskard DO, Kooner JS (2001) Vascular endothelial function and oxidative stress mechanisms in patients with Behçet's syndrome. J Am Coll Cardiol 37:517–520
31. Protogerou A, Lekakis J, Stamatelopoulos K et al (2003) Arterial wall characteristics in patients with Adamantiades-Behçet's disease. Adv Exp Med Biol 528:399–404
32. Ozdemir R, Barutcu I, Sezgin AT et al (2004) Vascular endothelial function and plasma homocysteine levels in Behçet's disease. Am J Cardiol 94:522–525
33. Oflaz H, Mercanoglu F, Karaman O et al (2005) Impaired endothelium-dependent flow-mediated dilation in Behçet's disease: more prominent endothelial dysfunction in patients with vascular involvement. Int J Clin Pract 59:777–781
34. Kayikcioglu M, Aksu K, Hasdemir C et al (2006) Endothelial functions in Behçet's disease. Rheumatol Int 26:304–308
35. Caliskan M, Gullu H, Yilmaz S et al (2008) Cardiovascular prognostic value of vascular involvement in Behçet's disease. Int J Cardiol 125:428–430
36. Ulusoy RE, Karabudak O, Kilicaslan F, Kirilmaz A, Us MH, Cebeci BS (2008) Noninvasive assessment of impaired endothelial dysfunction in mucocutaneous Behçet's disease. Rheumatol Int 28:617–621
37. Caliskan M, Yilmaz S, Yildirim E et al (2007) Endothelial functions are more severely impaired during active disease period in patients with Behçet's disease. Clin Rheumatol 26:1074–1078

38. Protogerou AD, Sfikakis PP, Stamatelopoulos KS et al (2007) Interrelated modulation of endothelial function in Behçet's disease by clinical activity and corticosteroid treatment. Arthritis Res Ther 9(5):R90
39. Alan S, Ulgen MS, Akdeniz S, Alan B, Toprak N (2004) Intima-media thickness and arterial distensibility in Behçet's disease. Angiology 55:413–419
40. Ikonomidis I, Lekakis J, Stamatelopoulos K, Markomihelakis N, Kaklamanis PG, Mavrikakis M (2004) Aortic elastic properties and left ventricular diastolic function in patients with Adamantiades-Behçet's disease. J Am Coll Cardiol 43:1075–1081
41. Ikonomidis I, Aznaouridis K, Protogerou A et al (2006) Arterial wave reflections are associated with left ventricular diastolic dysfunction in Adamantiades-Behçet's disease. J Card Fail 12:458–463
42. Protogerou AD, Achimastos A, Vlachopoulos C et al (2008) Reduced pressure wave reflections in patients with active clinical status of Adamantiades-Behçet's disease. Hellenic J Cardiol 49:408–414
43. Protogerou AD, Lekakis J, Ikonomidis I et al (2006) Pressure wave reflections, central blood pressure, and aortic stiffness in patients with Adamantiades-Behçet's disease: a cross-sectional case-control study underlining the role of chronic corticosteroid treatment. Am J Hypertens 19:660–666
44. Kurum T, Yildiz M, Soy M, Ozbay G, Alimgil L (2005) Tuzun B Arterial distensibility as determined by carotid-femoral pulse wave velocity in patients with Behçet's disease. Clin Rheumatol 24:134–138
45. Bacon PA, Stevens RJ, Carruthers DM, Young SP, Kitas GD (2002) Accelerated atherogenesis in autoimmune rheumatic diseases. Autoimmun Rev 1:338–347
46. Van Doornum S, McColl G, Wicks IP (2002) Accelerated atherosclerosis: an extraarticular feature of rheumatoid arthritis? Arthritis Rheum 46:862–873
47. Shoenfeld Y, Gerli R, Doria A et al (2005) Accelerated atherosclerosis in autoimmune rheumatic diseases. Circulation 112:3337–3347
48. Manzi S, Meilahn EN, Rairie JE et al (1997) Age-specific incidence rates of myocardial infarction and angina in women with systemic lupus erythematosus: comparison with the Framingham Study. Am J Epidemiol 145:408–415
49. van der Wal AC, Becker AE, van der Loos CM, Das PK (1994) Site of intimal rupture or erosion of thrombosed coronary atherosclerotic plaques is characterized by an inflammatory process irrespective of the dominant plaque morphology. Circulation 89:36–44
50. van der Wal AC, Das PK, Tigges AJ, Becker AE (1992) Adhesion molecules on the endothelium and mononuclear cells in human atherosclerotic lesions. Am J Pathol 141:1427–1433
51. Libby P, Ridker PM (2004) Inflammation and atherosclerosis: role of C-reactive protein in risk assessment. Am J Med 116(Suppl 6A):9S–16S
52. Seyahi E, Ugurlu S, Cumali R et al (2006) Atherosclerosis in Takayasu arteritis. Ann Rheum Dis 65:1202–1207
53. de Leeuw K, Sanders JS, Stegeman C, Smit A, Kallenberg CG, Bijl M (2005) Accelerated atherosclerosis in patients with Wegener's granulomatosis. Ann Rheum Dis 64:753–759
54. Cohen Tervaert JW (2009) Translational mini-review series on immunology of vascular disease: accelerated atherosclerosis in vasculitis. Clin Exp Immunol 156:377–385
55. Kural-Seyahi E, Fresko I, Seyahi N et al (2003) The long-term mortality and morbidity of Behçet's syndrome: a 2-decade outcome survey of 387 patients followed at a dedicated center. Medicine (Baltimore) 82:60–76
56. Urowitz MB, Bookman AA, Koehler BE, Gordon DA, Smythe HA, Ogryzlo MA (1976) The bimodal mortality pattern of systemic lupus erythematosus. Am J Med 60:221–225
57. Ugurlu S, Seyahi E, Yazici H (2008) Prevalence of angina, myocardial infarction and intermittent claudication assessed by Rose Questionnaire among patients with Behçet's syndrome. Rheumatology (Oxford) 47:472–475
58. Seyahi E, Memisoglu E, Hamuryudan V et al (2004) Coronary atherosclerosis in Behçet's syndrome: a pilot study using electron-beam computed tomography. Rheumatology (Oxford) 43:1448–1450

59. Manger K, Kusus M, Forster C et al (2003) Factors associated with coronary artery calcification in young female patients with SLE. Ann Rheum Dis 62:846–850
60. Chung CP, Oeser A, Avalos I, Raggi P, Stein CM (2006) Cardiovascular risk scores and the presence of subclinical coronary artery atherosclerosis in women with systemic lupus erythematosus. Lupus 15:562–569
61. Mishima Y, Ishikawa K, Ueno A (1973) Arterial involvement in Behçet's disease. Jpn J Surg 3:52–60
62. Chajek T, Fainaru M (1975) Behçet's disease. Report of 41 cases and a review of the literature. Medicine (Baltimore) 54:179–196
63. Shimizu T, Ehrlich GE, Inaba G, Hayashi K (1979) Behçet's disease (Behçet's syndrome). Semin Arthritis Rheum 8:223–260
64. Koc Y, Gullu I, Akpek G et al (1992) Vascular involvement in Behçet's disease. J Rheumatol 19:402–410
65. Kaklamani VG, Vaiopoulos G, Kaklamanis PG (1998) Behçet's disease. Semin Arthritis Rheum 27:197–217
66. Kaseda S, Koiwaya Y, Tajimi T et al (1982) Huge false aneurysm due to rupture of the right coronary artery in Behçet's syndrome. Am Heart J 103(4 Pt 1):569–571
67. Siepmann M, Kirch W (1997) Coronary anomaly in Behçet's syndrome. Rheumatol Int 17:39–42
68. Ipek G, Omeroglu SN, Mansuroglu D, Kirali K, Uzun K, Sismanoglu M (2001) Coronary artery bypass grafting in a 26-year-old man with total occlusion of the left main coronary artery related to Behçet's disease. J Thorac Cardiovasc Surg 122:1247–1249
69. Cevik C, Otahbachi M, Nugent K, Jenkins LA (2009) Coronary artery aneurysms in Behçet's disease. Cardiovasc Revasc Med 10:128–129
70. Jin SJ, Mun HS, Chung SJ, Park MC, Kwon HM, Hong YS (2008) Acute myocardial infarction due to sinus of Valsalva aneurysm in a patient with Behçet's disease. Clin Exp Rheumatol 26(4 Suppl 50):S117–S120
71. Porcu P, Chavanon O, Bertrand B et al (2008) Giant aneurysm of the proximal segment of the left anterior descending artery in a patient with Behçet's disease – a combined approach. Can J Cardiol 24:e73–e74
72. Lee S, Lee CY, Yoo KJ (2007) Acute myocardial infarction due to an unruptured sinus of Valsalva aneurysm in a patient with Behçet's syndrome. Yonsei Med J 48:883–885
73. Cuisset T, Quilici J, Bonnet JL (2007) Giant coronary artery aneurysm in Behçet's disease. Heart 93:1375
74. Huong DL, Wechsler B, Papo T et al (1997) Endomyocardial fibrosis in Behçet's disease. Ann Rheum Dis 56:205–208
75. Aouba A, Nebie L, Fabiani JN, Bruneval P, Patri B, De Bandt M (2004) Tricuspid aseptic endocarditis revealing right endomyocardial fibrosis during an unrecognized Behçet's disease. A case report. Presse Med 33(19 Pt 2):1367–1369
76. McDonald GS, Gad-Al-Rab J (1980) Behçet's disease with endocarditis and the Budd-Chiari syndrome. J Clin Pathol 33:660–669
77. Lee I, Park S, Hwang I, Kim MJ, Nah SS, Yoo B, Song JK (2008) Cardiac Behçet's disease presenting as aortic valvulitis/aortitis or right heart inflammatory mass: a clinicopathologic study of 12 cases. Am J Surg Pathol 32:390–398
78. Lakhanpal S, Tani K, Lie JT, Katoh K, Ishigatsubo Y, Ohokubo T (1985) Pathologic features of Behçet's syndrome: a review of Japanese autopsy registry data. Hum Pathol 16:790–795
79. Ozkan M, Emel O, Ozdemir M et al (1992) M-mode, 2-D and Doppler echocardiographic study in 65 patients with Behçet's syndrome. Eur Heart J 13:638–641
80. Tunc SE, Dogan A, Gedikli O, Arslan C, Sahin M (2005) Assessment of aortic stiffness and ventricular diastolic functions in patients with Behçet's disease. Rheumatol Int 25:447–451
81. Bozkurt A, Akpinar O, Uzun S, Akman A, Arslan D, Birand A (2006) Echocardiographic findings in patients with Behçet's disease. Am J Cardiol 97:710–715
82. Calguneri M, Erbas B, Kes S, Karaaslan Y (1993) Alterations in left ventricular function in patients with Behçet's disease using radionuclide ventriculography and Doppler echocardiography. Cardiology 82:309–316

83. Komsuoglu B, Goldeli O, Kulan K et al (1994) Doppler evaluation of left ventricular diastolic filling in Behçet's disease. Int J Cardiol 47:145–150

84. Gemici K, Baran I, Gullulu S, Kazazoglu AR, Cordan J, Ozer Z (2000) Evaluation of diastolic dysfunction and repolarization dispersion in Behçet's disease. Int J Cardiol 73:143–148

85. Gullu IH, Benekli M, Muderrisoglu H et al (1996) Silent myocardial ischemia in Behçet's disease. J Rheumatol 23:323–327

86. Turkolmez S, Gokcora N, Alkan M, Gorer MA (2005) Evaluation of myocardial perfusion in patients with Behçet's disease. Ann Nucl Med 19:201–206

87. Gullu H, Caliskan M, Erdogan D et al (2007) Patients with Behçet's disease carry a higher risk for microvascular involvement in active disease period. Ann Med 39:154–159

88. Keser G, Aksu K, Tamsel S et al (2005) Increased thickness of the carotid artery intima-media assessed by ultrasonography in Behçet's disease. Clin Exp Rheumatol 23(4 Suppl 38):S71–S76

89. Ozturk MA, Oktar SO, Unverdi S et al (2006) Morphologic evidence of subclinical atherosclerosis obtained by carotid ultrasonography in patients with Behçet's disease. Rheumatol Int 26:867–872

90. Rhee MY, Chang HK, Kim SK (2007) Intima-media thickness and arterial stiffness of carotid artery in Korean patients with Behçet's disease. J Korean Med Sci 22:387–392

91. Hong SN, Park JC, Yoon NS et al (2008) Carotid artery intima-media thickness in Behçet's disease patients without significant cardiovascular involvement. Korean J Intern Med 23:87–93

92. Seyahi E, Ugurlu S, Cumali R et al (2008) Atherosclerosis in Behçet's Syndrome. Semin Arthritis Rheum 38:1–12

93. Belcaro G, Nicolaides AN, Laurora G et al (1996) Ultrasound morphology classification of the arterial wall and cardiovascular events in a 6-year follow-up study. Arterioscler Thromb Vasc Biol 16:851–856

94. Ebrahim S, Papacosta O, Whincup P et al (1999) Carotid plaque, intima media thickness, cardiovascular risk factors, and prevalent cardiovascular disease in men and women: the British Regional Heart Study. Stroke 30:841–850

95. Adams MR, Nakagomi A, Keech A et al (1995) Carotid intima-media thickness is only weakly correlated with the extent and severity of coronary artery disease. Circulation 92:2127–2134

96. del Sol AI, Moons KG, Hollander M et al (2001) Is carotid intima-media thickness useful in cardiovascular disease risk assessment? The Rotterdam Study. Stroke 32:1532–1538

97. Johnsen SH, Mathiesen EB (2009) Carotid plaque compared with intima-media thickness as a predictor of coronary and cerebrovascular disease. Curr Cardiol Rep 11:21–27

98. Del Porto F, Lagana B, Lai S et al (2007) Response to anti-tumour necrosis factor alpha blockade is associated with reduction of carotid intima-media thickness in patients with active rheumatoid arthritis. Rheumatology (Oxford) 46:1111–1115

99. Ferrante A, Giardina AR, Ciccia F, et al (2009) Long-term anti-tumour necrosis factor therapy reverses the progression of carotid intima-media thickness in female patients with active rheumatoid arthritis. Rheumatol Int [Epub ahead of print]

100. Leiba M, Seligsohn U, Sidi Y et al (2004) Thrombophilic factors are not the leading cause of thrombosis in Behçet's disease. Ann Rheum Dis 63:1445–1449

101. Orem A, Yandi YE, Vanizor B, Cimsit G, Uydu HA, Malkoc M (2002) The evaluation of autoantibodies against oxidatively modified low-density lipoprotein (LDL), susceptibility of LDL to oxidation, serum lipids and lipid hydroperoxide levels, total antioxidant status, antioxidant enzyme activities, and endothelial dysfunction in patients with Behçet's disease. Clin Biochem 35:217–224

102. Orem A, Efe H, Deger O, Cimsit G, Uydu HA, Vanizor B (1997) Relationship between lipid peroxidation and disease activity in patients with Behçet's disease. J Dermatol Sci 16:11–16

103. Karakucuk S, Baskol G, Oner AO, Baskol M, Mirza E, Ustdal M (2004) Serum paraoxonase activity is decreased in the active stage of Behçet's disease. Br J Ophthalmol 88:1256–1258

104. Mungan AG, Can M, Acikgöz S, Estürk E, Altinyazar C (2006) Lipid peroxidation and homocysteine levels in Behçet's disease. Clin Chem Lab Med 44:1115–1118

105. Sandikci R, Türkmen S, Güvenen G et al (2003) Lipid peroxidation and antioxidant defence system in patients with active or inactive Behçet's disease. Acta Derm Venereol 83:342–346
106. Köse K, Yazici C, Cambay N, Aşcioğlu O, Doğan P (2002) Lipid peroxidation and erythrocyte antioxidant enzymes in patients with Behçet's disease. Tohoku J Exp Med 197:9–16
107. Esmat S, El Sherif H, Anwar S, Fahmy I, Elmenyawi M, Shaker O (2006) Lipoprotein (a) and nitrites in Behçet's disease: relationship with disease activity and vascular complications. Eur J Dermatol 16:67–71
108. Musabak U, Baylan O, Cetin T et al (2005) Lipid profile and anticardiolipin antibodies in Behçet's disease. Arch Med Res 36:387–392
109. Gürbüz O, Ozdemir Y, Cosar CB, Kural G (2001) Lipoprotein (a) in Behçet's disease as an indicator of disease activity and in thrombotic complications. Eur J Ophthalmol 11:62–65
110. Orem A, Deger O, Memiş O, Caliskan K, Cimşit G (1994) High lipoprotein (a) levels as a thrombogenic risk factor in Behçet's disease. Ann Rheum Dis 53:351–352
111. Orem A, Cimsit G, Deger O, Vanizor B, Karahan SC (1999) Autoantibodies against oxidatively modified low-density lipoprotein in patients with Behçet's disease. Dermatology 198:243–246
112. Müftüoglu AU, Yazici H, Yurdakul S et al (1986) Behçet's disease. Relation of serum C-reactive protein and erythrocyte sedimentation rates to disease activity. Int J Dermatol 25:235–239
113. Yazici H (1997) The place of Behçet's syndrome among the autoimmune diseases. Int Rev Immunol 14:1–10

Chapter 9
Locomotor System Disease in Behçet's Syndrome

Sebahattin Yurdakul and Gülen Hatemi

Keywords Arthralgia • Arthritis • Azathioprine • Behçet's disease • Behçet's syndrome • Colchicine • Fibromyalgia • Joint involvement • Myositis • Osteonecrosis • Synovial fluid • Synovial histology

Hulusi Behçet described three patients with aphthous stomatitis, genital ulceration, and uveitis as well as erythema nodosum lesions in 1937 [1, 2]. One year after the original description, he also wrote about "rheumatoid pains" [3] and then expanded the clinical spectrum of the disease to other, now well-known features such as acneiform lesions, thrombophlebitis, myositis, and hemoptysis, all associated with acute exacerbations of the disease [4, 5].

This chapter will review the locomotor system involvement seen in Behçet's syndrome. Joint involvement is an essential part of Behçet's syndrome occurring in the form of either arthritis or arthralgia in half of the patients. Fibromyalgia can be an accompanying feature especially among the females. Generalized or localized myositis and osteonecrosis are quite infrequent.

Joint Involvement

The frequency of joint involvement can vary greatly depending upon where the patients were seen. As expected this was quite low, 9–12% in the reports from dermatology departments [6, 7] and rather high, up to 68–70% in those from rheumatology departments [8, 9]. The most quoted figure is around 50%, in the form of either arthritis or arthralgia [10–37].

S. Yurdakul (✉)
Department of Medicine, Division of Rheumatology, Cerrahpasa Medical Faculty, University of Istanbul, Turkey
e-mail: profsyurdakul@yahoo.com

Y. Yazıcı and H. Yazıcı (eds.), *Behçet's Syndrome*,
DOI 10.1007/978-1-4419-5641-5_9, © Springer Science+Business Media, LLC 2010

We observed that among 184 patients 71 (39%) had arthritis and 29 (16%) patients had arthralgia alone in our dedicated multidisciplinary weekly Behçet's syndrome outpatient clinic [38]. We had the opportunity to determine the characteristics of arthritis, such as the distribution, symmetry, and the number of the joints involved, and the duration of an arthritic episode in our prospective study. Among 71 patients, 47 (66%) had a total of 80 episodes of arthritis during a mean follow-up period of 19 ± 14 (SD) months [38]. The usual clinical course of Behçet's syndrome with recurrent and unpredictable episodes of exacerbation and remissions in the many organ systems involved is also true for joint involvement. Although oral and genital ulcers are the most frequently presenting symptoms, articular involvement may occur as the first symptom in 9–23% of patients [9, 17, 18, 25, 27, 30, 33, 34]. When joint manifestations antedate other features of Behçet's syndrome by months or years it is quite difficult to differentiate the clinical picture from other inflammatory arthritides. The involvement of wrists and elbows with a subacute or chronic course, and even in a symmetrical fashion may mimic seronegative rheumatoid arthritis (RA).

Affected joints are usually swollen and may be warm but redness of the overlying skin is unusual [12, 38] except when associated with erythema nodosum. In many series joint deformity was not observed even in patients with chronic arthritis [8–11, 14, 16–22, 38]. However, mild deformity in elbows and ankles has been reported in a small number of patients [26, 27, 35].

Joints Involved

Based on the arthritic episodes in our prospective study, the most commonly involved joints were knees, followed by ankles, wrists, elbows, and hands. The other joints such as hips and shoulders were less likely affected [38] (Fig. 9.1). While a similar pattern of joint involvement has been observed in the vast majority of the studies [10–35] shoulders were the main affected joints in a few reports [8, 9, 17, 31]. However, almost all these were retrospective studies, and the number and distribution of the joints involved per patient had not been reported except in one [26].

Some years ago there used to be a major controversy about whether sacroiliitis was part of Behçet's syndrome. While some authors had not reported any sacroiliitis [8, 17] one author had reported a high rate of both sacroiliitis (grade I–III sacroiliitis in 63%) and ankylosing spondylitis (20%) among 106 patients [18]. In 1974, Behçet's syndrome was classified along the seronegative spondylarthritides in the seminal Moll et al. paper [39]. However, in reports describing sacroiliitis there had been no blind reading or the inclusion of control groups. Later our group studied radiographic sacroiliitis in a blind protocol among 37 patients with Behçet's syndrome along with 28 age- and sex-matched healthy controls, and 4 patients with ankylosing spondylitis as positive controls [40]. In this study, we found no evidence of an increased frequency of sacroiliitis among the patients with Behçet's syndrome compared with healthy controls [41]. Subsequent reports were also confirmatory [41–44]. Furthermore, back pain is not a part of this syndrome.

Fig. 9.1 Distribution of the joints involved (Permission from the editor of the Annals of the Rheumatic Diseases [38])

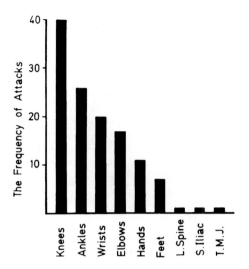

In addition to the methodological problems of presence of blind reading and the inclusion of healthy and diseased controls a further and important issue is the high observer variation in interpreting pelvis radiographs for sacroiliitis as we had reported some years ago [45]. Furthermore, when we recently looked at a group of Behçet's syndrome patients with acne, arthritis, and enthesopathy, the frequency of sacroiliitis was 20% in Behçet's syndrome patients with acne and arthritis, 7% in Behçet's syndrome patients without arthritis, 25% in RA, and 100% in ankylosing spondylitis [46]. HLA B27 was positive in two of these Behçet's syndrome patients with sacroiliitis. Finally it is worth remembering, as we have just pointed out that the frequency of sacroiliitis is also increased among RA patients as well – in fact one study reports a figure as high as 33% [47] – and one would hardly include RA among the seronegative spondylarthritides. Table 9.1 summarizes the clinical differences of Behçet's syndrome from seronegative spondylarthritides.

Enthesopathy

There are conflicting reports regarding the frequency of enthesopathy in Behçet's syndrome. This might be due to the different methods of evaluation and different patient populations studied. Hamza et al. showed enthesopathy by physical examination and radiography in 5 among 174 patients [48]. In Caporn et al. series five among fourteen (36%) patients had enthesopathy [19]. Chang et al. in physical examination, reported 2 patients with enthesitis among 58 patients with Behçet's syndrome [43]. In another study, bony spurs were detected in 3 of 59 patients [9]. A survey revealed 1 patient with tendinitis among 65 patients [49]. Finally, among

Table 9.1 Differences
between Behçet's syndrome
and seronegative spondylarthritides (SNSA)

Behçet's syndrome
Systemic vasculitis
Back pain rare
Sacroiliitis not increased
No familial association with the diseases of SNSA
Close association with HLA B5 (51)
"Shared" clinical signs in Behçet's syndrome (BS) different from SNSA:
Genital ulceration usually scrotal
Urogenital infection absent
Nail changes not present
Different pattern of eye involvement

the 47 Behçet's syndrome patients with arthritis, we had reported 2 patients had Achilles tendinitis and 1 had calcaneal erosions [38].

We had previously proposed the presence of clusters of disease expression of Behçet's syndrome [50]. Acne and arthritis was one of these distinct clusters [51]. We went on to test the hypothesis that enthesopathy was specifically increased in this cluster. We studied 35 Behçet's syndrome patients with acne and arthritis, 38 Behçet's syndrome patients without arthritis, 37 patients with ankylosing spondylitis, 25 with RA and 25 healthy controls by ultrasonograhy [52]. On physical examination 69% of Behçet's syndrome patients with acne and arthritis had tender/painful enthesis and 17% had swollen enthesis while these frequencies were 54 and 16% for ankylosing spondylitis patients, and 48 and 16% for RA patients. The frequency of tender/painful enthesis was 26% among Behçet's syndrome patients without arthritis and 12% in healthy controls while none of the patients in these two groups had swollen enthesis. On ultrasonographic examination ankylosing spondylitis patients had the highest enthesopathy score followed by Behçet's syndrome patients with acne and arthritis while the mean enthesopathy scores among the remaining three groups were similar. Power Doppler score was highest among Behçet's syndrome patients with acne and arthritis followed by ankylosing spondylitis, RA, Behçet's syndrome patients without arthritis and healthy controls [52]. This association of enthesopathy with acne and arthritis supports the contention that one of the pathogenetic mechanisms underlying Behçet's syndrome may be similar to that of acne-associated reactive arthritis.

Number of Joints Involved

In our series (38) the arthritis was monoarticular in 54 of the 80 attacks (68%) among our 47 patients during the follow-up (Fig. 9.2). In the remainder the mean number of joints involved per patient was 3. The maximum number of joints involved during an attack was five, occurring in only two patients [38]. Similarly,

Fig. 9.2 Number of joints
involved during an attack
(Permission from the editor of
the Annals of the Rheumatic
Diseases [38])

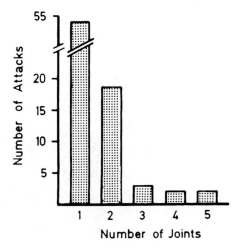

63%, 58/92 attacks were also reported as monoarticular by Calguneri et al. [26]. Monoarthritis was also usually the most frequent involvement in some reports [23, 27, 28, 36] while oligoarthritis [9, 19, 21, 22, 24, 25, 30, 33, 35] and polyarthritis were reported by others [8, 11, 14, 15, 18, 29].

Symmetry

Joint involvement was usually symmetrical when it was even oligoarticular or polyarticular in our experience [38] and in three other studies [8, 24, 29]. On the other hand, mainly asymmetrical involvement has been noted in some series [17, 26, 28, 35].

Duration

We analyzed the duration of 56 attacks of arthritis in 37 patients. Forty-six (82%) attacks lasted for 2 months or less although chronic arthritis lasting from several months to 4 years occurred in a few cases [38] (Fig. 9.3) as well as in others [9, 18, 21, 33]. Subacute or chronic course was usual in Mason and Barnes' patients [8] and in others [15, 27].

Morning Stiffness

Morning stiffness was mild, lasting up to a maximum of half an hour in 16/47 (34%) patients in our study [38]. Kim mentioned that it lasted more than 30 min,

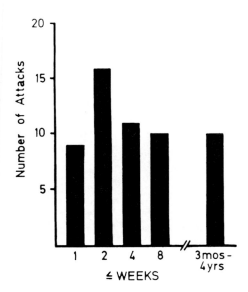

Fig. 9.3 Duration of the arthritic attacks (Permission from the editor of the Annals of the Rheumatic Diseases [38])

typical for RA in 60% of 59 patients [9]. Mason and Barnes described "significant" morning stiffness in 80% (15/19) of patients [8] and Mousa et al. mentioned arthralgia and morning stiffness in 17 patients [21], but both studies did not give any duration [8, 21]. However, Ek reported no morning stiffness among seven patients with arthritis [23].

Subcutaneous Nodules

Subcutaneous rheumatoid-like nodules are rare. Chamberlain reported two patients with Behçet's syndrome who had subcutaneous nodules [17]. However, one of these patients had concomitant seropositive RA and the other had only "possible" Behçet's disease. Histological examination of the nodules was not available in these patients [17]. We had also seen a definite Behçet patient with arthritis and a subcutaneous rheumatoid-like nodule at elbow [53]. Histology showed that polymorphonuclear cells predominated in the superficial areas and lymphocytes at the deep zones. There was granulation tissue rich in fibrin with inflammatory cells around the vessels. Abundant fibrin and fibrinoid was present especially at the surface of the nodule. This histology clearly differed from that of the classical rheumatoid nodule with its distinct zones and palisading. The histology in our patient was rather more like nodules seen in rheumatic fever.

Pseudothrombophlebitis (Baker's Cyst Rupture) and Pseudoseptic Arthritis

Knee synovitis may be associated with a synovial cyst in the popliteal fossa behind the knee (Baker's cyst) similar to what can be observed in other inflammatory arthritides. This cyst may rupture and cause tenderness, swelling, and a positive Homans' test in the calf, thus easily mimicking acute deep vein thrombophebitis (pseudothrombophlebitis) [15, 54, 55]. Ultrasonographic examination is helpful to differentiate one from the other.

A pseudoseptic arthritis has also been described with intense inflammation in the affected joint. In this instance synovial fluid leukocyte counts are very high. This condition may occur spontaneously, after joint aspiration or arthroscopic synovial biopsy of the knee suggesting a local pathergy response of the synovium [56–58].

Laboratory Findings

Acute phase reactants like erythrocyte sedimentation rate (ESR) and C-reactive protein are usually increased during the arthritis attacks [8, 9, 21, 26–28, 33–35, 38]. ESR was 30.8 ± 21.9 (SD) mm/h in patients with active arthritis, 18.7 ± 14.9 in remission while it was 18.7 ± 14.9 in patients without joint involvement [38]. In addition, in a prospective study of 150 patients, erythema nodosum, thrombophlebitis, and arthritis, in that order, were the manifestations of the disease most closely associated with ESR and C-reactive protein elevations [59], but these may not correlate with the severity of arthritic attacks [38, 59].

Rheumatoid factor and antinuclear antibodies are negative [8, 9, 22, 27, 33–35, 38] as well as anticyclic citrullinated peptide (antiCCP) antibodies [60].

We found that HLA B5 was more frequent among the patients with joint involvement (65/78, 83%) than among those without (43/67, 64%) ($x^2 = 5.99$, $p < 0.02$) and proposed that this was further evidence that joint involvement was an integral part of Behçet's syndrome [38].

Synovial Fluid

Synovial fluid was of inflammatory type with a predominance of polymorphonuclear leucocytes [9, 13, 15, 26, 38, 61]. However, a good mucin clot was formed in the majority (59%, 19/32) of the specimens [38]. Synovial glucose levels were within normal limits [26, 38]. Complement levels were usually elevated in synovial fluids and this differs from depressed levels that can be seen in RA. Complement blood levels are normal in Behçet's syndrome [15, 62] (Table 9.2).

Radiological Changes

Radiographical erosions of peripheral joints are infrequent, even in patients with chronic arthritis. Series with sizeable number of patients mention either no radiological changes [10, 11, 13, 15–17, 20–23, 33, 34] or some erosions in a few patients [8, 9, 11, 19, 25–27, 35, 38]. However, a Japanese study of hand radiographs in 20 patients with arthritis for more than 5 years showed juxta-articular demineralization in 11 patients, carpal rotation in 9, narrowing of the joint space in 3, and

Table 9.2 Synovial fluid in Behçet's syndrome[a]

White cell count: mm^3
  15,000 ± 10,000; 75% PMN (n = 32) [38]
  4,900 ± 3,400; 75% PMN (n = 18) [26]
Good mucin clot: 19/32, (59 %) specimens [38]
Glucose levels usually normal:
  Synovial fluid: 70.3 ± 34.5 mg/dl (n = 9)
  Simultaneous blood: 82.2 ± 30.5 mg/dl (n = 9) [38]
Complement levels usually elevated [62]

	CH50 (U/ml)	C3 (mg/dl)	C4 (mg/dl)
Behçet's syndrome (n = 17)	30.2 ± 6.9	76.1 ± 25.9	32.3 ± 15.1
Rheumatoid arthritis (n = 15)	11.5 ± 7.8	43.7 ± 32.4	14.6 ± 11.5

[a]PMN = Polymorphonuclear; mean ± SD

asymmetrical bone destruction in 2 [63]. Various types of erosions including a "pencil in cup" pattern have been reported at different joints in case reports [64–70]. One report mentions multiple and reversible osteolytic lesions as well [71].

Synovial Histology

The synovial histology shows a nonspecific synovitis. A wide range of changes including pannus formation with erosive changes have been reported.

Vernon-Roberts et al. studied eight specimens of synovial membrane from six patients [72]. Only the superficial zones of the synovium were affected and seven of eight specimens were replaced by dense inflamed granulation tissue composed of lymphocytes intermingled with macrophages, vascular elements, fibroblasts, and neutrophils. There was a marked plasma cell infiltrate and lymphoid follicle formation in one specimen only. Pannus and erosive changes were present in three specimens.

Gibson et al. compared the synovial tissue of seven patients with Behçet's syndrome and seven patients with early RA [73]. They could not distinguish any features between the two conditions either by ordinary light or electron microscopic examinations. However, immunofluorescent studies indicated consistent deposition of IgG in Behçet's syndrome. In another study, the histology in surgical specimens of synovial tissues from five affected joints of three patients was quite similar to what has previously been observed [72]. Furthermore, not only the superficial zone but also the deeper layer was affected by inflammatory changes and with lymphoid cells. One patient had marked plasma cell infiltration and a lymphoid follicle formation like in RA [74].

We also observed the loss of the superficial cell layer of the synovium, which was replaced by inflammatory granulation tissue in half of 12 needle biopsy specimens. There was paucity of plasma cells, and in five instances lymphoid follicle formation was noted. There was no involvement of the deeper layers of synovium in our series [38].

Fibromyalgia

Our group investigated the frequency of fibromyalgia among 108 consecutive patients with Behçet's syndrome, 64 with RA, 54 systemic lupus erythematosus, and 50 age and sex-matched healthy controls [75]. One observer gave the questionnaire and the other one who was blinded to diagnoses examined their tender points as described originally in the 1990 ACR criteria for classification for fibromyalgia. Overall ten (9.2%) patients with Behçet's syndrome vs. one (2%) healthy controls fulfilled the fibromyalgia criteria. This overall higher frequency was statistically significant only among the females (9/56, 16.1% versus 1/40, 2.5%, $x^2 = 4.6$, $p = 0.042$) [75]. A similar study from Iraq showed that there were 53/90 (58.9%) patients with Behçet's syndrome with widespread pain compared with 6/40 (15%) healthy controls ($p < 0.001$). However, only eight (8.9%) (seven female and one male) patients with Behçet's syndrome vs. one healthy control (2.5%) had well-defined fibromyalgia ($x^2 = 1.75$, $p = $ NS) [76]. On the other hand, a Korean study also reported that patients with Behçet's syndrome indeed had significantly more frequent fibromyalgia compared to what was seen in both systemic lupus erythematosus patients, and in healthy controls (26/70, 37.1% vs. 14/90, 15.6%; $p = 0.003$, and vs. 2/100, 2%; $p < 0.001$, respectively). Furthermore, it was associated with the presence of anxiety and depression, and not with the disease activity [77].

Myositis

Myositis has been described in Behçet's syndrome but is rare. It may be local or generalized. There may be minimal to severe muscle weakness on physical examination and serum muscle enzymes may be elevated in the generalized form. The muscle both at biopsies and autopsy examination show typical changes of myositis with marked inflammatory cellular infiltration and muscle fiber changes, similar to what is seen in polymyositis or dermatomyositis [78–80]. Similar histologic changes have also been reported in patients with localized myositis. This is characterized by pain and swelling in affected region with and without elevation of serum muscle enzymes. Both children and adults can be affected [81–84].

In one study, despite normal findings in light microscopy, electron microscopy revealed alterations in the muscle of all seven patients, two with mild muscle weakness and five without neuromuscular symptoms and signs [85]. These alterations were capillary basement membrane thickening, varying degrees of myoflamenteous disarray and loss, aggregation of mitochondria and lysosomes in subsarcolemmal sites, central nucleation in areas lacking contractile material, and most strikingly the presence of cytoplasmic inclusions. As there were no control groups in the study the clinical significance of these findings remain unclear [85]. Neurogenic muscular atrophy has also been reported in a child with Behçet's syndrome [86].

Osteonecrosis

Osteonecrosis is a rare manifestation. Virtually no general series mention it [9–38] except one in which one patient developed osteonecrosis of both femoral and humeral heads among 29 patients [8]. Weight-bearing joints such as hips and knees are the most frequently affected and the observed osteonecrosis was usually attributed to large doses of systemic corticosteroids in case reports and small series [87–90]. In a retrospective chart review 14/4,150 (0.03%) patients had osteonecrosis. Similarly, the most common site was the hip, and all but one had been on corticosteroids [91]. Osteonecrosis and bone infarction in association with anticardiolipin antibodies were present in two Behçet's syndrome patients [88].

Functional Outcome Measures in Locomotor System Disease

Recently, various outcome measures have been developed for rheumatic diseases. These tools assess many component of the patient status such as pain, function, and mental well-being. Although there are limited number of studies they have revealed increased disability scores, mainly among patients with joint involvement. Quality of life (QoL) and life satisfaction (LS) assessments showed a poor QoL and diminished LS in 41 patients with Behçet's syndrome compared with 40 healthy controls assessed by the Nottingham Health Profile (NHP) and Life Satisfaction Index (LSI). Joint involvement was one of the important components related to decreased QoL and LS in Behçet's syndrome [92]. In another study, arthritis considerably affected levels of pain, QoL, and health status of the patients [35].

A recent comparative work from USA between 129 patients with Behçet's syndrome and 116 with early RA using the Multidimensional Health Assessment Questionnaire (MDHAQ) has shown similar results for pain and the physician global assessment of disease activity, but Behçet's syndrome patients reported significantly higher levels of functional disability, fatigue, and patient assessment of global disease activity [93]. Moreover, Behçet's syndrome patients with arthritis ($n = 68$) exhibited significantly higher functional disability scores, fatigue, and patient global values than the RA patients, while results for pain and the physician global assessment were similar. Furthermore, those patients with arthritis had significantly higher scores for function, pain, fatigue, and patient and physician global assessment compared to Behçet's syndrome patients without arthritis [93].

Treatment (See Also Chap. 19)

The arthritis of Behçet's syndrome is self-limited and can be usually managed with colchicine. Colchicine was beneficial for preventing the episodes of joint involvement in a double-blind, placebo-controlled study [94]. Although nonsteroidal anti-inflammatory drugs have used widely for arthritis our double-blind, placebo-controlled study with azapropazone was disappointing [95]. Azapropazone was not superior compared with placebo except for pain only at day 7 [95]. The efficacy of intra-articular corticosteroids has been equivocal in anecdotal reports.

Azathioprine is the treatment of choice in the patients with recurrent arthritis or resistant cases. Azathioprine 2.5 mg/kg/day were significantly effective for eye, mucocutaneous lesions as well as arthritis in a double-blind placebo-controlled study. Furthermore, at least 3 months is required for a beneficial response [96].

Benzathine penicillin in addition to colchicine suggests a beneficial effect for arthritis in an open study [97]. In an uncontrolled experience d-penicillamine did not result any effect in controlling the chronic arthritis of Behçet's syndrome [98].

Interferon α [99–101] and antiTNF-α drugs [102] may be tried in even more resistant patients but such cases are rare.

References

 1. Behçet H (1937) Über rezidivierende aphthöse, durch ein Virus verursachte Geschwüre am Mund, am Auge und an den Genitalien. Dermatol Monatsschr 105:1152–1157
 2. Behçet H (1937) Agız ve tenasül uzuvlarında husule gelen aftöz tegayyürlerle, ayni zamanda gözde görünen virütik olması muhtemel tesevvüsler üzerine mülahazalar, ve mihrakı intan hakkında süpheler. Deri Hastaliklari ve Frengi Arsivi 4:1369–1378, in Turkish
 3. Behçet H, Gözcü N (1938) Üc nahiyede nüksi tavazzular yapan, ve hususi bir virus tesirile umumi intan hasil ettigine kanaatimiz artan (Entite morbide) hakkinda. Deri Hastaliklari ve Frengi Arsivi 5:1863–1873, in Turkish
 4. Behçet H (1940) Some observations on the clinical picture of the so-called triple symptom complex. Dermatologica 81:73–83
 5. Behçet H (1942) Trisentomkompleks veya sendrom veyahut morbus Behçet nasil tespit edilmistir? Deri Hastaliklari ve Frengi Arsivi 9:2663–2673, in Turkish
 6. Haim S, Sherf K (1966) Behçet's disease: presentation of 11 cases and evaluation of treatment. Isr J Med 2:69–74
 7. Tursen U, Gurler A, Boyvat A (2003) Evaluation of clinical findings according to sex in 2313 Turkish patients with Behçet's disease. Int J Dermatol 42:346–351
 8. Mason RM, Barnes CG (1969) Behçet's syndrome with arthritis. Ann Rheum Dis 28:95–103
 9. Kim HA, Choi KW, Song YW (1997) Arthropathy in Behçet's disease. Scand J Rheumatol 26:125–129
10. Oshima Y, Shimizu T, Yokohari R et al (1963) Clinical studies on Behçet's syndrome. Ann Rheum Dis 22:36–45
11. Strachan RW, Wigzell FW (1963) Polyarthritis in Behçet's multiple symptom complex. Ann Rheum Dis 22:26–35
12. Mamo GJ, Baghdassarian A (1964) Behçet's disease: a report of 28 cases. Arch Ophtalmol 71:38–48
13. O'Duffy JD, Carney A, Deodhar S (1971) Behçet's disease, report of 10 cases, 3 with new manifestations. Ann Intern Med 75:561–570
14. Cooper DA, Penny R (1974) Behçet's syndrome: clinical, immunological and therapeutic evaluation of 17 patients. Aust NZ J Med 4:585–596
15. Zizic MT, Stevens MB (1975) The arthropathy of Behçet's disease. Johns Hopkins Med J 136:243–250
16. Chajek T, Fainaru M (1975) Behçet's disease: report of 41 cases and a review of the literature. Medicine 54:179–196

17. Chamberlain MA (1977) Behçet's syndrome in 32 patients in Yorkshire. Ann Rheum Dis 36:491–499
18. Dilsen N, Koniçe M, Övül C (1979) Arthritic patterns in Behçet's disease. In: Dilşen N, Konice M, Övül C (eds) Behçet's disease: proceedings of an international symposium on Behçet's disease. Excerpta Medica, Amsterdam, pp 145–155
19. Caporn N, Higgs RE, Dieppe PA, Watt I (1983) Arthritis in Behçet's syndrome. Br J Radiol 56:87–91
20. Oto A, Oktay A, Dündar S et al (1985) Behçet's disease: an analysis of 190 cases. Asian Med J 28:580–589
21. Mousa AR, Marafie AA, Rifai KM, Dajani AI, Mukhtar MM (1986) Behçet's disease in Kuwait, Arabia: a report of 29 cases and a review. Scand J Rheumatol 15:310–332
22. Al-Rawi ZS, Sharquie KE, Khalifa SJ, Al-Hadithi FM, Munir JJ (1986) Behçet's disease in Iraqi patients. Ann Rheum Dis 45:987–990
23. Ek L, Hedfors E (1993) Behçet's disease: a review and a report of 12 cases from Sweden. Acta Derm Venereol 73:251–254
24. Pande I, Uppal SS, Kailash S, Kumar A, Malaviya AN (1995) Behçet's disease in India: a clinical, immunological, immunogenetic and outcome study. Br J Rheumatol 34:825–830
25. Zierhut M, Saal J, Player U, Kotter I, Durk H, Fierlbeck G (1995) Behçet's disease: epidemiology and eye manifestations in German and Mediterranean patients. Ger J Opthalmol 4:246–251
26. Çalgüneri M, Kiraz S, Ertenli İ, Erman M, Karaaslan Y, Celik İ (1997) Characteristics of peripheral arthritis in Behçet's disease. N Z Med J 110:80–81
27. Benamour S, Zeroual B, Alaoui FZ (1998) Joint manifestations in Behçet's disease: a review of 340 cases. Rev Rhum Engl Ed 65:299–307
28. Chang HK, Kim JW (2002) The clinical features of Behçet's disease in Yongdong districts: analysis of a cohort followed from 1997 to 2001. J Korean Med Sci 17:784–789
29. Mok CC, Cheung TC, Ho CT et al (2002) Behçet's disease in southern Chinese patients. J Rheumatol 29:1689–1693
30. Cheng YK, Tong BY, Chng HH (2004) Behçet's disease: experience in a tertiary rheumatology centre in Singapore and a review of the literature. Ann Acad Med Singapore 33:510–514
31. Hamdan A, Mansour W, Uthman I, Masri AF, Nasr F, Arayssi T (2006) Behçet's disease in Lebanon: clinical profile, severity and two-decade comparison. Clin Rheumatol 25:364–367
32. Salvarani C, Pipitone N, Catanoso MG et al (2007) Epidemiology and clinical course of Behçet's disease in the Reggio Emilia area of Northern Italy: a seventeen-year population-based study. Arthritis Rheum 57:171–178
33. Ait Badi MA, Zyani M, Kaddouri S, Niamane R, Hda A, Algayres JP (2008) Les manifestations articulaires de la maladie de Behçet. A propos de 79 cas. Rev Med Interne 29:277–282
34. Bono W, Khammar Z, Lamchachti L, Lahlou M, Rabbi S, Harzy T (2008) Joint involvement of Behçet's disease: review study of 62 cases in 5 years. Clin Exp Rheumatol 26:S17, abstract
35. Gur A, Sarac AJ, Burkan YK, Nas K, Cevik R (2006) Arthropathy, quality of life, depression, and anxiety in Behçet's disease: relationship between arthritis and these factors. Clin Rheumatol 25:524–531
36. B'chir Hamzaoui S, Harmel A, Bouslama K, Abdallah M, Ennafaa M, M'rad S, Ben Dridi M (2006) le groupe tunisien d'étude sur la maladie de Behçet. La maladie de Behçet en Tunisie. Étude clinique de 519 cas [Behçet's disease in Tunisia. Clinical study of 519 cases]. Rev Med Interne 27:742–750
37. Houman MH, Neffati H, Braham A et al (2007) Behçet's disease in Tunisia. Demographic, clinical and genetic aspects in 260 patients. Clin Exp Rheumatol 25:S58–S64
38. Yurdakul S, Yazici H, Tüzün Y et al (1983) The arthritis of Behçet's disease: a prospective study. Ann Rheum Dis 42:505–515
39. Moll JM, Haslock I, Macrae IF, Wright V (1974) Associations between ankylosing spondylitis, psoriatic arthritis, Reiter's disease, the intestinal arthropathies, and Behçet's syndrome. Medicine 53:343–364

40. Yazici H, Tuzlaci M, Yurdakul S (1981) A controlled survey of sacroiliitis in Behçet's disease. Ann Rheum Dis 40:558–559
41. Chamberlain MA, Robertson RJ (1993) A controlled study of sacroiliitis in Behçet's disease. Br J Rheumatol 32:693–698
42. Maghraoui AE, Tabache F, Bezza A et al (2001) A controlled study of sacroiliitis in Behçet's disease. Clin Rheumatol 20:189–191
43. Chang HK, Lee DH, Jung SM et al (2002) The comparison between Behçet's disease and spondyloarthritides: does Behçet's disease belong to the spondyloarthropathy complex? J Korean Med Sci 17:524–529
44. Olivieri I, Salvarani C, Cantini F (1997) Is Behçet's disease part of the spondyloarthritis complex? J Rheumatol 24:1870–1871
45. Yazici H, Turunc M, Ozdogan H, Yurdakul S, Akinci A (1987) Observer variation in grading sacroiliac radiographs might be cause of sacroiliitis reported in certain disease states. Ann Rheum Dis 46:1439–1445
46. Hatemi G, Fresko I, Yurdakul S et al (2010) Sacroiliitis and HLA B27 positivity in Behçet's syndrome patients with acne, arthritis and enthesopathy. Arthritis Rheum 62:305–306
47. Martel W, Duff I (1961) Pelvo-spondylitis in rheumatoid arthritis. Radiology 77:744–755
48. Hamza M (1993) Enthesitis in Behçet's disease. In: Wechsler B, Godeau P (eds) Behçet's disease. Excerpta Medica, Amsterdam, pp 251–253
49. Imbert I, Legros P, Prigent D et al (1987) Articular manifestations of Behçet's disease. Apropos of 65 cases. Rev Rhum Mal Osteoartic 54:93–96
50. Tunc R, Keyman E, Melikoglu M, Fresko I, Yazici H (2002) Target organ associations in Turkish patients with Behçet's disease: a cross sectional study by exploratory factor analysis. J Rheumatol 29:2393–2396
51. Diri E, Mat C, Hamuryudan V, Yurdakul S, Hizli N, Yazici H (2001) Papulopustular skin lesions are seen more frequently in patients with Behçet's syndrome who have arthritis: a controlled and masked study. Ann Rheum Dis 60:1074–1076
52. Hatemi G, Fresko I, Tascilar K, Yazici H (2008) Increased enthesopathy among Behçet's syndrome patients with acne and arthritis: an ultrasonography study. Arthritis Rheum 58:1539–1545
53. Yurdakul S, Yazici H, Tüzüner N, Aytac S, Müftüoglu A (1981) Olecranon nodules in a case of Behçet's disease. Ann Rheum Dis 40:182–184
54. Mulhern LM, Pollock BH (1980) Pseudothrombophlebitis and Behçet's syndrome. Arthritis Rheum 25:477–478
55. Dawes PT, Raman D, Haslock I (1983) Acute synovial rupture in Behçet's syndrome. Ann Rheum Dis 42:591–592
56. Giacomello A, Taccari E, Zoppini A (1980) Marked synovial sensitivity to pricking in Behçet's syndrome. Arthritis Rheum 23:259–260
57. Volpe A, Caramaschi P, Marchetta A, Desto E, Arcar G (2006) Pseudoseptic arthritis in a patient with Behçet's disease. Clin Exp Rheumatol 24:S123
58. Humby F, Gullick N, Kelly S, Pitzalis C, Oakley SP (2008) A synovial pathergy reaction leading to a pseudo-septic arthritis and a diagnosis of Behçet's disease. Rheumatology 47:1255–1256
59. Müftüoglu A, Yazici H, Yurdakul S et al (1986) Behçet's disease: Relation of serum C-reactive protein and erythrocyte sedimentation rate to disease activity. Int J Dermatol 25:235–239
60. Koca SS, Akbulut H, Dag S, Artas H, Isik A (2007) Anti-cyclic citrullinated peptide antibodies in rheumatoid arthritis and Behçet's disease. Tohoku J Exp Med 213:297–304
61. El-Ramahi KM, Al-Dalaan A, Al-Balaa S, Al-Kawi MZ, Bohlega S (1993) Joint fluid analysis in Behçet's disease. In: Wechsler B, Godeau P (eds) Behçet's disease. Excerpta Medica, Amsterdam, pp 279–282
62. Hamza M, Ayed K, el Euch M, Moalla M, Ben Ayed H (1984) Synovial fluid complement levels in Behçet's disease. Ann Rheum Dis 43:767
63. Takeuchi A, Mori M, Hashimoto A (1984) Radiographic abnormalities in patients with Behçet's disease. Clin Exp Rheumatol 2:259–262

64. Currey HLF, Elson RA, Mason RM (1968) Surgical treatment of manubriosternal pain in Behçet's syndrome: report of a case. J Bone Joint Surg Br 50:836–840
65. Jawad AS, Goodwill CJ (1986) Behçet's disease with erosive arthritis. Ann Rheum Dis 45:961–962
66. Takeuchi A, Hashimoto T (1989) Arthropathy of Behçet's disease: a case with "pencil-in-cup" deformities. Arthritis Rheum 32:1629–1630
67. Tan J, Gögüs F, Sepici V (1993) 'Pencil-in-cup' deformity in Behçet's disease. Br J Rheumatol 32:644–645
68. Crozier F, Arlaud J, Tourniaire P et al (2003) Arthrite manubrio-sternale et syndrome de Behçet: a propos de 3 observations. J Radiol 84:1978–1981
69. Düzgün N, Ates A (2003) Erosive arthritis in a patient with Behçet's disease. Rheumatol Int 23:265–267
70. Aydin G, Keles I, Atalar E, Orkun S (2005) Extensive erosive arthropathy in a patient with Behçet's disease: case report. Clin Rheumatol 24:645–647
71. Sciuto M, Porciello G, Occhipini G, Trippi D, Cagno MC, Vitali C (1996) Multiple and reversible osteolytic lesions: an unusual manifestation of Behçet's disease. J Rheumatol 23:564–566
72. Vernon-Roberts B, Barnes CG, Revell PA (1978) Synovial pathology in Behçet's syndrome. Ann Rheum Dis 37:139–145
73. Gibson T, Laurent R, Highton J, Wilton M, Dyson M, Millis R (1981) Synovial histopathology of Behçet's syndrome. Ann Rheum Dis 40:376–381
74. Nanke Y, Kotake S, Momohara S, Tateishi M, Yamanaka H, Kamatani N (2002) Synovial histology in three Behçet's disease patients with orthopedic surgery. Clin Exp Rheumatol 20:S35–S39
75. Yavuz Ş, Fresko I, Hamuryudan V, Yurdakul S, Yazici H (1998) Fibromyalgia in Behçet's syndrome. J Rheumatol 25:2219–2220
76. Al-Izzi MK, Jabber AS (2004) Fibromyalgia in Iraqi patients with Behçet's syndrome. J Med Liban 52:86–90
77. Lee SS, Yoon HJ, Chang HK, Park KS (2005) Fibromyalgia in Behçet's disease is associated with anxiety and depression, and not with disease activity. Clin Exp Rheumatol 23:S15–S19
78. Arkin CR, Rothschild BM, Florendo NT, Popoff N (1980) Behçet's syndrome with myositis: a case report with pathologic findings. Arthritis Rheum 23:600–604
79. Finucane P, Doyle CT, Ferriss JB, Molloy M, Murnaghan D (1985) Behçet's syndrome with myositis and glomerulonephritis. Br J Rheumatol 24:372–375
80. Lingenfelser T, Duerk H, Stevens A, Grossmann T, Knorr M, Saal JG (1992) Generalized myositis in Behçet's disease: treatment with cyclosporine. Ann Intern Med 116:651–653
81. Yazici H, Tuzuner N, Tuzun Y et al (1982) Localized myositis in Behçet's disease. Arthritis Rheum 24:636
82. Di Giacomo V, Carmenini G, Meloni F, Valesini G (1982) Myositis in Behçet's disease. Arthritis Rheum 25:1025
83. Sarui H, Maruyama T, Ito I et al (2002) Necrotizing myositis in Behçet's disease: characteristic features on magnetic resonance imaging and a review of the literature. Ann Rheum Dis 61:751–752
84. Lang BA, Laxer RM, Thorner P, Greenberg M, Silverman ED (1990) Pediatric onset of Behçet's syndrome with myositis: case report and literature review illustrating unusual features. Arthritis Rheum 33:418–425
85. Frayha R (1982) Muscle involvement in Behçet's disease. Arthritis Rheum 24:636–637
86. Frayha RA, Afifi AK, Bergman RA, Nader S, Bahuth NB (1985) Neurogenic muscular atrophy in Behçet's disease. Clin Rheumatol 4:202–211
87. Ronco P, Wechsler B, Saillant G, Godeau P (1981) Aseptic osteonecrosis during corticosteroid treatment of Behçet's disease. Nouv Presse Med 10:1707–1710
88. Chang HK, Choi YJ, Baek SK, Lee DH, Won KS (2001) Osteonecrosis and bone infarction in association with Behçet's disease: report of two cases. Clin Exp Rheumatol 19:S51–S54

89. Yapar Z, Kibar M, Soy M, Ozbek S (2001) Osteonecrosis in Behçet's disease seen on bone scintigraphy. Clin Nucl Med 26:267–268
90. Jäger M, Thorey F, Wild A, Voede M, Krauspe R (2003) Osteonekrosen bei morbus Adamantiades-Behçet: diagnostik, therapie und verlauf. Z Rheumatol 62:390–394
91. Gogus F, Fresko I (2006) Avascular necrosis in Behçet's syndrome. Clin Exp Rheumatol 24:S44, abstract
92. Bodur H, Borman P, Ozdemir Y, Atan C, Kural G (2006) Quality of life and life satisfaction in patients with Behçet's disease: relationship with disease activity. Clin Rheumatol 25:329–333
93. Moses AN, Fisher M, Yazici Y (2008) Behçet's syndrome patients have high levels of functional disability, fatigue and pain as measured by a Multi-dimensional Health Assessment Questionnaire (MDHAQ). Clin Exp Rheumatol 26:S110–S113
94. Yurdakul S, Mat C, Tüzün Y et al (2001) A double blind study of colchicine in Behçet's syndrome. Arthritis Rheum 44:2686–2692
95. Moral F, Hamuryudan V, Yurdakul S, Yazici H (1995) Inefficacy of azapropazone in the acute arthritis of Behçet's syndrome: a randomized, double blind, placebo controlled study. Clin Exp Rheumatol 13:493–495
96. Yazici H, Pazarlı H, Barnes CG et al (1990) A controlled trial of azathioprine in Behçet's syndrome. N Engl J Med 322:281–285
97. Çalguneri M, Kiraz S, Ertenli I, Benekli M, Karaarslan Y, Celik I (1996) The effect of prophylactic penicillin treatment on the course of arthritis of Behçet's disease: a randomised clinical trial. Arthritis Rheum 39:2062–2065
98. Yurdakul S, Ozdogan H, Yazici H (1986) D-Penillamine therapy in the arthritis of Behçet's syndrome. In: Lehner T, Barnes CG (eds) Behçet's disease. Royal Society of Medicine Services International Congress and Symposium Series No 103. Royal Society of Medicine Services, London, p 315, abstract
99. Hamuryudan V, Moral F, Yurdakul S et al (1994) Systemic interferon α2b treatment in Behçet's syndrome. J Rheumatol 21:1098–1100
100. Kötter I, Vonthein R, Zierhut M et al (2004) Differential efficacy of human recombinant interferon-alpha2a on ocular and extraocular manifestations of Behçet's disease: results of an open 4-center trial. Semin Arthritis Rheum 33:311–319
101. Calgüneri M, Oztürk MA, Ertenli I, Kiraz S, Apraş S, Ozbalkan Z (2003) Effects of interferon alpha treatment on the clinical course of refractory Behçet's disease: an open study. Ann Rheum Dis 62:492–493
102. Sfikakis PP, Markomichelakis N, Alpsoy E et al (2007) Anti-TNF therapy in the management of Behçet's disease – review and basis for recommendations. Rheumatology 46:736–741

Chapter 10
Behçet's Disease: Gastrointestinal Involvement

Jae Hee Cheon, Aykut Ferhat Çelik, and Won Ho Kim

Keywords Anastomotic site ulcers • Azatihoprine • Behçet's disease • Crohn's disease • Diagnostic criteria for GIBD • Enteroclysis • Esophageal disease • Fistulas • Gastrointestinal involvement • Ileocecal disease • Inflammatory bowel disease • Intestinal pathology • Intestinal ulcers • NSAID entero-colitis • Prognosis • Radiology • Rectal involvement • Recto-sigmeodoscopy • Smoking • Stomach involvement • Surgical management • Top–down therapy

Introduction

Gastrointestinal (GI) tract involvement in Behçet's disease (BD) was first described by Bechgaard in 1940 [1]. It often leads to severe complications such as perforation or massive bleeding. As such it is a major cause of morbidity and mortality.

Epidemiology

A substantial number of BD patients complain of GI symptoms [2–5], present in at least 50% of BD patients in Japan [2]. On the other hand, GI complaints are rather common in the general population and it is difficult to discern whether a GI symptom in a BD patient is actually related directly to BD. The reported frequency of gastrointestinal Behçet's disease (GIBD) shows wide variation (Table 10.1). There is a list of issues to consider:

A.F. Çelik (✉)
Division of Gastroenterology, Department of Internal Medicine, University of Istanbul, Istanbul, Turkey
e-mail: afcelik@superonline.com

Y. Yazıcı and H. Yazıcı (eds.), *Behçet's Syndrome*,
DOI 10.1007/978-1-4419-5641-5_10, © Springer Science+Business Media, LLC 2010

Table 10.1 Frequency of BD gastrointestinal involvement in different studies

References	Country	Year	Number of patients with BD	GI involvement (%)
Shimizu et al.[a] [2]	Japan	1971	?	50
O'Duffy et al.[b] [6]	USA	1971	10	30
Yamamato et al.[a] [144]	Japan	1974	2,031	25
Chamberlain et al.[b] [8]	UK	1977	32	6
Eun et al.[b] [7]	Korea	1984	114	5.3
Jankowski et al.[a] [10]	UK	1992	15	40
Dilsen et al.[a] [9]	Turkey	1993	496	5
Yurdakul et al.[b] [12]	Turkey	1996	1,000	0.7
Gürler et al.[b] [13]	Turkey	1997	2,147	2.8
Bang D et al.[b] [14]	Korea	1997	1,155	4
Bang D et al.[a] [11]	Korea	2001	3,497	7.3
Chang et al.[b] [16]	Korea	2002	73	15
Bang DS et al.[b] [37]	Korea	2003	1,901	3.2
Tursen et al.[b] [18]	Turkey	2003	2,313	1.4
Seyahi et al.[b,c] [15]	Turkey	2003	121	0.8
Yi et al.[c] [19]	Korea	2008	842	15[a]/8[b]

[a] GI involvement diagnosed according to GI symptoms

[b] GI involvement diagnosed according to GI symptoms and endoscopic/radiologic documentations

[c] Pediatric data

1. Practically all the available data about the frequency of GIBD are based on the experience of different and separate clinical disciplines, like gastroenterology, dermatology, etc. This has the potential of considerably over- or underestimating the true frequency.
2. Different reports have used differing diagnostic criteria to diagnose the primary illness. For example, the presence of GI lesions is one of the items in the Japanese criteria [20]. This makes a patient with GI involvement more likely to be diagnosed with BD by the said criteria.
3. It might be said that in order to make a firm diagnosis of intestinal BD, the intestinal lesions must be identified by an objective method. However, in some studies (Table 10.1), the mere presence of GI symptoms has been used to make the diagnosis. For example, one study from Istanbul [12] did not have the specialty bias since it came from a multidisciplinary unit. On the other hand, the authors only considered the GI symptoms in assessing the frequency of GIBD. This was not backed by endoscopy or radiology. A recent Korean study [19] reported that 125/842 (15%) patients experienced GI symptoms and 69 (8%) of these were found to have GI involvement by endoscopic examination. However, even endoscopic observation of GI lesions might not strictly indicate GIBD because of the specificity issues (see section Differential Diagnosis). Furthermore, intestinal involvement may not receive much attention, unless sporadic cases present with severe inflammation, intestinal ulcers, or bleeding. This may seemingly increase the prevalence of GIBD [6, 8, 10], especially in low prevalence countries, where the mucocutaneous cases without GI involvement are more easily missed.

4. Although intestinal BD usually presents with lesions in the small and large intestine, on rare occasions it manifests in the esophagus and the stomach and may not be recognized.
5. Gastrointestinal endoscopic lesions in patients with BD may be explained by other reasons, like non-steroidal anti-inflammatory drug (NSAID) related GI lesions, (see differential diagnosis). This point was paid nearly no attention in previous GIBD prevalence discussions.

Some distinct and reproducible real geographic trends in incidence, however, have been discerned. Despite a high prevalence of BD, intestinal involvement has been reported to be rare in Mediterranean BD patients, ranging from 0 to 5% [12, 13, 21–23]. However, in East Asia, including Korea and Japan, where BD is also highly prevalent, intestinal involvement is relatively common (5–25%) [14, 16].

Data on esophageal involvement are scarce and mostly based on patient symptoms. The quoted prevalence of 11 and 66% is likely to be unduly high [24, 25]. A recent Korean endoscopic survey found the frequency to be quite low (0.7%) [19].

According to two surveys in surgical patients, the frequency of gastroduodenal involvement was reported to be as low as esophageal involvement [26, 27]. However, an endoscopic study in BD patients with upper GI symptoms [19] showed three times more gastric and duodenal ulcers (14%) than esophageal ulcerations (4.7%). NSAID use might at least partially explain these findings. While BD is diagnosed frequently among patients aged 20–30 years [28, 29], the onset of GIBD is in the fourth or early fifth decade [4, 30–32]. On the other hand, no age group is immune [33] and GIBD has even been reported in an 11-month old baby [34]. According to one report, juvenile BD accounts for 3–7% of all cases of GIBD [35]. Interestingly, the rate of intestinal involvement has been reported higher (69%) among Japanese children with BD as compared to that found among the adults (25–50%) [36].

The male/female ratio of GIBD was found 1:1 in one Turkish study [18]. In contrast, studies throughout Korea [30–32] and Japan [26] have shown a slight preponderance for males (1.2–2.0:1). Whether males with GIBD have more severe disease, as is the case for many other manifestations of BD, needs to be further assessed. However, in another Korean study, the frequency of severe GI disease was not found to be similar between males and females [37].

Clinical Manifestations

GI Manifestations

Symptoms of GIBD can vary from mild GI discomfort to more severe symptoms with complications, such as bleeding, fistula, or perforation [2, 21]. The most common symptom is abdominal pain followed by diarrhea, bleeding, vomiting, bowel habit changes, and weight loss. This is similar to what is usually observed in inflammatory bowel disease (IBD) [2, 30–32]. The location and pattern of pain often correlates

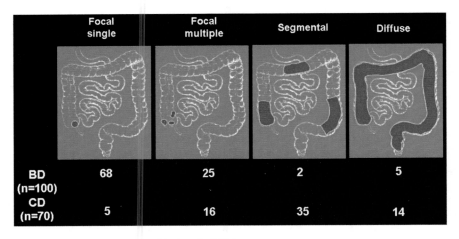

	Focal single	Focal multiple	Segmental	Diffuse
BD (n=100)	68	25	2	5
CD (n=70)	5	16	35	14

Fig. 10.1 Distribution pattern of lesions in GIBD

with the location of the pathology. As in Crohn's disease (CD), one common pain pattern of GIBD is cramps in the right lower quadrant in patients with ulcers in the ileocecal area. Deep, penetrating ulcers increase the complication rate [21, 26]. Perforating ulcers tend to occur repeatedly, and at multiple sites [17, 38, 39].

GI involvement in BD may affect all areas from the lips to the anus. The ulcers are most commonly found in the terminal ileum and the cecum and less frequently in the colon, sparing the rectum [26, 40]. Less than 15% of cases diffusely involve the colon (Fig. 10.1) [31]. Perianal ulcers, like orogenital ulcers, may rarely accompany GIBD [41]. Bleeding can be life threatening in some patients [42, 43]. The GI manifestations usually appear 4–6 years after the onset of the oral ulcers. Constipation or tenesmus is not usual. Similar to what is seen in other IBDs, the clinical features in GIBD vary considerably over time [44–46].

Esophageal involvement occurs more frequently in males [47], causing substernal pain, dysphagia, and hematemesis. Esophageal lesions are most frequently located in the middle esophagus and are nonspecific. Various other forms of esophageal lesions including erosions, aphthous, linear, or perforating ulcers, widely spreading esophagitis, dissection of the mucosa, varices, and stenosis [19, 48–50] have been reported. Usually, biopsy and cultures are required to differentiate this condition from infectious or malignant conditions. Moreover, involvement may not be correlated with systemic disease activity, disease duration, or any other disease aspect. In more than 50% of the cases, esophageal involvement is accompanied by other GI manifestations, mainly jejunal and ileocolonic ulcers [19]. In addition, rare, serious complications such as stricture, bleeding, fistula, or perforations have been described [51].

The gastroduodenal mucosa appears to be the least frequently involved segment in GI tract. Aphthous ulcers can occur in the duodenum [27]. Differentiating between gastric involvement of GIBD and gastric or duodenal ulcer may be difficult.

Finally, possible involvement of other intra-abdominal organs including liver, pancreas, or spleen, has also been reported [21]. However, it is difficult to say that they are causally related to BD [52].

Extraintestinal Manifestations

Many of these manifestations are shown in Table 10.2. Budd–Chiari syndrome is an important extraintestinal manifestation carrying a grave prognosis [61].

Laboratory Findings

In a prospective study, ESR and CRP showed poor performance as markers of disease activity in patients with complete and possible types of GIBD [62]. Moreover, CRP is not usually markedly elevated in BD in general [63]. Therefore, very high levels of

Table 10.2 Comparison of GIBD and CD characteristics

	GIBD	CD
Extraintestinal involvement [15, 53–55]		
Oral ulcer	100%[a]	20%
Genital ulcer/Genital scar	95%/~60%[a]	4%[c]/No case
Nodular lesion	50%[a]	2–10%
Arthritis	20%	5%
Venous thrombosis	15%[a]	<1%
Eye involvement	45%[a]	3–6%[d]
Neurologic involvement	5%[a]	<1%
Intestinal involvement [26, 40, 56]		
Ileocecal	50–90%	40–60%
Rectal	<1%	10%
Upper GI	1%	5%
Perianal	1%[b]	10–15%
Complications [21, 26, 56]		
Perforation/fistula/stricture	25–50%/5–10%[b]/8%	2%/(20–30%)/17%
Pyoderma gangrenosum	<1%	1–10%
Laboratory assessment [56–60, 145]		
ASCA (IgA or IgG)	28–49%	62–41%
Distribution and endoscopic morphology of intestinal ulcers	Round, focal, isolated	Longitudinal, diffuse segmental
Granuloma (in mucosal biopsy)	<1%	10–15%

[a] Prominently less in females
[b] No anal fistula formation
[c] History based; no real description of typical genital ulcer
[d] Rarely progress to blindness

CRP in a patient with GIBD indicate complications like, stricture, fistula, and abscess formation. These pathologies as well as distinctly high CRP levels, on the other hand, are more common in CD, and can help in differential diagnosis of this condition from GIBD (Table 10.2). A specific laboratory marker that accurately reflects the involvement of the GI tract in BD is yet to be found. It has been proposed that anti-*Saccharomyces cerevisiae* antibodies (ASCA), a well known hall mark of CD [64] could be also high in patients with BD and GIBD [57, 58, 65, 66]. Intestinal tuberculosis, on the other hand, can also be associated with high ASCA levels (I-TBC) [67].

Endoscopic and Radiologic Findings

Radiological and endoscopic findings of GIBD are very similar to what is seen in CD. When intestinal involvement is suspected, colonoscopy is necessary. To identify possible small intestine lesions proximal to the terminal ileum, small bowel barium follow-through or enteroclysis are required. Recently, entire direct small bowel evaluation has been feasible using wireless capsule endoscopy or double balloon endoscopy [68]. A case series showed that capsule endoscopy is also promising in patients with GIBD [69, 70].

Well-demarcated punched-out ulcers, or aphthoid ulcers are the most common lesions of GIBD [31, 40]. The smaller ulcers have been considered histologically and perhaps pathogenetically to be similar to the oral aphthous ulcers [71]. Larger ulcers usually have an oval or irregular configuration. The depth of ulcer penetration varies. Superficial ulcers have occasionally been shown to resolve, but deeper ulcers often extend through the bowel wall [59, 72, 73]. It has been reported that the typical colonoscopic findings in GIBD are single or a few deep round/oval ulcers with a discrete elevated margin in the ileocecal area or anastomotic site (Fig. 10.2) [3, 4, 31]. Although the ulcers are found most frequently in the ileocecal area, they may be present

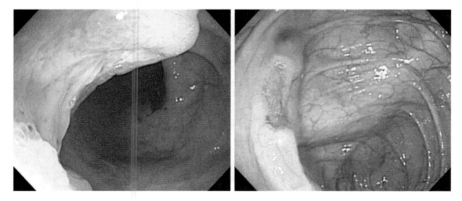

Fig. 10.2 Colonoscopic findings. Single or a few deep round/oval ulcers with a discrete elevated margin are observed in the ileocecal area

at any site throughout the digestive system. Enteroclysis findings among Turkish BD patients with GI involvement showed intestinal ulcerations that were usually shallow, multiple, and commonly localized to the terminal ileum [74]. This contrasted with the findings in the colonoscopic study from Korea, in which large isolated ulcers were more prominently seen [59]. More recently, a 10-year colonoscopy experience from Turkey (Celik, unpublished data), however, is more in line with the Korean data. It might be enteroclysis had overestimated intestinal disease.

Radiological findings of GIBD parallel endoscopic findings. Barium study is useful for demonstrating the characteristic features of BD involving the GI tract, and in determining the extent of these lesions. With barium study, the characteristic radiological findings include single or multiple discrete, collar button-shaped or ring-shaped lesions with considerable thickening of the surrounding mucosal folds (Fig. 10.3) [75, 76]. The double contrast technique is considered to be more valuable in diagnosis.

CT is useful in demonstrating bowel wall thickening and lesions in the extraluminal space. It is recommended for early detection of complications as well as for the exclusion of other abdominal pathologic conditions [77]. Sometimes, GIBD presents as an ileocecal mass, or obstructed and conglomerated bowel loops, requiring surgical resection to differentiate an inflammatory mass from a neoplasm [75].

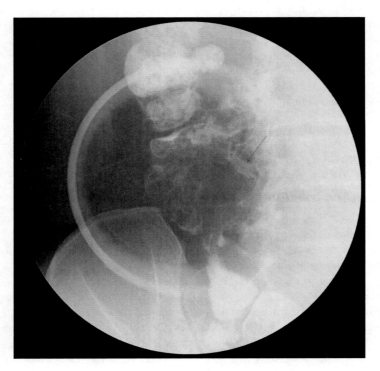

Fig. 10.3 Barium enema findings. About 2-cm sized geographic ulcer is seen at ileocecal valve (*arrow*)

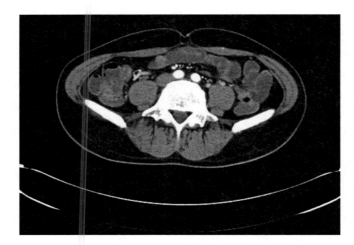

Fig. 10.4 CT enterography shows focal wall thickening involving ileocecal valve and terminal ileum

It is particularly useful in assessing lesions proximal to the ileocecal valve. CT may be necessary and enough tool to localize the lesion before doing barium follow through or enteroclysis, especially in case of obstruction and/or localized abdominal pain companion. Finally, it also helps to assess the possibility of an abscess or perforation.

Although CT and MR enterographies/enterocolysis are promising techniques (Fig. 10.4) in diagnosing of IBD and GIBD, they are not yet in routine use except in some experienced radiology clinics. The abdominal ultrasonography has limited usefulness for bowel evaluation.

Pathogenesis

Immune Abnormalities

Much remains unknown about the pathogenesis of BD and GIBD (see Chap. 14). The GI tract is one of the major ports of entry for a variety of environmental, immune-provoking agents, so one hypothesis is that GIBD represents an intestinal immune response to possible infectious agents. M cells, which are optimized for antigen adherence and transport, play a pivotal role as a portal of entry for potentially pathogenic agents in gut-associated lymphoid tissue [78] and ileal lesions in BD frequently coincide with Peyer's patches [79, 80]. A recent study indicated that TLR (toll-like receptor)-2- and TLR-4-expressing cells accumulated in the intestinal lesions of BD, suggesting that IL-12 produced by TLR-2-expressing cells may contribute to the induction of a Th1-dominant immune response in GIBD. Expression of both TLR-2 and TLR-4 mRNAs was detected in BD intestinal lesions [81]. A yet unidentified pathogen might stimulate both TLR-2 and TLR-4 in GIBD. Changes in vascular endothelial cells and neutrophil hyperfunction, triggered by signal transduction from TLR-2 or TLR-4 and exemplified by increased chemotaxis and hydroxyl radical production, are thought to be involved in the pathological mechanisms of intestinal BD [82–84]. Adhesion molecules on leukocytes and endothelial cells may also play important roles in pathogenesis [84, 85]. Intercellular adhesion molecule (ICAM)-1 is strongly expressed in the majority of venules with inflammatory changes in GIBD. These LFA-1/ICAM-1 interactions might result in the transmission of neutrophils through the endothelial cells of postcapillary or collective venules [82]. In the active stage, inflammatory cells that are mainly infiltrating neutrophils are found principally in intestinal BD lesions in the absence of infection [26, 82, 86], and histological studies have found neutrophil-mediated vasculitis in the intestinal area [21, 40]. The association of neutrophils with GI ulcer formation or vasculitis has also been convincingly demonstrated in BD. Chronic, persistent hypoxia from the intestinal wall has been implicated as the cause of ulcer formation [21]. The exact underlying mechanisms of abnormal neutrophil hyperactivity are still under investigation and the enhanced spontaneous neutrophil function has been observed particularly in HLA B51-positive BD patients [87]. Moreover, activated CD8[+] T cell participation in the pathogenesis of GIBD was reported in a study of peripheral blood lymphocytes [88]. Recent reports have shown that T cell immune responses were skewed toward Th1 dominance in GIBD and Txk-expressing Th1 cells, and suggested that Th1-associated cytokines may play a critical role in the pathogenesis of this disease [89]. Cytokines such as INF-α, IL-12, TNF-α, IL-2, and IL-18 are released by Th1 cells in BD patients. Among these, TNF-α plays a pivotal role in BD, and anti-TNF-α therapy both reduces TNF-α production and modulates the functional activity of Th1 cells. This provides an immunological background for using thalidomide or anti-TNF-α therapy, such as infliximab, in treatment [22].

Genetics

The association of CARD15/NOD2 polymorphisms are well established in CD but not in ulcerative colitis (UC). Two separate studies did not find an association with CARD15/NOD2 variant in BD patients from Turkey [142] and the UK [90]. On the other hand, CARD15/NOD2 polymorphisms were also not found to be associated with CD either, in Turkey [91, 92]. The association of GIBD with the CARD15/NOD2 polymorphism among patients in regions where this association with CD is well established has thus far not been studied.

A possible association has been reported between the development of gastroduodenal ulcers and the A2/B46/Cw1 or A11/B46/Cw1 genotypes in Taiwanese BD patients [27].

Finally, there are two case reports indicating concordance of GI involvement between monozygotic twins [93, 94].

Environment

It has been shown that the cessation of smoking may cause flares in oral ulcers, [95] and nicotine patches reduce their frequency and severity in BD [96]. On the other hand, there is no formal information about the possible effects of smoking on intestinal disease in BD, as is the case in IBD [97, 98].

Intestinal Permeability

Increased intestinal permeability was described in two reports [99, 100]. The relevance of this finding to the disease mechanism remains to be seen.

Diagnosis

The diagnosis of GIBD usually requires two steps: (1) The patient should have BD; (2) Intestinal lesions for which no other explanation can be discerned must be identified. For example, GIBD can be diagnosed if there is a large, typically shaped ulcer in the small or large intestine, and clinical findings meet the BD diagnostic criteria, with the exclusion of infectious enterocolitis, intestinal tuberculosis (I-TBC), CD, and other possible causes, including NSAID colitis. Some GI ulcers in BD patients are difficult to differentiate from those seen in IBD and I-TBC (Fig. 10.5). The latter point is especially important in geographies in which BD and TBC are both common.

To aid in the differential diagnosis, formal guidelines have been proposed. One such set is a consensus-based practice guideline for the diagnosis and treatment of GIBD using a modified Delphi approach, as proposed in Japan (Table 10.3) [101].

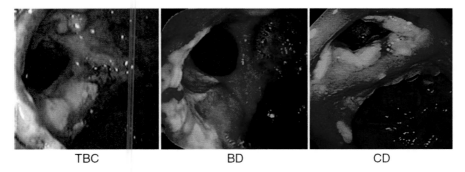

TBC   BD   CD

Fig. 10.5 Behçet's disease (BD), Crohn's disease (CD), and Intestinal tuberculosis (I-TBC); they are three similar inflammatory pathology with common ileocecal localization and mostly undistinguishable morphology (From Dr. Çelik's personal archive)

Table 10.3 Guideline statements for diagnosis of intestinal Behçet's disease (Japan)

Diagnosis of intestinal Behçet's disease can be made if:
A. There is a typical oval-shaped large ulcer in the terminal ileum, OR
B. There are ulcerations or inflammation in the small or large intestine,
AND clinical findings meet the diagnostic criteria of Behçet's disease

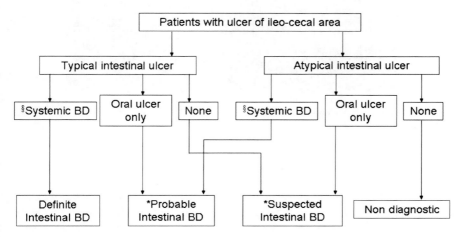

Fig. 10.6 Algorithm for the diagnosis of intestinal Behçet's disease based on the type of ileo-colonic ulcerations and clinical manifestations. *Section*: complete, incomplete, and suspected subtypes of systemic Behçet's disease were classified according to the diagnostic criteria of the Research Committee of Japan. *Asterisk*: close follow-up is necessary

On the other hand, not all patients with GIBD satisfy the systemic BD criteria at the time of colonoscopic evaluation, and systemic manifestations may sequentially develop over a period of many years [102, 103]. Based on this, new diagnostic criteria for GIBD were developed, reflecting temporal changes in systemic manifestations of BD [104]. In this scheme, the patients are categorized into four groups for the diagnosis of GIBD: definite, probable, suspected, and nondiagnostic (Fig. 10.6). The sensitivity for the combined definite, probable, and suspected groups was 99% while the specificity was 83.0%. Further prospective studies with international validation are needed.

Differential Diagnosis

Inflammatory Bowel Disease

IBD and BD may be closely related, and some authors have reported that they are part of a spectrum of diseases rather than distinct disease entities [105]. Both commonly

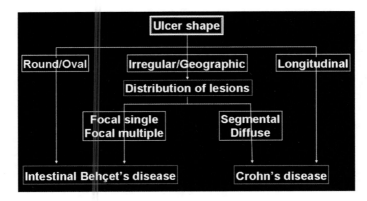

Fig. 10.7 Classification analysis regression tree for the differential diagnosis between GIBD and Crohn's disease

have a young age of onset, nonspecific GI manifestations, similar extraintestinal manifestations, and a chronic, waxing and waning course. GIBD has similar findings with CD in many aspects, including intestinal, extraintestinal involvement, complications, and laboratory parameters (Table 10.2) [53]. It is generally regarded that GIBD has a more guarded prognosis when compared to CD or UC. BD patients with longitudinal colonic ulcers with or without granuloma, more typical of CD, have also been described [106, 107]. Moreover, there are several reports on the coexistence of BD and CD [108]. It is difficult to distinguish whether these patients did in fact have BD or CD with extraintestinal complications, or both BD and CD. UC may also resemble BD with colonic lesions [109]. As mentioned above, rectal involvement is rare in GIBD [56].

In a study from a tertiary dedicated center, both for IBD and BD, the performance of ISGBD criteria [110] was tested in differentiating IBD from BD [53]. The performance of the ISGBD criteria was quite satisfactory, however, whether these results would remain robust in a nontertiary or low BD-prevalent setting needs to be further looked at.

According to a recent endoscopic report, GIBD and CD could be differentiated in more than 90% of the cases by the shape and the distribution patterns of ulcers by endoscopy [56] (Fig. 10.7). A classification tree was proposed as a simple and accurate method for differentiation (Fig. 10.7) [56]. However, lacking of the gold standard for discrimination of both disease may have some influence on the results of this study.

Intestinal Tuberculosis

I-TBC must also be differentiated from GIBD (Fig. 10.5). Patients with I-TBC lack extraintestinal features of BD, and they often have a previous history of pulmonary tuberculosis. The presence of bowel wall thickening in short segments especially in the ileocecal region, multiple enlarged lymph nodes with central low attenuation or calcification in CT, favor the diagnosis of I-TBC [111]. In suspected cases, endoscopic punch biopsy culture and tissue PCR for *Mycobacterium tuberculosis* help diagnosis.

NSAID (Nonsteroidal Antiinflammatory Drugs) Enterocolitis

Although large series are lacking, case reports and uncontrolled endoscopic cohorts [112, 113] clearly indicate the existence of an NSAID-related enterocolitis. BD patients frequently use NSAIDs for control of arthralgia or arthritis. In a multidisciplinary Behçet's center in Turkey, one-third of BD patients with colonoscopic lesions suggestive of GIBD were decided not to have GIBD [114] in that their intestinal ulcerations healed 2–3 months after stopping NSAIDs. This observation is quite in line with the endoscopic findings in patients under NSAID treatment for other reasons [115]. In the late 1960s and early 1970s, extensive use of flexible colonoscopic procedures, for which the Japanese were the pioneers, made us to recognize NSAID-related lower GI pathologies and ulcerations. Perhaps this was why the reported GIBD frequency from Japan was rather high in these earlier years (Table 10.1).

Simple Ulcer Syndrome

A disease entity has been described with deep discrete, punched-out, ulcerations of round or oval appearance in the ileocecal region, histologically showing nonspecific inflammation [116]. These simple ulcers of the colon, also known as a nonspecific or idiopathic ulcers, is a well-recognized clinical entity showing macroscopic and microscopic similarities to GIBD as well as to CD. Whether GIBD and simple ulcer represent the same disease or separate disease entity is controversial [82, 103, 116]. Simple ulcers, especially in the ileocecal area, at the onset may be followed by the systemic manifestations of either BD or CD suggesting that they might represent incomplete forms of either disease. Because of similar pathology with NSAID's, a careful history is also important.

Malignancy

Infiltrative GI lymphoma involving the terminal ileum with bowel wall may resemble GIBD. However, by contrast enhanced CT, pathological segment of the bowel appears to be much less pronounced in lymphoma [77] than GIBD. Giant, bulky, postinflammatory polyps may occasionally form in the colon and simulate carcinoma. Endoscopy with biopsy is necessary to differentiate these from malignancy.

Other Enterocolitides

Appendicitis or diverticulitis must also be differentiated from GIBD. CT is useful in making this differentiation. In appendicitis, the perienteric or pericolonic infiltration is usually more severe than the changes observed in the bowel wall [77].

Disease Activity Index/Inflammatory Bowel Disease Questionnaire

Even though the clinical disease activity in patients with GIBD fluctuate considerably over time, similar to what is seen in GIBD, there are currently no specific disease activity indexes for GIBD. Some physicians adopt Crohn's Disease Activity Index (CDAI) [44, 45, 101].

The Inflammatory Bowel Disease Questionnaire (IBDQ) is frequently used to evaluate therapeutic efficacy of medical or surgical interventions in patients with IBD [117]. Similar to its use in UC or CD, the IBDQ has been shown to be a stable and useful instrument in assessing health-related quality of life. Similar to what is observed in CD, it strongly correlated with disease activity index, among BD patients in a Korean study [44].

Pathology (See Chap. 13)

Treatment (See Also Chap. 19)

Although usually having an undulating course, GIBD may be intractable, and due to complications, it can be the direct cause of death, as in CD [118]. The goal of management is to treat early to avoid recurrences, surgical procedures, and irreversible damage [5]. No controlled trials are available. Similar to IBD treatment protocols, 5-aminosalicylic acid (5-ASA), immunosuppressives, and biological agents, either used singly or in combination, are the three main modalities of medical treatment [28].

Medical Management

5-ASA or Sulfasalazine

Sulfasalazine or 5-ASA has been shown to be effective in treating intestinal or esophageal BD in some uncontrolled studies and case series [119–121], while it was not reported as effective in others [122]. The therapeutic effects of mesalazine on oral and esophageal ulcers [121] may be explained by the systemic antiinflammatory effect of the active form of 5-ASA in the peripheral blood, which is unacetylated

5-ASA. The usual dose of 5-ASA is 2–4 g/day. When sulfasalazine is used, the optimal dose is 3–4 g/day. Authors agree that unless clinical and endoscopic activity is mild, 5-ASA in GIBD is not warranted.

Glucocorticoids

Glucocorticoids have also been reported to be effective in treating GIBD [28, 109]. They often reduce the size of ulcerations and are used as a first-line drug during the acute phase of the disease. They are usually used in 5-ASA-refractory cases or those with severe systemic symptoms, recurrent GI bleeding, or moderate or severe disease activity. The dosage depends on severity. The initial dose is 0.5–1 mg/kg/day of prednisolone for 1–2 weeks [28]. Intravenous pulse therapy with methyl-prednisolone (1 g/day) is sometimes used [28]. Dose reduction often results in recurrent symptoms.

Immunomodulators

Immunosuppressive agents are indicated when patients are corticosteroid-dependent or -resistant [4]. Azathioprine, as in IBD, at 2–2.5 mg/kg/day, is the recommended first line agent. In a Korean retrospective study, maintenance therapy with azathioprine had a beneficial effect on the reoperation rate after surgery [30] and the authors recommended that azathioprine be included in the maintenance treatment regimen at least in patients undergoing operations.

Thalidomide

Thalidomide is known to be effective in mucocutaneous BD [123] and IBD [124]. Similarly, a recent Japanese case series reported that seven patients with resistant GIBD achieved complete remission with thalidomide at an initial dose of 2 mg/kg/day [125]. In another case series from Turkey, 4/5 patients with GIBD responded well to this same dose thalidomide [143].

Biological Agents

Several case reports and case series have suggested that infliximab could be useful in inducing [126–129] and maintaining remission in GIBD [130]. To prevent surgery, infliximab should be used before severe or extended intestinal lesions are observed. This strategy is consistent with the results of recent studies in CD and is called top–down therapy [131]. Esophageal ulcer perforation in BD was successfully treated with a simple drainage operation in combination with infliximab [132]. Moreover, infliximab use was reported to treat massive bleeding from an ileal ulcer in a BD patient [133]. Treatment is usually instituted as outlined for CD, i.e., a 0-week, 2-weeks, and 6-weeks regimen.

Autologous Hematopoietic Stem Cell Transplantation

In two case reports, patients with severe refractory GIBD were successfully treated with lymphocyte-depleted autologous stem cell transplantation following high-dose immunosuppressive therapy [134, 135]. The rationale for this therapy is the assumption that a vigorous immunoablative regimen can delete autoaggressive lymphocyte clones, thus allowing a reset of the immune system.

Endoscopic Therapy

Obstruction and fibrotic strictures rarely occur and can be adequately treated using balloon dilation. GI bleeding is a serious and common complication of GIBD. The spraying of absolute ethanol has been shown to be effective in a case series from Japan [122]. The effect of ethanol is thought to be achieved through the decrease or disappearance of neutrophils or mononuclear cells from ulcer surface.

Surgical Treatment

Surgery is considered in patients who are unresponsive to medical treatment or those with bowel complications such as perforation or persistent bleeding [12]. Optimal surgical procedures and the length of normal bowel to be resected are still controversial. Some reports suggest that a more extensive surgical resection such as hemicolectomy with as much as 60–100 cm of ileal resection is preferable [26, 136]. However, others recommended a more conservative approach, resecting only grossly involved segments of bowel [30, 137], since there seems to be no difference in the rate of recurrences after either modality. Intestinal lesions, usually at the ileocecal area, tend to recur at the anastomosis site, and often require multiple operations because of perforations and fistula formation [72]. Because of mechanical trauma induced inflammation, the pathergy phenomenon might be important here [138]. To prevent this, authors do not agree on the value of short term corticosteroids use [28, 139]. The type of operation, the location of lesion, and the number of ulcers did not appear to be related to the recurrence in one surgical case series [72]. The recurrence rate of intestinal lesions was approximately 50% at 2 years postoperatively [88]. Several types of postoperative recurrence exist, with the most common type being one or two new deep ulcers, followed by multiple aphthous ulcers and enterocutaneous fistulas. Lesions were found at or near the anastomotic site in 80% of recurrent cases. The usual practice is to examine the bowel during surgery, and bowel resection should include a generous normal resection margin as well as skip lesions. Since preoperative diagnosis is difficult and the recurrence rate is high, postoperative periodic follow-up with endoscopy is strongly recommended, with special attention to the anastomosis site.

Prognosis

The prognosis in GIBD appears to be more guarded than in CD. Medical treatment for GIBD is rather effective in initially inducing remission [140]. This was 67% within 8 weeks in a Korean retrospective survey [140]. In other studies, which included patients with previous abdominal surgery, the initial response rate to medical treatment was lower, 38–46% [30, 88].

The eventual recurrence rates, however, are high. Intestinal lesions recur frequently (25–78%) after medical treatment. In one study, GIBD patients had a poor clinical outcome, with a cumulative recurrence rate of 25% and 43% and cumulative surgery rate of 7% and 15% after 2 and 5 years of diagnosis [140]. According to another Korean study, the overall recurrence rate after successful treatment was 28%; 13% after remission with medical treatment and 50% after surgery [59]. A Japanese survey reported cumulative recurrence rates of 25% and 49%, and cumulative operation rates of 28% and 32% after 2 and 5 years of diagnosis [88]. The cumulative probabilities of reoperation were 18% at 2 years, and 38% at 5 years.

A list of poor prognostic factors have been proposed including, the absence of remission after initial medical treatment and apparent GI symptoms at the time of diagnosis [140]. Furthermore, the shape of intestinal ulcer correlates with prognosis, with typical volcano type ulcers necessitating more frequent surgery [59]. Extensive disease involving the ileum along with the presence of ocular disease and the presence of ASCA were also proposed as poor prognostic markers [65]. The recurrence rates are also relatively high in patients who undergo surgery as a result of perforation or fistula formation.

We do not have much information about the postsurgical follow-up data beyond 10 years. As in other manifestations of BD [141], the GIBD burden may be confined to the early years of the disease course.

Summary

BD commonly involves the GI tract with clinical manifestations similar to those in IBD. Although the true frequency of GIBD is still a matter of debate, it probably is not more than 10–15% in patients with BD. Despite recent advances in diagnosis and treatment, the prognosis remains unsatisfactory.

References

1. Bechgaard P (1940) Et tilfaelds af recidiverende aphtos stomatitis ledsaget af conjunctivitis og ulcerationer paa genitalia og hud. Ugeskr Laeger 102:1019–1023
2. Shimizu T, Ehrlich GE, Inaba G, Hayashi K (1979) Behçet's disease (Behçet syndrome). Semin Arthritis Rheum 8(4):223–260
3. Lee SK, Kim WH (2006) Diagnostic challenges in Asia: intestinal Behçet's disease. Falk Symp 151:1–13
4. Yang SK (2005) Intestinal Behçet's disease. Intest Res 3(1):1–10
5. Kaklamani VG, Vaiopoulos G, Kaklamanis PG (1998) Behçet's disease. Semin Arthritis Rheum 27(4):197–217
6. O'Duffy JD, Carney A, Deodhar S (1971) Behçet's disease: report of 10 cases, 3 with new manifestation. Ann Intern Med 75:561–570
7. Eun HC, Chung H, Choi SJ (1984) Clinical analysis of 114 patients with Behçet's disease. J Korean Med Assoc 27:933–939
8. Chamberlain MA (1977) Behçet's syndrome in 32 patients in Yokshire. Ann Rheum Dis 36:491–499
9. Dilsen N, Konice M, Aral O et al (1993) Risk factors of vital organ involvement in Behçet's disease. In: Weschler B, Godeau F (eds) Behçet's disease, Proceedings of the Sixth International Conference on Behçet's Disease. Excerpta Medica, Amsterdam, pp 165–169
10. Jankowski J, Crombi I, Jankowski R (1992) Behçet's syndrome in Scotland. Post Med J 68:566–570
11. Bang D, Lee JH, Lee ES et al (2001) Epidemiologic and clinical survey of Behçet's disease in Korea: the first multicenter study. J Korean Med Sci 16:615–618
12. Yurdakul S, Tuzuner N, Yurdakul I, Hamuryudan V, Yazici H (1996) Gastrointestinal involvement in Behçet's syndrome: a controlled study. Ann Rheum Dis 55(3):208–210
13. Gurler A, Boyvat A, Tursen U (1997) Clinical manifestations of Behçets disease: an analysis of 2147 patients. Yonsei Med J 38(6):423–427
14. Bang D, Yoon KH, Chung HG, Choi EH, Lee ES, Lee S (1997) Epidemiological and clinical features of Behçet's disease in Korea. Yonsei Med J 38(6):428–436
15. Kural-Seyahi E, Ozdogan H, Yurdakul S, Ugurlu S, Ozyazgan Y, Mat C et al (2004) The outcome of the children with Behçet's syndrome. Clin Exp Rheumatol 22(Suppl 34):116a
16. Chang HK, Kim JW (2002) The clinical features of Behçet's disease in Yongdong district: analysis of a cohort followed from 1997 to 2001. J Korean Med Sci 17:784–789
17. Ng FH, Cheung TC, Chow KC, Wong SY, Ng WF, Chan HC et al (2001) Repeated intestinal perforation caused by an incomplete form of Behçet's syndrome. J Gastroenterol Hepatol 16(8):935–939
18. Tursen U, Gurler A, Boyvat A (2003) Evaluation of clinical findings according to sex in 2313 Turkish patients with Behçet's disease. Int J Dermatol 42(5):346–351
19. Yi SW, Cheon JH, Kim JH, Lee SK, Kim TI, Lee YC et al (2009) The prevalence and clinical characteristics of esophageal involvement in patients with Behçet's disease: a single center experience in Korea. J Korean Med Sci 24(1):52–56
20. Mizushima Y, Inaba G, Mimura Y, Ono S (1988) Diagnostic criteria for Behçet's disease in 1987, and guidelines for treating Behçet's disease. Saishin Igaku 43:382–391
21. Bayraktar Y, Ozaslan E, Van Thiel DH (2000) Gastrointestinal manifestations of Behçet's disease. J Clin Gastroenterol 30(2):144–154
22. Sfikakis PP (2002) Behçet's disease: a new target for anti-tumour necrosis factor treatment. Ann Rheum Dis 61(Suppl 2):ii51–ii53
23. Yazici H, Tuzun Y, Pazarli H, Yurdakul S, Yalcin B, Muftuoglu A (1980) Behçet's disease as seen in Turkey. Haematologica 65(3):381–383
24. Bottomley WW, Dakkak M, Walton S, Bennett JR (1992) Esophageal involvement in Behçet's disease. Is endoscopy necessary? Dig Dis Sci 37(4):594–597

25. Houman MH, Ben Ghorbel I, Lamloum M, Khanfir M, Braham A, Haouet S et al (2002) Esophageal involvement in Behçet's disease. Yonsei Med J 43(4):457–460
26. Kasahara Y, Tanaka S, Nishino M, Umemura H, Shiraha S, Kuyama T (1981) Intestinal involvement in Behçet's disease: review of 136 surgical cases in the Japanese literature. Dis Colon Rectum 24(2):103–106
27. Ning-Sheng L, Ruay-Sheng L, Kuo-Chih T (2005) High frequency of unusual gastric/duodenal ulcers in patients with Behçet's disease in Taiwan: a possible correlation of MHC molecules with the development of gastric/duodenal ulcers. Clin Rheumatol 24(5):516–520
28. Sakane T, Takeno M, Suzuki N, Inaba G (1999) Behçet's disease. N Engl J Med 341(17):1284–1291
29. Yazici H, Tuzun Y, Pazarli H, Yurdakul S, Ozyazgan Y, Ozdogan H et al (1984) Influence of age of onset and patient's sex on the prevalence and severity of manifestations of Behçet's syndrome. Ann Rheum Dis 43(6):783–789
30. Choi IJ, Kim JS, Cha SD, Jung HC, Park JG, Song IS et al (2000) Long-term clinical course and prognostic factors in intestinal Behçet's disease. Dis Colon Rectum 43(5):692–700
31. Lee CR, Kim WH, Cho YS, Kim MH, Kim JH, Park IS et al (2001) Colonoscopic findings in intestinal Behçet's disease. Inflamm Bowel Dis 7(3):243–249
32. Kim DK, Yang SK, Byeon JS, Myung SJ, Jo JY, Choi KD et al (2005) Clinical manifestations and course of intestinal Behçet's disease: an analysis in relation to disease subtypes. Intest Res 3(1):48–54
33. Lang BA, Laxer RM, Thorner P, Greenberg M, Silverman ED (1990) Pediatric onset of Behçet's syndrome with myositis: case report and literature review illustrating unusual features. Arthritis Rheum 33(3):418–425
34. Wu PS, Chen HL, Yang YH, Jeng YM, Lee PI, Chang MH (2005) Intestinal Behçet's disease presenting as neonatal onset chronic diarrhea in an 11-month-old male baby. Eur J Pediatr 164(8):523–525
35. Fujikawa S, Suemitsu T (1997) Behçet's disease in children: a nationwide retrospective survey in Japan. Acta Paediatr Jpn 39(2):285–289
36. Tabata M, Tomomasa T, Kaneko H, Morikawa A (1999) Intestinal Behçet's disease: a case report and review of Japanese reports in children. J Pediatr Gastroenterol Nutr 29(4):477–481
37. Bang DS, Oh SH, Lee KH, Lee ES, Lee SN (2003) Influence of sex on patients with Behçet's disease in Korea. J Korean Med Sci 18(2):231–235
38. Isik B, Ara C, Kirimlioglu H, Sogutlu G, Yilmaz M, Yilmaz S et al (2005) Single or multiple perforations with varying locations as a complication of intestinal Behçet's disease: report of three cases. Scand J Gastroenterol 40(5):599–603
39. Pirildar T, Keser G, Tunc E, Alkanat M, Tuncyurek M, Doganavsargil E (2001) An unusual presentation of Behçet's disease: intestinal perforation. Clin Rheumatol 20(1):61–62
40. Lee RG (1986) The colitis of Behçet's syndrome. Am J Surg Pathol 10(12):888–893
41. Iwama T, Utzunomiya J (1977) Anal complication in Behçet's syndrome. Jpn J Surg 7(3):114–117
42. Kim SU, Cheon JH, Lim JS, Paik SH, Kim SK, Lee SK et al (2007) Massive gastrointestinal bleeding due to aneurysmal rupture of ileo-colic artery in a patient with Behçet's disease. Korean J Gastroenterol 49(6):400–404
43. Smith JA, Siddiqui D (2002) Intestinal Behçet's disease presenting as a massive acute lower gastrointestinal bleed. Dig Dis Sci 47(3):517–521
44. Kim WH, Cho YS, Yoo HM, Park IS, Park EC, Lim JG (1999) Quality of life in Korean patients with inflammatory bowel diseases: ulcerative colitis, Crohn's disease and intestinal Behçet's disease. Int J Colorectal Dis 14(1):52–57
45. Best WR, Becktel JM, Singleton JW, Kern F Jr (1976) Development of a Crohn's disease activity index. National cooperative Crohn's disease study. Gastroenterology 70(3):439–444
46. Cheon JH, Han DS, Park JY, Ye BD, Jung SA, Young Sook Park, You Sun Kim, Joo Sung Kim, Chung Mo Nam, Youn Nam Kim, Suk-Kyun Yang, Won Ho Kim (2010). Development,

Validation, and Responsiveness of a Novel Disease Activity Index for Intestinal Behçet's Disease. Inflamm Bowel Dis (in press)

47. Mori S, Yoshihira A, Kawamura H, Takeuchi A, Hashimoto T, Inaba G (1983) Esophageal involvement in Behçet's disease. Am J Gastroenterol 78(9):548–553

48. Yashiro K, Nagasako K, Hasegawa K, Maruyama M, Suzuki S, Obata H (1986) Esophageal lesions in intestinal Behçet's disease. Endoscopy 18(2):57–60

49. Anti M, Marra G, Rapaccini GL, Barone C, Manna R, Bochicchio GB et al (1986) Esophageal involvement in Behçet's syndrome. J Clin Gastroenterol 8(5):514–519

50. Brodie TE, Ochsner JL (1973) Behçet's syndrome with ulcerative oesophagitis: report of the first case. Thorax 28(5):637–640

51. Morimoto Y, Tanaka Y, Itoh T, Yamamoto S, Kurihara Y, Nishikawa K (2005) Esophagobronchial fistula in a patient with Behçet's disease: report of a case. Surg Today 35(8):671–676

52. Celik AF, Hatemi I (2005) Gastrointestinal involvement of Behçet's syndrome. Turkiye Klinikleri J Int Med Sci 1:48–54

53. Hatemi I, Hatemi G, Celik AF, Melikoglu M, Arzuhal N, Mat C et al (2008) Frequency of pathergy phenomenon and other features of Behçet's syndrome among patients with inflammatory bowel disease. Clin Exp Rheumatol 26(Suppl 50):S91–95

54. Iscimen A, Imren S, Serdaroglu S, Kutlar M et al (1987) The significance of genital scars in the diagnosis of Behçet's syndrome. In: 11th European congress of rheumatology, Athens, Greece, June 28 to July 4, p F327

55. Mat CM, Goksungur N, Engin B, Yurdakul S, Yazici H (2006) The frequency of scarring after ulcers in Behçet's syndrome: a prospective study. Int J Dermatol 45:554–556

56. Lee SK, Kim BK, Kim TI, Kim WH (2009) Differential diagnosis of intestinal Behçet's Disease and Crohn's disease by colonoscopic findings. Endoscopy 41(1):9–16

57. Fresko I, Ugurlu S, Ozbakır F, Celik A, Yurdakul S, Hamuryudan V et al (2005) Anti-Saccharomyces cerevisiae antibodies (ASCA) in Behçet's syndrome. Clin Exp Rheumatol 23(Suppl 38):S67–S70

58. Byeong GK, You SK, Joo SK, Hyun CJ, In SS (2002) Diagnostic role of anti-Saccharomyces cerevisiae mannan antibodies combined with anti-neutrophil cytoplasmic antibodies in patients with inflammatory bowel diseases. Dis Colon Rectum 45:1062–1069

59. Kim JS, Lim SH, Choi IJ, Moon H, Jung HC, Song IS et al (2000) Prediction of the clinical course of Behçet's colitis according to macroscopic classification by colonoscopy. Endoscopy 32(8):635–640

60. Pulimood AB, Ramakrishna BS, Kurian G, Peter S, Mathan MM (1999) Endoscopic mucosal biopsies are useful in distinguishing granulomatous colitis due to Crohn's disease from tuberculosis. Gut 45:537–541

61. Ben Ghorbel I, Ennaifer R, Lamloum M, Khanfir M, Miled M, Houman MH (2008) Budd–Chiari syndrome associated with Behçet's disease. Gastroenterol Clin Biol 32(3):316–320

62. Park JJ, Cheon JH, Kim TI, Kim WH (2009) Correlation of erythrocyte sedimentation rate and C-reactive protein with clinical disease activity in intestinal Behçet's disease. Gut58 (suppl 2):A461

63. Muftuoglu AU, Yazici H, Yurdakul S, Tuzun Y, Pazarli H, Gungen G et al (1986) Behçet's disease. Relation of serum C-reactive protein and erythrocyte sedimentation rates to disease activity. Int J Dermatol 25(4):235–239

64. Quinton J-F, Sendid B, Reumaux D, Cortot A, Grandbastien B, Charrier G et al (1988) Anti-Saccharomyces cerevisiae mannan antibodies combined with antineutrophil cytoplasmic auto-antibodies in inflammatory bowel disease: prevalence and diagnostic role. Gut 42:788–791

65. Choi CH, Kim TI, Kim BC, Shin SJ, Lee SK, Kim WH et al (2006) Anti-Saccharomyces cerevisiae antibody in intestinal Behçet's disease patients: relation to clinical course. Dis Colon Rectum 49(12):1849–1859

66. Krause I, Monselise Y, Milo G, Weinberger A (2002) Anti-Saccharomyces cerevisiae antibodies – a novel serologic marker for Behçet's disease. Clin Exp Rheumatol 20(Suppl 26):S21–S24

67. Makharia GK, Sachdev V, Gupta R, Lal S, Pandey RM (2007) Anti-*Saccharomyces cerevisiae* antibody does not differentiate between Crohn's disease and intestinal tuberculosis. Dig Dis Sci 52(1):33–39, Epub 2006 Dec 8
68. Chang DK, Kim JJ, Choi H, Eun CS, Han DS, Byeon JS et al (2007) Double balloon endoscopy in small intestinal Crohn's disease and other inflammatory diseases such as cryptogenic multifocal ulcerous stenosing enteritis (CMUSE). Gastrointest Endosc 66(Suppl 3):S96–S98
69. Hamdulay SS, Cheent K, Ghosh C, Stocks J, Ghosh S, Haskard DO (2008) Wireless capsule endoscopy in the investigation of intestinal Behçet's syndrome. Rheumatology (Oxford) 47(8):1231–1234
70. Gubler C, Bauerfeind P (2005) Intestinal Behçet's disease diagnosed by capsule endoscopy. Endoscopy 37(7):689
71. Thach BT, Cummings NA (1976) Behçet's syndrome with "aphthous colitis". Arch Intern Med 136(6):705–709
72. Lee KS, Kim SJ, Lee BC, Yoon DS, Lee WJ, Chi HS (1997) Surgical treatment of intestinal Behçet's disease. Yonsei Med J 38(6):455–460
73. Lebwohl O, Forde KA, Berdon WE, Morrison S, Challop R (1977) Ulcerative esophagitis and colitis in a pediatric patient with Behçet's syndrome. Response to steroid therapy. Am J Gastroenterol 68(6):550–555
74. Korman U, Cantasdemir M, Kurugoglu S, Mihmanli I, Soylu N, Hamuryudan V et al (2003) Enteroclysis findings of intestinal Behçet's disease: a comparative study with Crohn disease. Abdom Imaging 28(3):308–312
75. Kim JH, Choi BI, Han JK, Choo SW, Han MC (1994) Colitis in Behçet's disease: characteristics on double-contrast barium enema examination in 20 patients. Abdom Imaging 19(2):132–136
76. Chung SY, Ha HK, Kim JH, Kim KW, Cho N, Cho KS et al (2001) Radiologic findings of Behçet's syndrome involving the gastrointestinal tract. Radiographics 21(4):911–924, discussion 24–26
77. Ha HK, Lee HJ, Yang SK, Ki WW, Yoon KH, Shin YM et al (1998) Intestinal Behçet's syndrome: CT features of patients with and patients without complications. Radiology 209(2):449–454
78. Gullberg E, Soderholm JD (2006) Peyer's patches and M cells as potential sites of the inflammatory onset in Crohn's disease. Ann N Y Acad Sci 1072:218–232
79. Isomoto H, Shikuwa S, Suematsu T, Migita K, Ito M, Kohno S (2008) Ileal lesions in Behçet's disease originate in Peyer's patches: findings on magnifying endoscopy. Scand J Gastroenterol 43(2):249–250
80. Takada Y, Fujita Y, Igarashi M, Katsumata T, Okabe H, Saigenji K et al (1997) Intestinal Behçet's disease pathognomonic changes in intramucosal lymphoid tissues and effect of a "rest cure" on intestinal lesions. J Gastroenterol 32(5):598–604
81. Nara K, Kurokawa MS, Chiba S, Yoshikawa H, Tsukikawa S, Matsuda T et al (2008) Involvement of innate immunity in the pathogenesis of intestinal Behçet's disease. Clin Exp Immunol 152(2):245–251
82. Hayasaki N, Ito M, Suzuki T, Ina K, Ando T, Kusugami K et al (2004) Neutrophilic phlebitis is characteristic of intestinal Behçet's disease and simple ulcer syndrome. Histopathology 45(4):377–383
83. Kobayashi M, Ito M, Nakagawa A, Matsushita M, Nishikimi N, Sakurai T et al (2000) Neutrophil and endothelial cell activation in the vasa vasorum in vasculo-Behçet disease. Histopathology 36(4):362–371
84. Zimmerman GA, Prescott SM, McIntyre TM (1992) Endothelial cell interactions with granulocytes: tethering and signaling molecules. Immunol Today 13(3):93–100
85. Senturk T, Aydintug O, Kuzu I, Duzgun N, Tokgoz G, Gurler A et al (1998) Adhesion molecule expression in erythema nodosum-like lesions in Behçet's disease. A histopathological and immunohistochemical study. Rheumatol Int 18(2):51–57
86. Lakhanpal S, Tani K, Lie JT, Katoh K, Ishigatsubo Y, Ohokubo T (1985) Pathologic features of Behçet's syndrome: a review of Japanese autopsy registry data. Hum Pathol 16(8):790–795

87. Direskeneli H (2001) Behçet's disease: infectious aetiology, new autoantigens, and HLA-B51. Ann Rheum Dis 60(11):996–1002
88. Naganuma M, Iwao Y, Inoue N, Hisamatsu T, Imaeda H, Ishii H et al (2000) Analysis of clinical course and long-term prognosis of surgical and nonsurgical patients with intestinal Behçet's disease. Am J Gastroenterol 95(10):2848–2851
89. Imamura Y, Kurokawa MS, Yoshikawa H, Nara K, Takada E, Masuda C et al (2005) Involvement of Th1 cells and heat shock protein 60 in the pathogenesis of intestinal Behçet's disease. Clin Exp Immunol 139(2):371–378
90. Ahmad T, Zhang L, Gogus F, Verity D, Wallace G, Madanat W et al (2005) CARD15 polymorphisms in Behçet's disease. Scand J Rheumatol 34:233–237
91. Ozen SC, Dagli U, Kilic MY, Toruner M, Celik Y, Ozkan M et al (2006) NOD2/CARD15, NOD1/CARD4, and ICAM-1 gene polymorphism in Turkish patients with inflammatory bowel disease. J Gastroenterol 41:304–310
92. Uyar FA, Over-Hamzaoglu H, Ture F, Gul A, Tozun N, Saruhan-Direskeneli G (2006) Distribution of common CARD15 variants in patients sporadic Crohn's disease cases from Turkey. Dig Dis Sci 51(4):706–710
93. Kobayashi T, Sudo Y, Okamura S, Ohashi S, Urano F, Hosoi T et al (2005) Monozygotic twins concordant for intestinal Behçet's disease. J Gastroenterol 40(4):421–425
94. Hamuryudan V, Yurdakul S, Ozbakir F, Yazici H, Hekim H (1991) Monozygotic twins concordant for Behçet's syndrome. Arthritis Rheum 34(8):1071–1072
95. Soy M, Erken E, Konca K, Ozbek S (2000) Smoking and Behçet's disease. Clin Rheumatol 19:508–509
96. Kaklamani VG, Markkomichelakis N, Kaklamanis PG (2002) Could nicotine be beneficial for Behçet's disease. Clin Rheumatol 21:341–342
97. Edward JB, Koepsell TD, Prera DR, Inuni TS (1987) Risk of ulcerative colitis among former and current cigarette smokers. N Engl J Med 316:707–710
98. Somerville KW, Logan RFA, Edmond M, Langman MJS (1984) Smoking and Crohn's disease. Br Med J 289:954–956
99. Fresko I, Hamuryudan V, Demir M, Hizli N, Sayman H, Melikoglu M et al (2001) Intestinal permeability in Behçet's syndrome. Ann Rheum Dis 60(1):65–66
100. Koc B, Aymelek S, Sonmez A, Yilmaz MI, Kocar H (2004) Increased sucrose permeability in Behçet's disease. Rheumatol Int 24(6):347–350
101. Kobayashi K, Ueno F, Bito S, Iwao Y, Fukushima T, Hiwatashi N et al (2007) Development of consensus statements for the diagnosis and management of intestinal Behçet's disease using a modified Delphi approach. J Gastroenterol 42(9):737–745
102. Shin SJ, Kim BC, Park SY, Kim TI, Kim WH (2005) Systemic manifestations of Behçet's disease in diagnosis of intestinal Behçet's disease. Gut 55:A120
103. Jung HC, Rhee PL, Song IS, Choi KW, Kim CY (1991) Temporal changes in the clinical type or diagnosis of Behçet's colitis in patients with aphthoid or punched-out colonic ulcerations. J Korean Med Sci 6(4):313–318
104. Cheon JH, Kim ES, Shin SJ et al (2009) Development and Validation of Novel Diagnostic Criteria for Intestinal Behçet's Disease in Korean Patients with Ileo-colonic Ulcers. Am J Gastroenterol 104(10):2492–2499
105. Yim CW, White RH (1985) Behçet's syndrome in a family with inflammatory bowel disease. Arch Intern Med 145(6):1047–1050
106. Kim ES, Chung WC, Lee KM, Lee BI, Choi H, Han SW et al (2007) A case of intestinal Behçet's disease similar to Crohn's colitis. J Korean Med Sci 22(5):918–922
107. Naganuma M, Iwao Y, Kashiwagi K, Funakoshi S, Ishii H, Hibi T (2002) A case of Behçet's disease accompanied by colitis with longitudinal ulcers and granuloma. J Gastroenterol Hepatol 17(1):105–108
108. Tolia V, Abdullah A, Thirumoorthi MC, Chang CH (1989) A case of Behçet's disease with intestinal involvement due to Crohn's disease. Am J Gastroenterol 84(3):322–325
109. Smith GE, Kime LR, Pitcher JL (1973) The colitis of Behçet's disease: a separate entity? Colonoscopic findings and literature review. Am J Dig Dis 18(11):987–1000

110. International Study Group for Behçet's Disease (1990) Criteria for diagnosis of Behçet's disease. Lancet 335(8697):1078–1080
111. Balthazar EJ, Gordon R, Hulnick D (1990) Ileocecal tuberculosis: CT and radiologic evaluation. AJR Am J Roentgenol 154(3):499–503
112. Puspok A, Keiner H, Oberhuber G (2000) Clinical, endoscopic, and histologic spectrum of nonsteroidal anti-inflammatory drug-induced lesions in the colon. Dis Colon Rectum 43:685–691
113. Laine L, Connors LG, Reicin A, Hawkey CJ, Burgos-Vagas R, Schnitzer TJ et al (2003) Serious lower gastrointestinal clinical events with nonselective NSAID or Coxib use. Gastroenterology 124:288–292
114. Celik AF, Pamuk ON, Melikoglu M, Yazici H (2008) How to diagnose Behçet's and intestinal Behçet's disease? In: Tozun N, Mantzaris, Daglı U, Schölmerich J (eds) IBD 2007-achievements in research and clinical practice. Springer, Dordrecht, pp 118–128
115. Kurahara K, Matsumoto T, Iida M, Honda K, Yao T, Fujishima M (2001) Clinical and endoscopic features of nonsteroidal anti-inflammatory drug-induced colonic ulcerations. Am J Gastroenterol 96(2):473–480
116. Iida M (1992) Clinical course of intestinal lesions in patients with intestinal disease and simple ulcer. Stomach Intestine 27:287–302
117. Pallis AG, Mouzas IA, Vlachonikolis IG (2004) The inflammatory bowel disease questionnaire: a review of its national validation studies. Inflamm Bowel Dis 10(3):261–269
118. Park KD, Bang D, Lee ES, Lee SH, Lee S (1993) Clinical study on death in Behçet's disease. J Korean Med Sci 8(4):241–245
119. Yoo HM, Han KH, Kim PS, Kim WH, Kang JK, Park IS et al (1997) Clinical features of intestinal Behçet's disease and therapeutic effects of sulfasalazine. Korean J Gastroenterol 29:465–472
120. Houman MH, Hamzaoui K (2006) Promising new therapies for Behçet's disease. Eur J Intern Med 17(3):163–169
121. Sonta T, Araki Y, Koubokawa M, Tamura Y, Ochiai T, Harada N et al (2000) The beneficial effect of mesalazine on esophageal ulcers in intestinal Behçet's disease. J Clin Gastroenterol 30(2):195–199
122. Matsukawa M, Yamasaki T, Kouda T, Kurihara M (2001) Endoscopic therapy with absolute ethanol for postoperative recurrent ulcers in intestinal Behçet's disease, and simple ulcers. J Gastroenterol 36(4):255–258
123. Hamuryudan V, Mat C, Saip S, Ozyazgan Y, Siva A, Yurdakul S et al (1998) Thalidomide in the treatment of the mucocutaneous lesions of the Behçet's syndrome. A randomized, double-blind, placebo-controlled trial. Ann Intern Med 128(6):443–450
124. Bariol C, Meagher AP, Vickers CR, Byrnes DJ, Edwards PD, Hing M et al (2002) Early studies on the safety and efficacy of thalidomide for symptomatic inflammatory bowel disease. J Gastroenterol Hepatol 17(2):135–139
125. Yasui K, Uchida N, Akazawa Y, Nakamura S, Minami I, Amano Y et al (2008) Thalidomide for treatment of intestinal involvement of juvenile-onset Behçet's disease. Inflamm Bowel Dis 14(3):396–400
126. Travis SP, Czajkowski M, McGovern DP, Watson RG, Bell AL (2001) Treatment of intestinal Behçet's syndrome with chimeric tumour necrosis factor alpha antibody. Gut 49(5):725–728
127. Kram MT, May LD, Goodman S, Molinas S (2003) Behçet's ileocolitis: successful treatment with tumor necrosis factor-alpha antibody (infliximab) therapy: report of a case. Dis Colon Rectum 46(1):118–121
128. Lee JH, Kim TN, Choi ST, Jang BI, Shin KC, Lee SB et al (2007) Remission of intestinal Behçet's disease treated with anti-tumor necrosis factor alpha monoclonal antibody (Infliximab). Korean J Intern Med 22(1):24–27
129. Byeon JS, Choi EK, Heo NY, Hong SC, Myung SJ, Yang SK et al (2007) Antitumor necrosis factor-alpha therapy for early postoperative recurrence of gastrointestinal Behçet's disease: report of a case. Dis Colon Rectum 50(5):672–676

130. Naganuma M, Sakuraba A, Hisamatsu T, Ochiai H, Hasegawa H, Ogata H et al (2008) Efficacy of infliximab for induction and maintenance of remission in intestinal Behçet's disease. Inflamm Bowel Dis 14(9):1259–1264

131. Hanauer SB (2003) Crohn's disease: step up or top down therapy. Best Pract Res Clin Gastroenterol 17(1):131–137

132. Mussack T, Landauer N, Ladurner R, Schiemann U, Goetzberger M, Burchardi C et al (2003) Successful treatment of cervical esophageal perforation in Behçet's disease with drainage operation and infliximab. Am J Gastroenterol 98(3):703–704

133. Ju JH, Kwok SK, Seo SH, Yoon CH, Kim HY, Park SH (2007) Successful treatment of life-threatening intestinal ulcer in Behçet's disease with infliximab: rapid healing of Behçet's ulcer with infliximab. Clin Rheumatol 26(8):1383–1385

134. Rossi G, Moretta A, Locatelli F (2004) Autologous hematopoietic stem cell transplantation for severe/refractory intestinal Behçet's disease. Blood 103(2):748–750

135. Yamato K (2003) Successful cord blood stem cell transplantation for myelodysplastic syndrome with Behçet's disease. Int J Hematol 77(1):82–85

136. Sayek I, Aran O, Uzunalimoglu B, Hersek E (1991) Intestinal Behçet's disease: surgical experience in seven cases. Hepatogastroenterology 38(1):81–83

137. Lida M, Kobayayashi H, Matsumoto T, Okada M, Fuchigami T, Yao T et al (1994) Postoperative recurrence in patients with intestinal Behçet's disease. Dis Colon Rectum 37(1):16–21

138. Bozkurt M, Torin G, Aksakal B, Ataoglu O (1992) Behçet's disease and surgical intervention. Int J Dermatol 31(8):571–573

139. Bradbury AW, Milne AA, Murie JA (1994) Surgical aspects of Behçet's disease. Br J Surg 81(12):1712–1721

140. Chung MJ, Cheon JH, Kim SU, Park JJ, Kim TI, Kim NK (2010) Response rates to medical treatments and long-term clinical outcomes of non-surgical patients with intestinal Behçet's disease. J Clin Gastroenterol Jan 5 [Epub ehead of print]

141. Kural-Seyahi E, Fresko I, Seyahi N, Ozyazgan Y, Mat C, Hamuryudan V et al (2003) The long term mortality and morbidity of Behçet's syndrome. A 2-decade outcome survey of 387 patients followed at a dedicated center. Medicine (Baltimore) 82:60–76

142. Uyar FA, Saruhan-Direskeneli G, Gül A (2004) Common Crohn's disease predisposing variants of the CARD15/NOD2 genes are not associated with Behçet's disease in Turkey. Clin Exp Rheumatol 22(Suppl 34):S50–S52

143. Hatemi I, Hatemi G, Senateş, Baysal B, Erzin Y, Celik AF (2008) Low dose thalidomide in immunosuppressive unresponsive IBD; effectiveness and side effects. Gastroenterology 132:4(Suppl 2):A665

144. Yamamoto T, Toyokkawa H, Matsubara JT et al (1974) A nation-wide survey of Behçet's disease in Japan. I. Epidemiological survey. Jpn J Opthalmol 18:282–290

145. Cigerciogulları E, Goksel S, Dogusoy B, Erdamar S, Celik AF, Erzin Y et al (2005) An analysis of the reliability of detection and diagnostic value of various pathologic features in Crohn's disease. Virchows Arch 447(2):P5O7

Chapter 11
Miscellaneous Manifestations of Behçet's Disease

Kenneth T. Calamia and İzzet Fresko

Keywords Amyloidosis • Bladder • Epididymitis • Glomerulonephritis • Impotence • Myelodysplastic • Vestibular

Introduction

Behçet's disease (BD) is a vasculitis with protean manifestations. It was originally described as a triad of oral and genital ulcerations and uveitis but later work has shown that articular, neurological, gastrointestinal, and major vessel involvement may also be part of the clinical picture. Additional manifestations such as the myelodysplastic syndrome, hearing abnormalities, renal disease, amyloidosis, and urologic problems may also be encountered and cause difficulties in the differential diagnosis especially in geographies where the frequency of the disease is low and hence not well recognized.

Hematologic Associations of Behçet's Disease

Hematologic complications are uncommon. When cytopenias are found in a BD patient, the possibility of autoimmune destruction, bleeding, hypersplenism, marrow toxicity from chemotherapy [1, 2], or an associated bone marrow disorder should be considered. There are approximately 30 reported cases of BD associated with the myelodysplastic syndrome (MDS). Most of the individually reported patients have been Japanese [3] but Korean [4] and Chinese [5] patients have also been recognized suggesting more common occurrence along the East Asian rim. The features of these patients have been compared to BD patients without MDS.

I. Fresko (✉)
Department of Internal Medicine, Division of Rheumatology, Cerrahpasa Medical Faculty, Istanbul, Turkey
e-mail: izzetfresko@yahoo.com

Y. Yazıcı and H. Yazıcı (eds.), *Behçet's Syndrome*,
DOI 10.1007/978-1-4419-5641-5_11, © Springer Science+Business Media, LLC 2010

Conversely the characteristics of the MDS has also been examined in patients with and without BD. Intestinal ulceration, occasionally involving the esophagus, has been found in 61–65% of BD cases with MDS [4, 5]. While ileocolonic ulcers are common in Japanese patients with BD, the frequency of these lesions among the patients with BD and MDS is much more common than in Japanese patients without MDS. Severe ulcerations have been associated with massive bleeding in one BD patient with MDS [6]. Uveitis is less frequent (17%) and HLA-B51 is found less frequently (29%) in patients with MDS-associated BD. Many of the diagnosed cases are atypical or of the "incomplete" type.

MDS is associated with trilineage dysplasia in the bone marrow. At the same time intramedullary apoptosis is accelerated under the influence of tumor necrosis factor-α, resulting in peripheral cytopenias despite a normal or hypercellular marrow [7]. Myelodysplastic marrow changes without chromosomal abnormalities have been found in about half of 15 BD without MDS in one study. The rates of apoptosis in BD patients were significantly higher than controls but lower than MDS patients and there was no difference in BD patients with or without morphological abnormalities [7]. Most patients with BD-associated MDS have the trisomy 8 chromosomal abnormality and the incidence of this anomaly in BD-associated MDS is higher than in MDS without BD [8]. The presence of trisomy 8 was found in each of three patients with multiple intestinal ulcers from a series of 43 with MDS without BD [9], and in other MDS cases [10], suggesting that this chromosomal abnormality may have a permissive role in the development of such ulcers. Trisomy 8 is possibly thought to be a risk factor for the development of BD, but the mechanism of this has not been determined. Because of several cytokine and cytokine receptor genes located on chromosome 8, alterations in cytokine levels may be responsible for this association [9]. Like in MDS without BD, most reported cases of BD and MDS have been classified as refractory anemia [5], but other forms of MDS have also been described [4].

The temporal relationship of the development of BD and MDS is variable, but in the majority of patients MDS has preceded or was recognized at the same time as BD [11]. A history of the use of immunosuppressive agents, including azathioprine, chlorambucil, and cyclophosphamide, for treatment of BD may be a causative factor in the development of MDS in some patients [11–13].

Immunosuppressive treatment of BD with associated MDS may be difficult, especially with immunosuppressive agents, because of the limited bone marrow reserve. Successful treatment of both conditions has been reported with myeloablation together with cord blood transplantation to provide stem cells [14–16], and with peripheral stem cell transplantation or bone marrow transplantation [4].

Hematologic disorders may mimic BD and may be a source of diagnostic confusion. Aphthosis can occur in patients with idiopathic or cyclic neutropenia [17, 18] or as the presenting manifestation of the hypereosinophilic syndrome [19]. BD has been reported in patients with chronic myeloid leukemia (CML), especially after treatment with interferon α (INF-α), possibly by augmentation of neutrophil function, but the infrequent association suggests that this may be a coincidence [20, 21].

The pathergy reaction was present in 24% of 29 patients with CML treated with INF-α, studied prospectively, but neither in any of 15 patients prior to the start of treatment nor in patients taking interferon-α for other reasons [22]. The cause of pathergy in these patients has not been determined but altered neutrophil function in both conditions is suspected [22]. BD has developed in a patient with CML under treatment with hydroxyurea [23] and use of this agent has been associated with aggravation of genital lesions in a patient who developed BD and CML at the same time [24]. BD symptoms developed in a patient with CML who had undergone allogenic bone marrow transplantation and had symptoms of chronic graph-versus-host disease [25]. Continued investigations into cytokine aberrations, cellular dysfunction, and immunologic abnormalities in patients with hematologic malignancies and BD may lead to further understanding of the pathogenesis of the disorder. There has been little support for BD as a risk factor for developing solid tumors [26].

Auditory and Vestibular Dysfunction in Behçet's Disease

The prevalence of hearing loss in BD was estimated to be 59% in a recent study of 27 patients compared to 35 age- and sex-matched controls (20%, $P=0.002$) [27]. Other studies have shown a frequency of hearing loss in Behçet patients between 12 and 80%, but the definition of hearing loss and testing used has been variable. Hearing loss ≥30 dB on pure tone audiogram in at least two frequencies was found in 55% of 63 consecutive BD patients compared to 5% of the controls ($P=0.001$)[28]. Using a similar definition, 32% of BD patients among a study group of 62 had hearing loss compared to none of the control patients [29]. In contrast to these findings, other studies have not revealed significant differences between consecutive BD patients and controls in hearing tests using pure tone audiometry [30]. The audiometric findings in reported series have also been variable but bilateral high frequency sensorineural hearing loss, often with a downslope, was most common in larger series [27–29]. The occurrence of high frequency loss, rather than loss at speech frequencies, may result in the failure of the clinician to appreciate hearing difficulties among many other symptoms.

There has been no consistent relationship between hearing loss and the age of the patient or the duration of BD, although some studies suggest that older patients and those with longer disease duration are at greater risk [31, 32]. There has been a suggestion of an association between the presence of hearing loss and uveitis, but there has been little support for an association with disease at other sites [33]. HLA-B51 was found in a higher number of patients with hearing loss compared to BD patients without hearing loss [29, 34]. Pathergy testing was found to be less common in patients with hearing loss than control BD patients in one study [27].

Another test of cochlear function, while not a test of hearing, is the measurement of evoked otoacoustic emissions. These emissions are believed to result from the vibratory motion of the outer hair cells in the organ of Corti and are expected in patients with normal hearing. Sensitive analysis of hearing and cochlear function in BD patients has been accomplished by Transiently Evoked Otoacoustic Emission (TEOAE) and Distortion Product Otoacoustic Emission (DPOAE) [30, 35–37].

These tests detect responses after a sound stimulus. Different regions of the cochlea can be assessed by using different frequency stimuli. In a prospective study of 20 BD patients and 20 controls, pure tone testing was abnormal in 25% of ears and high frequency audiometry was abnormal in 60% among the patients, both more frequent than in control patients. Significant mean reductions were also found in TEOAE between patients and controls [36]. DPOAEs amplitudes were significantly higher at 1 and 2 kHz in a group of BD patients, all of whom had normal pure tone audiometry, than in control patients [30]. In another study, DPOAEs responses were significantly different in 26 BD patients compared to matched controls in all frequencies [35]. These data indicate the possibility of damage to the outer hair cells or to loss of nerve fibers or nerve function in the control of cochlear responses. The particular value of these tests may be in the early detection of subclinical auditory deficiency in BD [37].

Hearing loss has generally been mild in Behçet patients; however, in the earlier surveys moderate-to-severe loss had been recognized more frequently [34]. It is possible that more aggressive treatment of disease in other locations has been responsible for this difference. Hearing loss can be bilateral or unilateral but most typically is gradual in onset, with progression over months to years [31]. However, sudden deafness may be the presenting manifestation of ear involvement. Acute unilateral hearing loss has occurred [29, 34, 38], as well as bilateral sudden and profound hearing losses [34, 39].

Peripheral, rather than central, causes are thought to be responsible for hearing loss, including that seen in those patients with neuro-BD [37]. Support for cochlear involvement was found in all of 20 BD patients with hearing loss in one study [29]. These and the findings by others suggest that the cochlea is the primary site of the pathology [28, 29, 34, 37]. Careful testing is required to recognize other cases of hearing loss in BD patients. A central auditory defect may be responsible for hearing loss, with characteristic abnormalities of brainstem auditory evoked potentials, in patients with neuro-BD [37]. A case of endolymphatic hydrops with tinnitus and bilateral hearing loss in association with BD has been reported [40]. In other individuals, acoustic reflex testing, which measures the movement and stiffness of the tympanic membrane after a loud sound and is dependent on multiple nuclei in the brain stem, or brainstem-evoked response audiometry, which measures compound action potentials of the cochlear nerve and other brainstem and midbrain nuclei to sound, have supported retrocochlear involvement [37, 41].

Evidence for the efficacy of any treatment for hearing loss in BD is limited and anecdotal. Corticosteroids, including pulse steroids, cyclophosphamide, and chlorambucil have been used successfully in the treatment of progressive or abrupt hearing loss in patients with BD. Cyclosporine has been reported to be helpful, [42] but others have found the agent to be ineffective [33, 41].

Cochlear implantation has been used in the treatment of profound hearing loss in BD patients [39, 43], including patient with blindness from the disease [44]. Although the number of BD patients treated and reported is very small, the results of cochlear implantation seem to be similar to patients implanted for other causes. There have been no reports of pathergy-like complications resulting in treatment failure.

Symptoms of vestibular dysfunction include dizziness, vertigo, imbalance or dysequilibrium, and oscillopsia. Vestibular involvement in BD had been reported to occur in 20–40% of BD patients, but testing done to determine abnormalities varied in the reported series. Symptoms of dizziness were found to be very common in BD patients and abnormalities were detected on caloric testing in 29% of patients and on rotation chair testing in 59% of 17 consecutive BD patients but in none of the matched controls [39]. Unilateral peripheral dysfunction was the dominant cause of symptoms when patients were systemically studied [37]. Tests of peripheral vestibular dysfunction, including caloric testing has been normal in some patients with vestibular dysfunction, suggesting a central vestibular defect. These cases are best recognized with the help of a combination of tests of vestibular function. Abnormalities on electronystagmography, saccadic tests, and vestibuloocular reflex testing will support a central rather than a peripheral cause for symptoms [29, 37]. However, magnetic resonance imaging showed no evidence of midbrain or brainstem in 20 patients with evidence of central dysfunction [29]. Patients with isolated central vestibular involvement usually do not have other symptoms or findings that support a diagnosis of neuro-Behçet's syndrome. On the other hand, symptoms of a central vestibular defect can also be a part of more typical central nervous system involvement.

There is no data to support any association of vestibular dysfunction with other manifestations of BD and pathologic data is lacking. However, the association of audiovestibular dysfunction in other systemic vasculitic or autoimmune conditions such as systemic lupus erythematosis, Cogan's syndrome, and Wegener's granulomatosis [45], suggest that similar pathogenic mechanisms, specifically vascular occlusion, may be operative. In addition, there appears to be no strong association between auditory and vestibular dysfunction in BD patients with one or the other complications. The distinct blood supply to involved structures may allow for localized immune, inflammatory involvement that may result in dysfunction of a single process [37].

Renal Involvement and Amyloidosis

Contrary to the ANCA positive vasculitides and the other systemic vasculitides that affect the middle sized vessels, renal involvement is not usually part of BS. However, numerous case reports and several cohorts show that it may occasionally be encountered. A wide variation in frequency between <1 and 29% have been reported but the lack of systematization and standard definitions seem to account for this variability [46–48].

The most frequent mode of presentation is asymptomatic hematuria and/or proteinuria. However, the whole spectrum of renal disease including edema and the nephrotic syndrome, hypertension and renal failure may also be seen [49]. Amyloidosis, glomerulonephritis, renal vascular disease, and possible interstitial involvement are its major forms. Cyclosporine nephrotoxicity should also be considered in the differential diagnosis [50].

Amyloidosis (AA type) is one of the principle forms of renal involvement among patients with BS. It has a frequency that varies between 0.01 and 4.8% in various clinical series [51] and seems to have a geographical predilection centering along the Mediterranean and Middle Eastern countries. It seems to be more rare in the Far East.

Men largely outnumber females and the frequency of male patients are around 80% in most case series. Major vascular involvement in the form of venous thrombi, arterial aneurysms, and occlusions are the major risk factors underlying its development although the presence of arthritis has also been implicated as a predisposition [52–54]. The mean age at the time of its diagnosis was 36.5 years (range 13–70 years) in a literature survey and the mean interval between the first symptom of BS and the development of the complication was approximately 10 years [49]. This period was shorter in males compared to females (9 years vs. 13 years), which goes with the fact that males in general have more severe disease compared to females. It is one of the most lethal complications of BS and has a cumulative 5-year mortality rate of around 50% [54].

The most frequent presentation of amyloidosis is nephrotic syndrome with or without renal failure. A study conducted among the dialysis centers in Turkey showed that it was the most common reason underlying end-stage renal failure and dialysis among patients with BS [50]. Case reports of patients with amyloidosis with trace of proteinuria or without proteinuria have also been reported [55].

Some authors have proposed that amyloidosis is an intrinsic feature of BS not dependent on chronic inflammation or specific predisposing factors [56]. However, this has not been supported in larger studies and available data strongly reinforces major vascular disease as the main risk and a substantial interval of around 10 years between the first symptom and its development.

The geographical predilection for the development of amyloidosis has prompted research concerning various genetic factors that may account for this difference. Several MEVF (also implicated in Familial Mediterranean Fever) mutations including M680I homozygosity [51] and serum amyloid A gene polymorphisms such as SAA1 α/α genotype has been implicated in the pathogenesis [57] but the results were inconclusive.

Colchicine is beneficial in the secondary amyloidosis related to Familial Mediterranean Fever but its role in the amyloidosis of BS has not been evaluated in a formal study. Some case reports have shown an improvement in renal function, decrease in proteinuria and edema under colchicine [58], whereas others have claimed the lack of any effect whatsoever with the drug [54].

Glomerulonephritis

The frequency of glomerulonephritis was <1% in a large series [59]. Some question its relation to BD because of its rarity but its occurrence after the onset of the other manifestations of the syndrome in most of the cases suggests that it is perhaps an inherent part of the syndrome. A study compared the clinical features of patients with BD who had glomerulonephritis to those who did not have glomerulonephritis and did not find a significant difference between the two groups, suggesting the lack of a definite risk factor [60].

The clinical picture of the patients with glomerulonephritis shows a wide variation ranging from asymptomatic hematuria and/or proteinuria to rapidly progressive disease [48]. Hypertension is occasionally present. Acute glomerulonephritis, rapidly progressive glomerulonephritis, nephrotic syndrome and renal failure are also observed. However, some of the cases are clinically silent and are detected upon screening for urinary abnormalities [59]. There are occasional reports concerning progression of silent glomerular disease to overt glomerular involvement [61, 62]. Overall, the course is generally mild and only very few of the patients progress to end-stage renal disease.

Histopathological examination shows a wide variety of lesions ranging from minor glomerular changes to crescentic glomerulonephritis. Focal proliferative, mesangial proliferative, membranous, minimal change and glomerulosclerosis have also been reported. Immunofluorescence examination has shown the deposition of IgG, IgA, IgM, and C3 along the capillaries and the mesangium [63–68]. Pauci-immune and ANCA-associated cases are rare.

There are no formal studies that address the management of glomerulonephritis in BD. Corticosteroids, azathioprine, cyclophosphamide, cyclosporine, and plasmapheresis have been used, but the exact contribution of each of these drugs to the natural course is not known.

Renal Vascular Disease

Renal vascular pathologies as part of major vascular involvement in BD were found in <1% of the patients with vascular involvement, in a review [69].

The most common type is renal arterial aneurysms. They do not have a specific location and can be found anywhere along the renal arteries [70–72]. Rupture and infarcts are common and some cases are bilateral. The most frequent clinical manifestation associated is hypertension. They are mainly observed in males as with other major vascular diseases.

Intrarenal microaneurysms and infarctions are occasionally reported. They sometimes cause nosological problems since the Chapel Hill Classification System defines these types of lesions as classic polyarteritis nodosa but the other manifestations of BD usually aid in the differential diagnosis [73].

Renal vein thrombosis is another form of vascular involvement that is seen in BD and is almost always associated with another major vascular pathology or with the nephrotic syndrome [74].

A peculiar type of vascular involvement is the microvascular manifestations such as perivascular fibrosis around interlobular arteries and arterioles and fibrinoid deposits around vascular walls observed in the occasional patient with hematuria and mild proteinuria [75]. However, it is difficult to delineate a separate category consisting of microvascular changes due to the paucity of data.

Renal vascular involvement may be evaluated by ultrasonography, computed tomography, magnetic resonance angiography, and classical angiography. The best information can be gathered by classical angiography although problems of catheterization due to pathergy-like phenomena have been reported with this imaging technique.

The management of renal vascular involvement has largely been empirical. Corticosteroids along with cyclophosphamide and intravascular procedures such as insertion of stents have been utilized but the value of these therapeutic measures is not known due to the paucity of the cases [76].

End-Stage Renal Failure and BS

A survey performed in the dialysis centers of Turkey have demonstrated that the prevalence of BS was 0.07% among 20,596 patients undergoing hemo or peritoneal dialysis for various conditions [50]. These patients tended to have more vascular, ocular, and arthritic involvement compared to controls and their main risk factors associated with end-stage renal disease was amyloidosis, glomerulonephritis, and cyclosporine use. Vascular access problems such as thrombosis and excessive arterial dilatation were not rare.

Dialysis seemed to reduce the manifestations of BS although the exact contribution of the process itself and that due to the natural course of the syndrome could not be accounted for.

Cases of renal transplantation have also been reported [77] and their short-term prognoses were favorable.

Urologic Manifestations of Behçet's Disease

Aside from genital ulcers, epididymitis or orchitis the most common urological manifestations in males with BD, reported in 6% of 100 newly diagnosed BD patients in Turkey studied prospectively [78]. Surveys in other countries have found varying rates of testicular and peritesticular involvement, suggesting the possibility of geographic or ethnic differences. Differences may reflect different survey methods. The highest reported rate was 31% in a series of prospectively examined male BD patients from Iraq [79].

The clinical features of epididymitis and/or orchitis include the spontaneous occurrence of pain, tenderness, and swelling in the testicles, which is usually unilateral. Fever may accompany the acute inflammation. Symptoms are often present for a few days to 2 weeks before spontaneous resolution, but recurrences are common [80]. Localization of the primary site of inflammation to the epididymis or to the testicle may not be possible clinically if swelling is prominent. The use of the term epididymo-orchitis to describe the clinical presentation reflects this uncertainty. Imaging methods such as testicular ultrasound or scrotal magnetic resonance imaging may assist in accurate localization of the pathologic involvement as well as ruling out comorbid diagnoses. A history of recurrent epididymitis may be associated with findings of thickening and nodularity of the epididymis on physical examination [78]. Surgical removal of the testes for suspected infection or abscess has been reported [78].

The occurrence of epididymo-orchitis may rarely precede other symptoms and signs of BD [81], or be a part of the presenting manifestations, but the complication more typically occurs in patients with established disease [79, 80].

The pathogenesis of epididymo-orchitis in BD patients is unknown. Histology is not available either. Presumably, the inflammation results from vasculitis which is thought to underlie disease manifestations in other organ systems. The involvement of the testicle in other vasculitic syndromes [82], including polyarteritis nodosa [83], rheumatoid vasculitis [84], and the occurrence of isolated testicular vasculitis [85], speaks for a predilection of this organ to be involved in inflammatory vascular disease.

There has been no definite evidence for the participation of infectious agents in cases of epididymo-orchitis in BD patients. Prostatitis may occur in BD patients [86, 87] but the cause of this comorbidity is ill defined. Immunosuppressive agents used in the treatment of BD may predispose to infectious prostatitis, including infection with opportunistic organisms [88]. Sterile urethritis has also been observed [86, 89], in up to 3% of patients in one survey [78]. Relapsing salpingitis has been reported in BD [86], but is so unusual that the occurrence may be coincidental.

When considering symptoms or findings in atypical locations in the Behçet patient, the possibility of localized vascular involvement, especially venous thrombosis, may be responsible. Thrombosis of the veins of the penis has been recognized and thrombosis in the veins of the bladder associated with transmural inflammation and mucosal ulceration with secondary hydroureteronephrosis has been reported [90]. Thrombotic vascular involvement of tissues surrounding the ovaries with resulting inflammation has also been noted in a BD patient at autopsy [91]. Priapism has been reported in two patients with vasculo-BD. In one case, thrombotic obliteration of medium-sized arteries in the penis resulted in infarction of the penile body and corpus cavernosum, requiring distal penectomy. The patient was under treatment for widespread thrombophlebitis at the time with heparin, aspirin, and steroids [92]. In the second case, thrombophlebitis of the cavernous body resulted in vasogenic priapism [93].

Erectile dysfunction was found in up to 63% of patients with neurologic manifestations of BD studied prospectively [94]. In these cases, arterial, veno-occlusive, or mixed vasculogenic impotence was usually responsible.

Urological manifestations are recognized also in children with BD. In a collaborative study of 86 children from five countries, signs of urethritis were found in three cases and orchitis or epdidymitis in four males [95]. In a survey of Iranian children with BD, epidimo-orchitis was found in 7.7% of 52 males with the disease [96]. The occurrence of epididymo-orchitis may support the diagnosis of BD in children in whom fever is a dominant manifestation of BD [97].

Bladder involvement in BD has been reported. Symptoms and findings can result from direct involvement of the bladder by the inflammatory process or can be secondary to central nervous system involvement. Pathologic findings of cystitis were found in ten cases in a series of 170 postmortem examinations on BD patients in Japan and rupture of the bladder was found in one case [98]. Ulcerated bladder mucosa with transmural inflammation and a leukocytoclastic vasculitis was found at operation in a BD patient who presented with a pelvic mass [99]. Eight patients with lower urinary tract symptoms were evaluated at a Behçet center in Istanbul over a 5-year period. Histopathologic findings included thickening of bladder walls and mononuclear inflammatory cell infiltration suggesting ischemia, with a lymphocytic vasculitis in one patient [100]. The incidence of bladder involvement was calculated to be 0.07% of BD patients [100]. Vesicovaginal [101], enterovesical, and urethrovaginal fistulae have occurred in BD patients, presumably from extension of the inflammatory, necrotic process into adjacent tissue.

There are no controlled studies on the treatment of any of the urologic manifestation of BD. Empiric treatment of urogenital disease in Behçet's patients depends on the nature and severity of the complication as well as the presence of disease in other locations. Intra-scrotal inflammation usually subsides with administration of nonsteroidal anti-inflammatory agents but in refractory cases, other agents can be considered [80]. Azathioprine and cyclosporine, used primarily for the treatment of uveitis were both effective in the treatment of recurrent epididymo-orchitis in one reported patient [81]. Interferon-α was also effective in induction and maintenance of remission in patients with multiple disease manifestations including epididymitis [102].

Neurogenic bladder can occur in BD without definite evidence of central nervous system dysfunction [100, 103]. Characteristic urodynamic findings include detrussor hyperreflexia resulting in a failure to store urine as well as and detrusor-sphincter dyssenergia with secondary voiding dysfunction. Intrinsic sphincter deficiency, detrussor overactivity, or areflexia has also been reported. More typically, the neurogenic bladder in BD patients is associated with central nervous system involvement, but the temporal relationship between the development of voiding symptoms to the central nervous system process is quite variable [100]. Typical voiding symptoms are those of overactive bladder syndrome including urinary frequency, urgency, and urge incontinence. Pontine areas in the brainstem are believed to be involved in control of urinary bladder function [94, 104] and the frequent involvement of this area in patients with neuro-Behçet [105] likely explains the voiding dysfunction in these patients [94]. Spinal cord involvement on BD is characteristically associated sphincteric dyssenergia with voiding symptoms as well as sexual dysfunction [106]. The recognition of neurologic complications in BD should include consideration of voiding difficulties that may be associated and patients with voiding problems should be evaluated for the possibility of central nervous system disease.

Voiding dysfunction in BD patients can also result from diabetes insipidus (DI) occurring in association with central nervous system involvement [107, 108]. In reported cases, loss of the high signal intensity of the posterior pituitary gland on magnetic resonance imaging was found. Cerebral venous thrombosis has been found in association with DI, but pathologic studies are lacking and the mechanism for the loss of posterior pituitary function in these cases is not known.

Treatment of BD-associated voiding dysfunction with anti-cholinergic agents such as oxybutinin, combined with intermittent catheterization resulted in increased detrussor compliance and complete continence in 50% of patients [94]. When medical treatment is inadequate, surgical treatment with enterocystoplasty using ileum or sigmoid colon has been used with satisfactory results [109, 110] (see Fig. 11.1)

Bladder cancer has been reported in BD patients both with and without a history of the use of cyclophosphamide treatment [111, 112]. Alkylating agents are also known to have adverse effects on fertility in either sex. Colchicine has been associated with neurotoxic effects and should be considered in patients with voiding dysfunction, especially in the absence of central nervous system involvement. In addition, colchicine may also have an adverse effect on spermatogenesis [113].

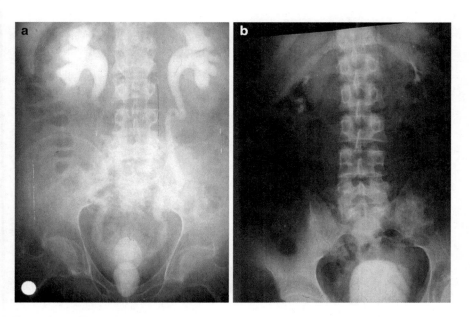

Fig. 11.1 (a) Hydronephrosis due to neurogenic bladder and increased intravesical pressure in a patient with BD (b) Disappearance of hydronephrosis after augmentation iliocystoplasty (Courtesy of B Cetinel)

Behçet's disease patients were used as diseased controls in an ultrasound study of the frequency of kidney stones in patients with ankylosing spondylitis [114]. Only 4 of 72 BD patients (5.5%) were found to have stones, slightly higher than healthy controls (3.3%). Both groups had lower percentage of patients with stones compared to patients with ankylosing spondylitis (25%).

References

1. Rosenthal NS, Farhi DC (1996) Myelodysplastic syndromes and acute myeloid leukemia in connective tissue disease after single-agent chemotherapy. Am J Clin Pathol 106(5):676–679
2. Lee KY, do Kim Y, Chang JY, Bang D (2008) Two cases of acute leukopenia induced by colchicine with concurrent immunosuppressants use in Behçet's disease. Yonsei Med J 49(1):171–173
3. Fine LA, Hoffman LD, Hoffman MD (2007) Aphthous ulcerations associated with trisomy 8-positive myelodysplastic syndrome. J Am Acad Dermatol 57(2 Suppl):S38–S41
4. Ahn JK, Cha HS, Koh EM et al (2008) Behçet's disease associated with bone marrow failure in Korean patients: clinical characteristics and the association of intestinal ulceration and trisomy 8. Rheumatology (Oxford) 47(8):1228–1230
5. Lin YC, Liang TH, Chang HN, Lin JS, Lin HY (2008) Behçet's disease associated with myelodysplastic syndrome. J Clin Rheumatol 14(3):169–174
6. Fujita H, Kiriyama M, Kawamura T et al (2002) Massive hemorrhage in a patient with intestinal Behçet's disease: report of a case. Surg Today 32(4):378–382
7. Arimura K, Arima N, Matsushita K et al (2007) High incidence of morphological myelodysplasia and apoptotic bone marrow cells in Behçet's disease. J Clin Immunol 27(2):145–151
8. Ohno E, Ohtsuka K, Watanabe K et al (1997) Behçet's disease associated with myelodysplastic syndromes. A case report and a review of the literature. Cancer 79(2):262–268
9. Kimura S, Kuroda J, Akaogi T, Hayashi H, Kobayashi Y, Kondo M (2001) Trisomy 8 involved in myelodysplastic syndromes as a risk factor for intestinal ulcers and thrombosis – Behçet's syndrome. Leuk Lymphoma 42(1–2):115–121
10. Kawabata H, Sawaki T, Kawanami T et al (2006) Myelodysplastic syndrome complicated with inflammatory intestinal ulcers: significance of trisomy 8. Intern Med 45(22):1309–1314
11. Eder L, Rozenbaum M, Boulman N et al (2005) Behçet's disease, myelodysplastic syndrome, trisomy 8, gastroenterological involvement – an association. Clin Exp Rheumatol 23(4 Suppl 38):S91–S95
12. Bangerter M, Griesshammer M, Tirpitz Cv et al (1999) Myelodysplastic syndrome with monosomy 7 after immunosuppressive therapy in Behçet's disease. Scand J Rheumatol 28(2):117–119
13. Michels SD, McKenna RW, Arthur DC, Brunning RD (1985) Therapy-related acute myeloid leukemia and myelodysplastic syndrome: a clinical and morphologic study of 65 cases. Blood 65(6):1364–1372
14. Nonami A, Takenaka K, Sumida C et al (2007) Successful treatment of myelodysplastic syndrome (MDS)-related intestinal Behçet's disease by up-front cord blood transplantation. Intern Med 46(20):1753–1756
15. Tomonari A, Tojo A, Takahashi T et al (2004) Resolution of Behçet's disease after HLA-mismatched unrelated cord blood transplantation for myelodysplastic syndrome. Ann Hematol 83(7):464–466
16. Yamato K (2003) Successful cord blood stem cell transplantation for myelodysplastic syndrome with Behçet's disease. Int J Hematol 77(1):82–85
17. Demiroglu H, Dundar S (1997) Behçet's disease and neutropenia. Int J Dermatol 36(7):557–559

18. Rogers RS 3rd (1997) Recurrent aphthous stomatitis: clinical characteristics and associated systemic disorders. Semin Cutan Med Surg 16(4):278–283
19. Leiferman KM, O'Duffy JD, Perry HO, Greipp PR, Giuliani ER, Gleich GJ (1982) Recurrent incapacitating mucosal ulcerations. A prodrome of the hypereosinophilic syndrome. JAMA 247(7):1018–1020
20. Budak-Alpdogan T, Demircay Z, Alpdogan O et al (1997) Behçet's disease in patients with chronic myelogenous leukemia: possible role of interferon-alpha treatment in the occurrence of Behçet's symptoms. Ann Hematol 74(1):45–48
21. Segawa F, Shimizu Y, Saito E, Kinoshita M (1995) Behçet's disease induced by interferon therapy for chronic myelogenous leukemia. J Rheumatol 22(6):1183–1184
22. Budak-Alpdogan T, Demircay Z, Alpdogan O et al (1998) Skin hyperreactivity of Behçet's patients (pathergy reaction) is also positive in interferon alpha-treated chronic myeloid leukaemia patients, indicating similarly altered neutrophil functions in both disorders. Br J Rheumatol 37(11):1148–1151
23. Vaiopoulos G, Terpos E, Viniou N, Nodaros K, Rombos J, Loukopoulos D (2001) Behçet's disease in a patient with chronic myelogenous leukemia under hydroxyurea treatment: a case report and review of the literature. Am J Hematol 66(1):57–58
24. Karincaoglu Y, Kaya E, Esrefoglu M, Aydogdu I (2003) Development of large genital ulcer due to hydroxyurea treatment in a patient with chronic myeloid leukemia and Behçet's disease. Leuk Lymphoma 44(6):1063–1065
25. Cakmak SK, Gul U, Kilic A, Gonul M, Soylu S, Demirel O (2006) Behçet's disease associated with chronic myelogenous leukemia and chronic graft-vs-host disease. Leuk Lymphoma 47(12):2674–2675
26. Kaklamani VG, Tzonou A, Kaklamanis PG (2005) Behçet's disease associated with malignancies. Report of two cases and review of the literature. Clin Exp Rheumatol 23(4 Suppl 38):S35–S41
27. Bakhshaee M, Ghasemi MM, Hatef MR, Talebmehr M, Shakeri MT (2007) Hearing loss in Behçet's syndrome. Otolaryngol Head Neck Surg 137(3):439–442
28. Ak E, Harputluoglu U, Oghan F, Baykal B (2004) Behçet's disease and hearing loss. Auris Nasus Larynx 31(1):29–33
29. Kulahli I, Balci K, Koseoglu E, Yuce I, Cagli S, Senturk M (2005) Audio-vestibular disturbances in Behçet's patients: report of 62 cases. Hear Res 203(1–2):28–31
30. Bayazit YA, Yilmaz M, Gunduz B et al (2007) Distortion product otoacoustic emission findings in Behçet's disease and rheumatoid arthritis. ORL J Otorhinolaryngol Relat Spec 69(4):233–238
31. Evereklioglu C, Cokkeser Y, Doganay S, Er H, Kizilay A (2001) Audio-vestibular evaluation in patients with Behçet's syndrome. J Laryngol Otol 115(9):704–708
32. Brama I, Fainaru M (1980) Inner ear involvement in Behçet's disease. Arch Otolaryngol 106(4):215–217
33. Soylu L, Aydogan B, Soylu M, Ozsahinoglu C (1995) Hearing loss in Behçet's disease. Ann Otol Rhinol Laryngol 104(11):864–867
34. Gemignani G, Berrettini S, Bruschini P et al (1991) Hearing and vestibular disturbances in Behçet's syndrome. Ann Otol Rhinol Laryngol 100(6):459–463
35. Dagli M, Eryilmaz A, Tanrikulu S et al (2008) Evaluation of cochlear involvement by distortion product otoacoustic emission in Behçet's disease. Auris Nasus Larynx 35(3):333–337
36. Muluk NB, Birol A (2007) Effects of Behçet's disease on hearing thresholds and transient evoked otoacoustic emissions. J Otolaryngol 36(4):220–226
37. Pollak L, Luxon LM, Haskard DO (2001) Labyrinthine involvement in Behçet's syndrome. J Laryngol Otol 115(7):522–529
38. Smith LN (1994) Unilateral sensorineural hearing loss in Behçet's disease. Am J Otolaryngol 15(4):286–288
39. Choung YH, Cho MJ, Park K, Choi SJ, Shin YR, Lee ES (2006) Audio-vestibular disturbance in patients with Behçet's disease. Laryngoscope 116(11):1987–1990

40. Igarashi Y, Watanabe Y, Aso S (1994) A case of Behçet's disease with otologic symptoms. ORL J Otorhinolaryngol Relat Spec 56(5):295–298
41. Adler YD, Jovanovic S, Jivanjee A, Krause L, Zouboulis CC (2002) Adamantiades–Behçet's disease with inner ear involvement. Clin Exp Rheumatol 20(4 Suppl 26):S40–S42
42. Elidan J, Levi H, Cohen E, BenEzra D (1991) Effect of cyclosporine A on the hearing loss in Behçet's disease. Ann Otol Rhinol Laryngol 100(6):464–468
43. Quaranta N, Bartoli R, Giagnotti F, Di Cuonzo F, Quaranta A (2002) Cochlear implants in systemic autoimmune vasculitis syndromes. Acta Otolaryngol Suppl 548:44–48
44. Szilvassy J, Czigner J, Jori J et al (1998) Cochlear implantation of a Hungarian deaf and blind patient with discharging ears suffering from Behçet's disease. J Laryngol Otol 112(2):169–171
45. Barna BP, Hughes GB (1988) Autoimmunity and otologic disease: clinical and experimental aspects. Clin Lab Med 8(2):385–398
46. Akpolat T, Dilek M, Aksu K, Keser G, Toprak O, Cirit M, Oğuz Y, Taşkapan H, Adibelli Z, Akar H, Tokgöz B, Arici M, Celiker H, Diri B, Akpolat I (2008) Renal Behçet's disease: an update. Semin Arthritis Rheum 38:241–248
47. Rosenthal T, Weiss P, Gafni J (1978) Renal involvement in Behçet's syndrome. Arch Intern Med 138:1122–1124
48. Kaklamani VG, Nikolopoulou N, Sotsiou F, Billis A, Kaklamanis P (2001) Renal involvement in Adamantiades–Behçet's disease. Case report and review of the literature. Clin Exp Rheumatol 19(5 Suppl 24):S55–S58
49. Akpolat T, Akkoyunlu M, Akpolat I, Dilek M, Odabas AR, Ozen S (2002) Renal Behçet's disease: a cumulative analysis. Semin Arthritis Rheum 31:317–337
50. Akpolat T, Diri B, Oğuz Y, Yilmaz E, Yavuz M, Dilek M (2003) Behçet's disease and renal failure. Nephrol Dial Transplant 18:888–891
51. Akpolat T, Yilmaz E, Akpolat I, Dilek M, Karagoz F, Balci B, Ozen S (2002) Amyloidosis in Behçet's disease and familial Mediterranean fever. Rheumatology (Oxford) 41:592–593
52. Dilsen N, Konice M, Aral O, Erbengi T, Uysal V, Kocak N, Ozdogan E (1988) Behçet's disease associated with amyloidosis in Turkey and in the world. Ann Rheum Dis 47:157–163
53. Yurdakul S, Tüzüner N, Yurdakul I, Hamuryudan V, Yazici H (1990) Amyloidosis in Behçet's syndrome. Arthritis Rheum 33:1586–1589
54. Melikoglu M, Altiparmak MR, Fresko I, Tunc R, Yurdakul S, Hamuryudan V, Yazici H (2001) A reappraisal of amyloidosis in Behçet's syndrome. Rheumatology (Oxford) 40:212–215
55. Chiba M, Inoue Y, Arakawa H, Masamune O, Ohkubo M (1987) Behçet's disease associated with amyloidosis. Gastroenterol Jpn 22:487–495
56. Rosenthal T, Bank H, Aladjem M, David R, Gafni J (1975) Systemic amyloidosis in Behçet's disease. Ann Intern Med 83:220–223
57. Utku U, Dilek M, Akpolat I, Bedir A, Akpolat T (2007) SAA1 alpha/alpha alleles in Behçet's disease related amyloidosis. Clin Rheumatol 26:927–929
58. Tasdemir I, Sivri B, Turgan C, Emri S, Yasavul U, Caglar S (1989) The expanding spectrum of a disease. Behçet's disease associated with amyloidosis. Nephron 52:154–157
59. Altiparmak MR, Tanverdi M, Pamuk ON, Tunc R, Hamuryudan V (2002) Glomerulonephritis in Behçet's disease: report of seven cases and review of the literature. Clin Rheumatol 21:14–18
60. Gürler A, Boyvat A, Türsen U (1997) Clinical manifestations of Behçet's disease: an analysis of 2147 patients. Yonsei Med J 38:423–427
61. Finucane P, Doyle CT, Ferriss JB, Molloy M, Murnaghan D (1985) Behçet's syndrome with myositis and glomerulonephritis. Br J Rheumatol 24:372–375
62. Tietjen DP, Moore WJ (1990) Treatment of rapidly progressive glomerulonephritis due to Behçet's syndrome with intravenous cyclophosphamide. Nephron 55:69–73
63. Fukuda Y, Hayashi H (1982) Renal involvement in Behçet's disease. Ensyo 2:545–548
64. Sugiyama E, Suzuki H, Akagawa N, Yamashita N, Yano S, Iida H, Kitagawa M (1984) [Behçet's disease associated with IgA nephropathy: report of a case]. Nippon Naika Gakkai Zasshi 73:1818–1822

65. Sudo J, Matsubara T, Iwai H, Ueda Y, Kameda S, Iwata T et al (1987) IgA nephropathy developed in a patient with Behçet's disease. Kidney dial 22:893–897

66. Donnelly S, Jothy S, Barré P (1989) Crescentic glomerulonephritis in Behçet's syndrome – results of therapy and review of the literature. Clin Nephrol 31:213–218

67. Hamuryudan V, Yurdakul S, Kural AR, Ince U, Yazici H (1991) Diffuse proliferative glomerulonephritis in Behçet's syndrome. Br J Rheumatol 30:63–64

68. El Ramahi KM, Al Dalaan A, Al Shaikh A, Al Meshari K, Akhtar M (1998) Renal involvement in Behçet's disease: review of 9 cases. J Rheumatol 25:2254–2260

69. Koç Y, Güllü I, Akpek G, Akpolat T, Kansu E, Kiraz S, Batman F, Kansu T, Balkanci F, Akkaya S et al (1992) Vascular involvement in Behçet's disease. J Rheumatol 19:402–410

70. Sueyoshi E, Sakamoto I, Hayashi N, Fukuda T, Matsunaga N, Hayashi K, Inoue K (1996) Ruptured renal artery aneurysm due to Behçet's disease. Abdom Imaging 21:166–167

71. Sherif A, Stewart P, Mendes DM (1992) The repetitive vascular catastrophes of Behçet's disease: a case report with review of the literature. Ann Vasc Surg 6:85–89

72. Han K, Siegel R, Pantuck AJ, Gazi MA, Burno DK, Weiss RE (1999) Behçet's syndrome with left ventricular aneurysm and ruptured renal artery pseudoaneurysm. Urology 54:162

73. Fukuda T, Hayashi K, Sakamoto I, Mori M (1995) Acute renal infarction caused by Behçet's disease. Abdom Imaging 20:264–266

74. Malik GH, Sirwal IA, Pandit KA (1989) Behçet's syndrome associated with minimal change glomerulonephritis and renal vein thrombosis. Nephron 52:87–89

75. Angotti C, D'Cruz DP, Abbs IC, Hughes GR (2003) Renal microinfarction in Behçet's disease. Rheumatology (Oxford) 42:1416–1417

76. Planer D, Verstandig A, Chajek-Shaul T (2001) Transcatheter embolization of renal artery aneurysm in Behçet's disease. Vasc Med 6:109–112

77. Apaydin S, Erek E, Ulkü U, Hamuryudan V, Yazici H, Sariyar M (1999) A successful renal transplantation in Behçet's syndrome. Ann Rheum Dis 58:719

78. Kirkali Z, Yigitbasi O, Sasmaz R (1991) Urological aspects of Behçet's disease. Br J Urol 67(6):638–639

79. Sharquie KE, Al-Rawi Z (1987) Epididymo-orchitis in Behçets disease. Br J Rheumatol 26(6):468–469

80. Kaklamani VG, Vaiopoulos G, Markomichelakis N, Kaklamanis P (2000) Recurrent epididymo-orchitis in patients with Behçet's disease. J Urol 163(2):487–489

81. Callejas-Rubio JL, Ortego N, Diez A, Castro M, De La Higuera J (1998) Recurrent epididymo-orchitis secondary to Behçets disease. J Urol 160(2):496

82. Pannek J, Haupt G (1997) Orchitis due to vasculitis in autoimmune diseases. Scand J Rheumatol 26(3):151–154

83. Eilber KS, Freedland SJ, Rajfer J (2001) Polyarteritis nodosa presenting as hematuria and a testicular mass. J Urol 166(2):624

84. Mayer DF, Matteson EL (2004) Testicular involvement in rheumatoid vasculitis. Clin Exp Rheumatol 22(6 Suppl 36):S62–S64

85. Joudi FN, Austin JC, Vogelgesang SA, Jensen CS (2004) Isolated testicular vasculitis presenting as a tumor-like lesion. J Urol 171(2 Pt 1):799

86. Ek L, Hedfors E (1993) Behçet's disease: a review and a report of 12 cases from Sweden. Acta Derm Venereol 73(4):251–254

87. Zouboulis CC, Kotter I, Djawari D et al (1997) Epidemiological features of Adamantiades–Behçet's disease in Germany and in Europe. Yonsei Med J 38(6):411–422

88. Fuse H, Ohkawa M, Yamaguchi K, Hirata A, Matsubara F (1995) Cryptococcal prostatitis in a patient with Behçet's disease treated with fluconazole. Mycopathologia 130(3):147–150

89. Chajek T, Fainaru M (1975) Behçet's disease. Report of 41 cases and a review of the literature. Medicine (Baltimore) 54(3):179–196

90. Carswell GF (1976) A case of Behçet's disease involving the bladder. Br J Urol 48(3):199–202

91. McDonald GS, Gad-Al-Rab J (1980) Behçet's disease with endocarditis and the Budd–Chiari syndrome. J Clin Pathol 33(7):660–669

92. Ates A, Aydintug OT, Duzgun N, Yaman O, Sancak T, Omur ND (2004) Behçet's disease presenting as deep venous thrombosis and priapism. Clin Exp Rheumatol 22(1):107–109
93. Moalla M, Gabsi M, el Ouakdi M, Zmerli S, Ben Ayed H (1990) Behçet disease and priapism. J Rheumatol 17(4):570–571
94. Erdogru T, Kocak T, Serdaroglu P, Kadioglu A, Tellaloglu S (1999) Evaluation and therapeutic approaches of voiding and erectile dysfunction in neurological Behçet's syndrome. J Urol 162(1):147–153
95. Kone-Paut I, Yurdakul S, Bahabri SA et al (1998) Clinical features of Behçet's disease in children: an international collaborative study of 86 cases. J Pediatr 132(4):721–725
96. Shaefei N, Shahram F, Davatchi F et al (1998) Comparison of juvenile with adult Behçet's disease (A). Arthritis Rheum 41(S124)
97. Pektas A, Devrim I, Besbas N, Bilginer Y, Cengiz AB, Ozen S (2008) A child with Behçet's disease presenting with a spectrum of inflammatory manifestations including epididymoorchitis. Turk J Pediatr 50(1):78–80
98. Lakhanpal S, Tani K, Lie JT, Katoh K, Ishigatsubo Y, Ohokubo T (1985) Pathologic features of Behçet's syndrome: a review of Japanese autopsy registry data. Hum Pathol 16(8):790–795
99. Dokmeci F, Cengiz B, Ortac F (1996) Pelvic mass in a patient with Behçet's disease. Obstet Gynecol 87(5 Pt 2):881
100. Cetinel B, Obek C, Solok V, Yaycioglu O, Yazici H (1998) Urologic screening for men with Behçet's syndrome. Urology 52(5):863–865
101. Monteiro H, Nogueira R, de Carvalho H (1995) Behçet's syndrome and vesicovaginal fistula: an unusual complication. J Urol 153(2):407–408
102. Aoki T, Tanaka T, Akifuji Y et al (2000) Beneficial effects of interferon-alpha in a case with Behçet's disease. Intern Med 39(8):667–669
103. Saito M, Miyagawa I (2000) Bladder dysfunction due to Behçet's disease. Urol Int 65(1): 40–42
104. Karandreas N, Tsivgoulis G, Zambelis T et al (2007) Urinary frequency in a case of Neuro-Behçet disease involving the brainstem - clinical, electrophysiological and urodynamic features. Clin Neurol Neurosurg 109(9):806–810
105. Akman-Demir G, Serdaroglu P, Tasci B (1999) Clinical patterns of neurological involvement in Behçet's disease: evaluation of 200 patients. The Neuro-Behçet Study Group. Brain 122(Pt 11):2171–2182
106. Yesilot N, Mutlu M, Gungor O, Baykal B, Serdaroglu P, Akman-Demir G (2007) Clinical characteristics and course of spinal cord involvement in Behçet's disease. Eur J Neurol 14(7):729–737
107. Szymajda A, Eledrisi MS, Patel R, Chaljub G, Cepeda E, Kaushik P (2003) Diabetes insipidus as a consequence of neurologic involvement in Behçet's syndrome. Endocr Pract 9(1): 33–35
108. Jin-No M, Fujii T, Jin-No Y, Kamiya Y, Okada M, Kawaguchi M (1999) Central diabetes insipidus with Behçet's disease. Intern Med 38(12):995–999
109. Cetinel B, Akpinar H, Tufek I, Uygun N, Solok V, Yazici H (1999) Bladder involvement in Behçet's syndrome. J Urol 161(1):52–56
110. Theodorou C, Floratos D, Hatzinicolaou P, Vaiopoulos G (1999) Neurogenic bladder dysfunction due to Behçet's disease. Int J Urol 6(8):423–425
111. Celik I, Altundag K, Erman M, Baltali E (1999) Cyclophosphamide-associated carcinoma of the urinary bladder in Behçet's disease. Nephron 81(2):239
112. Baltaci S, Gogus C, Karamursel T, Tulunay O (2003) Invasive bladder carcinoma in a patient with Behçet's disease. Int J Urol 10(12):669–671
113. Sarica K, Suzer O, Gurler A, Baltaci S, Ozdiler E, Dincel C (1995) Urological evaluation of Behçet patients and the effect of colchicine on fertility. Eur Urol 27(1):39–42
114. Korkmaz C, Ozcan A, Akcar N (2005) Increased frequency of ultrasonographic findings suggestive of renal stones in patients with ankylosing spondylitis. Clin Exp Rheumatol 23(3):389–392

Chapter 12
Juvenile Behçet's Syndrome

Emire Seyahi and Huri Özdoğan

Keywords Children • Family history • Juvenile Behçet's syndrome • Pediatric Behçet's syndrome • Puberty

Behçet's syndrome (BS) mostly affects adults, with a usual onset in the second and third decades [1]. It is rare in children. In the recent years, there have been a number of reports of childhood BS from various countries, as seen in Table 12.1 [2–13]. However, there is no general agreement on the definition of juvenile BS. Some centers consider the onset of initial symptom, yet others the fulfillment of diagnostic criteria before the age of 16. A significant number of adult patients experience their first symptom in early childhood but it may take years before the disease fully develops. Therefore, we strongly propose the term juvenile BS should cover only those patients who fulfill the ISG criteria for diagnosis [14] before the age of 16. This approach could help us understand and better define the features of childhood BS. Only then it will be possible to see the differences and similarities between adult and juvenile BS. In this chapter, we review the literature and present our findings.

Epidemiology

The prevalence of BS in children aged up to 15 years in France was found to be 1/600,000 [15]. Another field survey done in Turkey screened a total of 46,813 children and found no patients with BS [16]. The prevalence in the latter survey could be calculated as <6/100,000 (within the 95% confidence intervals) according to the zero patient formula [17]. However, pediatric BS registries report higher prevalence rates ranging between 2 and 5% among the whole Behçet population [2, 3, 6, 7, 10, 12]. Male-to-female ratio is almost equal to 1, ranging from 0.7 to 1.4.

E. Seyahi (✉)
Division of Rheumatology, Department of Medicine, Cerrahpasa Medical Faculty,
University of Istanbul, Istanbul, Turkey
e-mail: eseyahi@yahoo.com

Y. Yazıcı and H. Yazıcı (eds.), *Behçet's Syndrome*,
DOI 10.1007/978-1-4419-5641-5_12, © Springer Science+Business Media, LLC 2010

Table 12.1 Comparison of demographic and clinical features of patients with juvenile BS in various series [2–13]

Country of the study, year	Iran, 1993	Tunisia, 1993	Korea, 1994	S.Arabia, 1996	Turkey, 1996	Japan, 1997	Greece, 1998	Israel, 1999	Germany, 1999	France, 2002	Turkey, 2004	Turkey, 2008
References	[2]	[3]	[4]	[5]	[6]	[7]	[8]	[9]	[10]	[11]	[12]	[13]
Juvenile / Adult, n	67/2,175 (3%)	14/582 (2%)	40/–	12/–	95/1,784 (5%)	31/–	18/70	19/–	8/168 (5%)	55/–	121/5,000 (2%)	83/–
Male/ Female, n	33/34, 1	9/5, 1.8	16/24, 0.7	7/5, 1.4	51/44, 1.15	14/17, 0.8	11/7, 1.4	11/8, 1.4	1	21/24, 0.89	61/60, 1	38/45, 0.84
Mean age at onset, years	–	12	10.6	12	13±3	<16	15	7	10.5	12	12.9±2.3	12±4
Mean follow-up, years	–	6±4	–	6	13±7	–	4	10	–	–	Median 8 years	–
Family history (%)	–	14	23	0	9	–	–	–	25	9	19	19
Oral ulcers (%)	77	100	100	100	100	100	100	100	100	100	100	100
Genital ulcers (%)	26	64	83	91	92	58	67	32	82	79	65	82
Papulopustular lesions (%)	61	71	69	33	59	55	50	90	70	38	62	51
Erythema nodosum (%)	Not defined	14	59	25	48	Not defined	44	37	46	26	40	52
Arthritis (%)	2	21	28	75	24	Not defined	61	32	57	17	20	40
Vascular disease (%)	0	29	7	8	19	6	11	11	25	21	14	10
Eye disease (%)	70	14	28	50	27	29	67	47	48	36	60	35
Neurologic disease (%)	0	14	3	50	3	13	17	26	21	24	10	7
Gastrointestinal involvement (%)	0	0	5	0	2	39	11	37	19	2	0.8	5

Familial Aggregation

Interestingly, a higher incidence of familial aggregation has frequently been reported among pediatric patients (9–47%) [3, 4, 6, 10–13, 18]. Although no particular Mendelian inheritance pattern has been shown so far [19], there is strong evidence for a hereditary background in BS [19–21]. Association with HLA and peculiar geographic distribution are in favor of genetic role in the ethiopathogenesis [20]. A high rate of sibling recurrence rate (defined as the ratio of the risk of being affected among the siblings of patients and the risk of being affected in the general population) was also reported in BS [21]. Furthermore, genetic anticipation, in the form of earlier disease onset in children compared with their parents was found to be present in 84% of the families [22]. Some authors suggested that increased prevalence of familial aggregation in juvenile patients with BS may define a subgroup of patients with an autosomal recessive inheritance [23].

Age at Disease Onset and Mode of Onset

Mean age at disease onset has a wide range, starting from a few months to 16 years [2–13]. Studies from Israel, Japan, and Korea report a younger mean age at onset (7–9 years) [4, 7, 9]. Even neonatal, transient BS cases have been reported [24–26]. In all of these babies, mothers had BS and the disease was self-limited with lesions clearing after 6–8 weeks.

The initial symptom is usually recurrent oral ulcers (70–80%), followed by genital ulcers (20–30%), skin lesions (5–15%), and eye disease (5%) [4, 8, 10, 11, 13]. The time period between first manifestation and the evolution of the full disease complex can be quite long ranging between 2 and 8 years [6, 8, 9, 11–13]. In our study this was found to be a mean of 2 years [12]. However, one study found that there was no differing delay in diagnosis between juvenile and adult patients [13].

Puberty

Disease onset before puberty has been reported in a number of series and case reports [6, 9, 12, 27–31]. Sarica et al. noted that 26 (16 M/10 F) of 95 patients (27%) with juvenile BS patients had fulfilled all criteria before reaching puberty [6]. Information about the onset of puberty was present in 58 (28 M/30 F) (48%) of 121 (61 M/60 F) juvenile cases in our series [12]. Disease onset had occurred before puberty in 28 (14 M/14 F, 48%). Among the clinical manifestations, the frequency of erythema nodosum and genital ulceration differed in relation to puberty. While, erythema nodosum was more likely to be present before puberty (17/28 vs. 6/30, respectively $P=0.004$), genital ulcers were more likely to be present

after puberty (13/28 (22%) vs. 23/30 (40%), respectively, $P=0.03$) [12]. The high
frequency of erythema nodosum among prepubertal children has already been
reported [31].

Skin Mucosa Lesions and Arthritis

As seen in Fig. 12.1, skin mucosa lesions are the most commonly reported features
similar to what is observed in adults. Oral ulcers are present in almost all patients
in all series (Table 12.1) and are usually the first symptom. Borlu et al. defined
types and anatomical localization of skin mucosa lesion in juvenile BS patients
[18]. Minor ulcerations were detected in the majority and the common sites were
buccal mucosa, gingiva, inside the lips, and tongue. While major ulceration was
observed only in a few patients, herpetiform type oral ulceration was not detected
at all. Pharyngeal stenosis has been reported as a rare complication of healing
recurrent oral and retropharyngeal ulcers [3, 12].

Genital ulcers are the second most frequent lesions in most studies (Table 12.1)
[2–13, 18]. The most affected areas for genital ulcers are the scrotum and pubis for
boys and major labiae for girls. Scars from previous ulcers can be observed in about
one-third of the patients [18]. We and others observed that genital ulcers were significantly less common among juvenile patients compared to adults (Fig. 12.2)
[2, 9, 12, 13] and were more prevalent in girls (Fig. 12.3) [12]. Furthermore, the
frequency of genital scarring among adult patients is around 65% [32], and this is
considerably higher when compared to that found among children.

Papulopustular lesions is the third most common mucocutaneous manifestation,
present in about 50–60% of the cases with a predilection for upper and lower
extremities, buttocks, and face [2–4, 6–10, 12, 13, 18]. Erythema nodosum is the

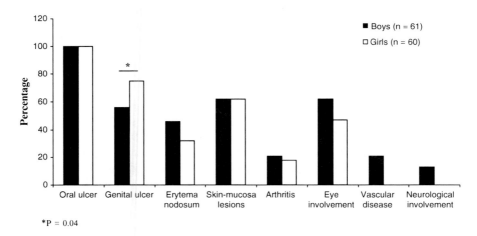

Fig. 12.1 Clinical characteristics at first visit among boys and girls [12]. *$P=0.04$

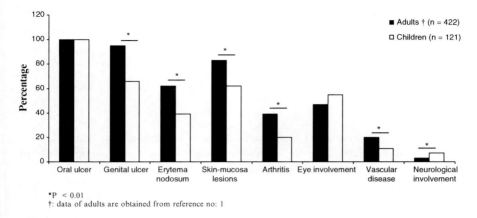

*P < 0.01
†: data of adults are obtained from reference no: 1

Fig. 12.2 Initial clinical characteristics of juvenile BS patients compared with adults†

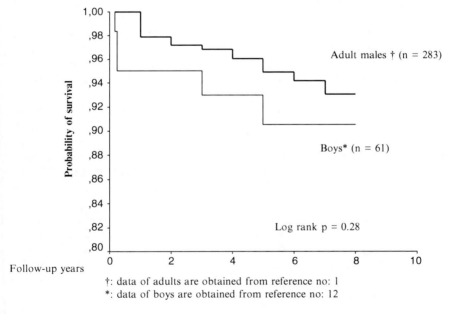

†: data of adults are obtained from reference no: 1
*: data of boys are obtained from reference no: 12

Fig. 12.3 Survival curves comparing adult males† with boys*

least common lesion, being present in 10–30% of the pediatric patients. It is most commonly seen on legs [18]. Peri-anal ulcers, extra-genital ulcers, and Sweet like lesions are other rare skin manifestations.

Episodic arthritis in the form of mono or oligoarthritis is seen in around 20% of the patients [12]. Arthralgias are far more frequent. The most affected joints are knees, elbows, and ankles. No joint deformities have been observed [33]. In our series, papulopustular lesions, erythema nodosum, and arthritis were seen less frequently among juvenile patients compared to the adults (Fig. 12.2) [12]. This was also noted by Shafaie et al. [2].

Eye Disease

In pediatric uveitis series, the prevalence of BS has been reported to be only 0.5–11% [34–37]. Unlike adults, juvenile idiopathic arthritis is the most common cause of uveitis in children, followed by idiopathic uveitis and pars planitis [34–37].

The frequency of eye disease in the published series of juvenile BS ranges between 14 and 70% [2–13]. Its frequency is similar to that reported in the adult case series [8–13]. On the other hand, a relatively lower prevalence (29%) of eye disease among juvenile population compared to adults is noted in Japan [7, 38].

Sungur et al. studied clinical features and complications of eye disease in 62 BS patients dividing them into age groups according to the age of onset [28]. They observed that anterior uveitis was the most common form of uveitis in patients younger than 10 years and that panuveitis with retinal vasculitis was seen frequently in patients older than 10 years [28].

In a retrospective analysis of a large series of Behçet patients with childhood onset uveitis no significant difference was observed, compared to adults with regard to gender predilection, presentation pattern, complications, or clinical outcome [39]. The mean age of uveitis was reported to be 14 years (range: 9–16). Patients were more mostly boys. The involvement was bilateral in the majority of the patients and panuveitis associated with retinal vasculitis was the most common type of involvement. By the end of follow-up (median 5 years), 17% of the patients with uveitis became legally blind [39]. In our series, after a median of 8 years of follow-up of 72 (39 M/33 F) patients with eye disease, the frequency of bilateral useful vision loss was present in 7 (5 M/2 F; 10%), while unilateral vision loss was present in 10 (8 M/2 F; 14%) [12]. The frequency of eye involvement and loss of useful vision among girls was not significantly different than what was observed among the boys [12]. Eye disease in the pediatric population seems to have a somewhat better outcome compared to what has been reported in adults [1, 40]. Recent outcome studies from USA and Israel showing less loss of vision in juvenile BS patients than adults are also in line with this observation [41, 42].

Vascular Involvement

Vascular involvement is seen almost exclusively in boys as in the adults. In our series no vascular disease was observed among girls [12]. It is less frequent among children compared to the adults [3–13]. Yet it may still run a severe unrelenting course with poor prognosis [3–13, 43–46]. Vascular involvement was present in

15% of boys (17/61) at initial visit and developed additionally in 13% (8/61) during the follow-up, in our study [12]. Large vessels were relatively more affected with the following frequencies: pulmonary artery aneurysms (4/17, 24%), vena cava thrombosis (3/17, 18%), Budd–Chiari syndrome (1/17, 6%), deep vein thrombosis of lower extremities (6/17, 35%), and superficial vein thrombosis (3/17, 18%) [12]. This has been also reported by others [3].

Neurological Involvement

There are mainly two types of neurological disease in BS: parenchymal CNS disease, and dural sinus thrombosis [47, 48]. Parenchymal CNS disease develops later during the follow-up and causes severe neurologic deficits. Dural sinus thrombi type of involvement is associated with venous thrombosis elsewhere in the body. It may cause intracranial hypertension with symptoms such as headache, nausea, vomiting and diplopia and has a better prognosis than parenchymal involvement. The frequency of neurological involvement is increased among juvenile population compared to the adults (Table 12.1 and Fig. 12.2). While, dural sinus thrombosis is the predominant type of neurological involvement especially in studies from Turkey [12], parenchymal type of involvement was the more dominant type in other juvenile series reported from France, Israel and Saudi Arabia [5, 9, 11, 49].

Intestinal Involvement

Intestinal disease is characterized by deep ulcers located commonly in the terminal ileum or the ileocecal region. They tend to perforate or penetrate the intestinal wall [50, 51]. The prevalence of the disease varies with geography; it is considered to be a common finding in the Far-East, in Japan and Korea, but rare in the Middle-East such as in Turkey [52]. Interestingly, intestinal involvement was reported to be more common in juvenile patients compared to the adults from countries of both geographical regions such as Japan, Korea, Israel and Turkey [4, 7, 9, 38]. In our series, only one boy (1/121, 0.8%) was found to have intestinal involvement [12].

Mortality and Outcome

As in adults, morbidities such as vascular and neurological disease and mortality are more pronounced among boys (Figs. 12.1–12.3). We observed five deaths (all males) among 121 juvenile patients (4%) during a follow-up of 8 years [12]. The causes of death were massive hemoptysis due to pulmonary artery aneurysms in two boys (both died at age 17), Budd–Chiari syndrome (1 boy died at age 10), suicide (1 boy died at age 20), and aspiration pneumonia caused by stricture due to healing recurrent oral and retropharyngeal ulcers (1 boy died at age 16). Mortality rates among boys [12] and adult males [1] were comparable (Fig. 12.3).

Management

Treatment principles are no different than that used in adults. Azathioprine, corticosteroids, colchicine, cyclosporine, cyclophosphamide, and interferon are used to treat juvenile BS patients [12]. In our series, while azathioprine and corticosteroids were used frequently among boys, colchicine followed by azathioprine were the main drugs for girls [12]. Reports suggest that interferon, infliximab, and thalidomide could be effective in treating resistant cases with juvenile BS [53–56]

References

1. Kural-Seyahi E, Fresko I, Seyahi N et al (2003) The long-term mortality and morbidity of Behçet's syndrome: a 2-decade outcome survey of 387 patients followed at a dedicated center. Medicine (Baltimore) 82:60–76
2. Shafaie N, Shahram F, Davatchi F et al (1993) Behçet's disease in children. In: Wechsler B, Odeau PG (eds) Behçet's disease. Excerpta Medica, Amsterdam, pp 381–383
3. Hamza M (1993) Juvenile Behçet's disease. In: Wechsler B, Odeau PG (eds) Behçet's disease. Excerpta Medica, Amsterdam, pp 377–380
4. Kim DK, Chang SN, Bang D, Lee ES, Lee S (1994) Clinical analysis of 40 cases of childhood-onset Behçet's disease. Pediatr Dermatol 11:95–101
5. Bahabri SA, al-Mazyed A, al-Balaa S, el-Ramahi L, al-Dalaan A (1996) Juvenile Behçet's disease in Arab children. Clin Exp Rheumatol 14:331–335
6. Sarica R, Azizlerli G, Köse A, Dişçi R, Ovül C, Kural Z (1996) Juvenile Behçet's disease among 1784 Turkish Behçet's patients. Int J Dermatol 35:109–111
7. Fujikawa S, Suemitsu T (1997) Behçet's disease in children: a nationwide retrospective survey in Japan. Acta Paediatr Jpn 39:285–289
8. Vaiopoulos G, Kaklamani VG, Markomichelakis N, Tzonou A, Mavrikakis M, Kaklamanis P (1999) Clinical features of juvenile Adamantiades–Behçet's disease in Greece. Clin Exp Rheumatol 17:256–259
9. Krause I, Uziel Y, Guedj D et al (1999) Childhood Behçet's disease: clinical features and comparison with adult-onset disease. Rheumatology (Oxford) 38:457–462
10. Treudler R, Orfanos CE, Zouboulis CC (1999) Twenty-eight cases of juvenile-onset Adamantiades–Behçet's disease in Germany. Dermatology 199:15–19
11. Koné-Paut I, Gorchakoff-Molinas A, Weschler B, Touitou I (2002) Paediatric Behçet's disease in France. Ann Rheum Dis 61:655–656
12. Seyahi E, Ozdogan H, Uğurlu S et al (2004) The outcome children with Behçet's syndrome. Clin Exp Rheumatol 22(4 Suppl 34):116
13. Karincaoglu Y, Borlu M, Toker SC et al (2008) Demographic and clinical properties of juvenile-onset Behçet's disease: a controlled multicenter study. J Am Acad Dermatol 58:579–584
14. International Study Group for Behçet's Disease (1990) Criteria for diagnosis of Behçet's disease. Lancet 335:1078–1080

15. Koné-Paut I, Bernard JL (1993) Behçet's disease in children: a French nationwide survey. Arch Fr Pediatr 50:145–154
16. Ozen S, Karaaslan Y, Ozdemir O et al (1998) Prevalence of juvenile chronic arthritis and familial Mediterranean fever in Turkey: a field study. J Rheumatol 25:2445–2449
17. Yazici H, Biyikli M, van der Linden S, Schouten HJ (2001) The 'zero patient' design to compare the prevalences of rare diseases. Rheumatology (Oxford) 40:121–122
18. Borlu M, Uksal U, Ferahbaş A, Evereklioglu C (2006) Clinical features of Behçet's disease in children. Int J Dermatol 45:713–716
19. Bird Stewart JA (1986) Genetic analysis of families of patients with Behçet's syndrome: data incompatible with autosomal recessive inheritance. Ann Rheum Dis 45:265–268
20. Gül A (2001) Behçet's disease: an update on the pathogenesis. Clin Exp Rheumatol 19(5 Suppl 24): S6–S12
21. Gül A, Inanc M, Ocal L, Aral O, Koniçe M (2000) Familial aggregation of Behçet's disease in Turkey. Ann Rheum Dis 59:622–625
22. Fresko I, Soy M, Hamuryudan V et al (1998) Genetic anticipation in Behçet's syndrome. Ann Rheum Dis 57:45–48
23. Molinari N, Kone Paut I, Manna R, Demaille J, Daures JP, Touitou I (2003) Identification of an autosomal recessive mode of inheritance in paediatric Behçet's families by segregation analysis. Am J Med Genet 122A(2):115–118
24. Stark AC, Bhakta B, Chamberlain MA, Dear P, Taylor PV (1997) Life-threatening transient neonatal Behçet's disease. Br J Rheumatol 36:700–702
25. Lewis MA, Priestley BL (1986) Transient neonatal Behçet's disease. Arch Dis Child 61:805–806
26. Fam AG, Siminovitch KA, Carette S, From L (1981) Neonatal Behçet's syndrome in an infant of a mother with the disease. Ann Rheum Dis 40:509–512
27. Yurdakul S, Ozdogan H, Kasapcopur O et al (1993) Behçet's syndrome with juvenile onset: report of 44 patients. Clin Exp Rheum 11(S9):71
28. Sungur GK, Hazirolan D, Yalvac I et al (2009) Clinical and demographic evaluation of Behçet's disease among different paediatric age groups. Br J Ophthalmol 93:83–87
29. Brik R, Shamali H, Bergman R (2001) Successful thalidomide treatment of severe infantile Behçet's disease. Pediatr Dermatol 18:143–145
30. Yuksel Z, Schweizer JJ, Mourad-Baars PE, Sukhai RN, Mearin LM (2007) A toddler with recurrent oral and genital ulcers. Clin Rheumatol 26:969–970
31. Ozdogan H (1996) Behçet's syndrome in children. In: Ansell BM, Bacon PA, Lie JT, Yazici H (eds) The vasculitides. Chapman & Hall, London, pp 416–424
32. Mat MC, Goksugur N, Engin B, Yurdakul S, Yazici H (2006) The frequency of scarring after genital ulcers in Behçet's syndrome: a prospective study. Int J Dermatol 45:554–556
33. Yurdakul S, Yazici H, Tüzün Y et al (1983) The arthritis of Behçet's disease: a prospective study. Ann Rheum Dis 42:505–515
34. Kanski JJ, Shun-Shin GA (1984) Systemic uveitis syndromes in childhood: an analysis of 340 cases. Ophthalmology 91:1247–1252
35. Tugal-Tutkun I, Havrlikova K, Power WJ, Foster CS (1996) Changing patterns in uveitis of childhood. Ophthalmology 103:375–383
36. Pivetti-Pezzi P (1996) Uveitis in children. Eur J Ophthalmol 6:293–298
37. Soylu M, Ozdemir G, Anli A (1997) Pediatric uveitis in southern Turkey. Ocul Immunol Inflamm 5:197–202
38. Tabata M, Tomomasa T, Kaneko H, Morikawa A (1999) Intestinal Behçet's disease: a case report and review of Japanese reports in children. J Pediatr Gastroenterol Nutr 29:477–481
39. Tugal-Tutkun I, Urgancioglu M (2003) Childhood-onset uveitis in Behçet's disease: a descriptive study of 36 cases. Am J Ophthalmol 136:1114–1119
40. Tugal-Tutkun I, Onal S, Altan-Yaycioglu R, Huseyin Altunbas H, Urgancioglu M (2004) Uveitis in Behçet's disease: an analysis of 880 patients. Am J Ophthalmol 138:373–380
41. Kesen MR, Goldstein DA, Tessler HH (2008) Uveitis associated with pediatric Behçet's disease in the American midwest. Am J Ophthalmol 146:819.e2–827.e2

42. Friling R, Kramer M, Snir M, Axer-Siegel R, Weinberger D, Mukamel M (2005) Clinical course and outcome of uveitis in children. J AAPOS 9:379–382

43. Koné-Paut I, Yurdakul S, Bahabri SA et al (1998) Clinical features of Behçet's disease in children: an international collaborative study of 86 cases. J Pediatr 132:721–725

44. Antar KA, Keiser HD, Peeva E (2005) Relapsing arterial aneurysms in juvenile Behçet's disease. Clin Rheumatol 24:72–75

45. Kutay V, Yakut C, Ekim H (2004) Rupture of the abdominal aorta in a 13-year-old girl secondary to Behçet's disease: a case report. J Vasc Surg 39:901–902

46. Besbas N, Ozyürek E, Balkanci F et al (2002) Behçet's disease with severe arterial involvement in a child. Clin Rheumatol 21:176–179

47. Akman-Demir G, Serdaroglu P, Tasci B (1999) Clinical patterns of neurological involvement in Behçet's disease: evaluation of 200 patients. The Neuro-Behçet Study Group. Brain 122:2171–2182

48. Siva A, Kantarci OH, Saip S et al (2001) Behçet's disease: diagnostic and prognostic aspects of neurological involvement. J Neurol 248:95–103

49. Kone-Paut I, Chabrol B, Riss JM, Mancini J, Raybaud C, Garnier JM (1997) Neurologic onset of Behçet's disease: a diagnostic enigma in childhood. J Child Neurol 12:237–241

50. Kasahara Y, Tanaka S, Nishino M, Umemura H, Shiraha S, Kuyama T (1981) Intestinal involvement in Behçet's disease: review of 136 surgical cases in the Japanese literature. Dis Colon Rectum 24:103–106

51. Yi SW, Cheon JH, Kim JH et al (2009) The prevalence and clinical characteristics of esophageal involvement in patients with Behçet's disease: a single center experience in Korea. J Korean Med Sci 24:52–56

52. Yurdakul S, Tüzüner N, Yurdakul I, Hamuryudan V, Yazici H (1996) Gastrointestinal involvement in Behçet's syndrome: a controlled study. Ann Rheum Dis 55:208–210

53. Guillaume-Czitrom S, Berger C, Pajot C, Bodaghi B, Wechsler B, Kone-Paut I (2007) Efficacy and safety of interferon-alpha in the treatment of corticodependent uveitis of paediatric Behçet's disease. Rheumatology (Oxford) 46:1570–1573

54. Saurenmann RK, Levin AV, Rose JB et al (2006) Tumour necrosis factor alpha inhibitors in the treatment of childhood uveitis. Rheumatology (Oxford) 45:982–989

55. Yasui K, Misawa Y, Shimizu T, Komiyama A, Kawakami T, Mizoguchi M (2003) Thalidomide therapy for juvenile-onset entero-Behçet's disease. J Pediatr 143:692–694

56. Kari JA, Shah V, Dillon MJ (2001) Behçet's disease in UK children: clinical features and treatment including thalidomide. Rheumatology (Oxford) 40:933–938

Chapter 13
Behçet's Disease: Pathology

Cuyan Demirkesen, Büge Öz, and Süha Göksel

Keywords Acne vulgaris • Behçet's disease • Behçet's syndrome • Brain edema • Cardiomegaly • Dural sinus thrombosis • Encephalomyelopathy • Endarteritis obliterans • Folliculitis • Gliosis • Immune complexes • Leukocytoclastic vasculitis • Lymphocytic vasculitis • Meningoencephalitis • Micro-abscess formation • Nodular opacities in the lung • Non-parenchymal CNS involvement • Parenchymal CNS involvement • Pathology • Pleural effusion • Pseudoaneursym • Pulmonary artery aneurysms • Pyloric metaplasia • Right ventricular thrombi • Sweet's syndrome • Toxic megacolon • Vasa brava • Vasa longa • Vasa recta • Vasculopathy

Behçet's disease (BD) has no strict pathognomonic features on histopathology, while it has a rather wide spectrum of microscopic changes which will be summarized and discussed.

Mucocutaneous Lesions

The mucocutaneous lesions are the hallmark of BD [1]. Oral and genital/extragenital ulcers, acneiform and papulopustular lesions, erythema nodosum (EN)-like lesions, superficial thrombophlebitis, and the pathergy reaction (test) are particularly important. Other rare manifestations are Sweet's syndrome-like lesions, pyoderma gangrenosum, erythema multiforme, pernio-like lesions, neutrophilic eccrine hidradenitis, bullous lesions due to necrotizing vasculitis, palpable purpura, and Kaposi sarcoma [2–10].

Oral Ulcers

The histopathology of oral aphthae in BD is quite similar to the lesions of idiopathic recurrent aphthous stomatitis (RAS).

C. Demirkesen (✉)
Pathology Department, Cerrahpaşa Medical Faculty, Istanbul University, Istanbul, Turkey
e-mail: cdemirkesen@yahoo.com

Y. Yazıcı and H. Yazıcı (eds.), *Behçet's Syndrome*,
DOI 10.1007/978-1-4419-5641-5_13, © Springer Science+Business Media, LLC 2010

The squamous epithelium, on the surface is replaced by a necrotic, fibrinopurulent exudate. Inflammatory cells, both lymphocytes and neutrophils, and regenerative changes in keratinocytes can be detected in the epithelium adjacent to the ulcer. The underlying mucosa is heavily infiltrated with neutrophils, lymphocytes, histiocytes, and plasma cells. There is prominent vascular proliferation, together with endothelial swelling. Partial occlusion of the vascular lumen and rarely leukocytoclastic vasculitis have been reported [11, 12]. The number of mast cells was found to be more than in RAS and controls [13]. In a recent study, upregulation of certain cytokeratin (CK) subtypes as well as apoptotic markers was observed along with a significant reduction in proliferative activity of the epithelium by the use of Ki-67. This is unusual for many other inflammatory skin lesions [14].

Genital Ulcers

The histopathology is similar to that in oral aphthous lesions. A neutrophil-predominating infiltrate is a feature of early lesions. In older lesions, the inflammatory cells are mostly lymphocytes, along with histiocytes and plasma cells. Chun reported lymphocytic vasculitis in almost half of the cases, while leukocytoclastic vasculitis was rare [12]. Other vascular changes such as thickening of the vessel walls, endothelial swelling, tendency for obliteration were reported particularly in small arteries and the capillaries [11].

Papulopustular and Acneiform Lesions

The histopathology of papulopustular lesions ranges from leukocytoclastic vasculitis to a lesser dense neutrophilic vascular reaction [15]. There may be findings of follicular involvement similar to those of deep suppurative folliculitis or acne vulgaris, as well. Some consider these follicular lesions nonspecific for BD and state that only papulopustular lesions with vessel-based histology should be considered as a criterion of BD [16] (see Chap. 4). There has been considerable discussion whether the dermal injury in BD is immune complex mediated [17, 18]. The weight of evidence, also in the light of more recent data, is that it is not immune complex mediated [19].

In follicular lesions, a neutrophil-predominating infiltrate around the hair follicle, with or without destruction of the follicular epithelium and sebaceous gland is the most common finding. There may be intrafollicular abscess formation along with infundibular plugging by keratin and sebaceous material (comedone). This is also what is seen in acne vulgaris [20]. There might be small vessel thickening and deposition of fibrinoid material in the vessel wall, more likely to be secondary to acute inflammation rather than a true neutrophilic vascular reaction [12].

Nonfollicular papulopustular lesions display both superficial and deep leukocyte, mononuclear cell or mixed cell infiltration mainly around vessels more likely representing a true vasculitis [21]. Sometimes, pustule formation without vasculitic changes may be seen.

EN-Like Nodular Lesions

The histopathological features of panniculitis due to BD, are mostly characterized by neutrophil-predominating infiltrate mainly in lobules, extending to septum of the subcutis (Figs. 13.1 and 13.2). A neutrophilic vasculitis, involving mostly arterioles and venules, can be detected in almost half of the cases [22, 23]. Chun et al.

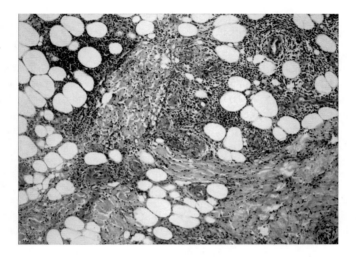

Fig. 13.1 EN-like nodular lesion: Panniculitis due to BD, involving mainly the lobules, extending to septum of the subcutis, together with vascular changes (HE×40)

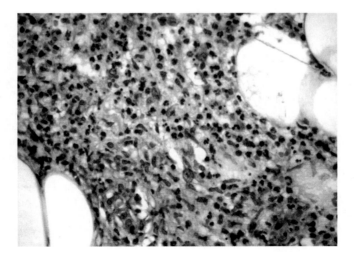

Fig. 13.2 Neutrophil predominating infiltrate in the lobulus of the subcutis (HE×400)

reported the presence of lymphocytic vasculitis, however, it may be a secondary phenomenon rather than a primary vasculitis [24]. Necrobiosis and leukocytoclasia are other common features seen in BD. Granuloma formation is infrequent. Nodular lesions of BD may resemble nodular vasculitis (NV) histologically, but can be distinguished from EN, associated with other diseases [25].

There have been several studies of adhesion molecules expressing the EN-like lesions [26–29]. No consistent pattern has yet been established.

Superficial Thrombophlebitis

These lesions clinically resemble EN-like lesions and, being more common in men, are clinically important in that they are frequently associated with other forms of vascular disease in BD (see Chap. 4). Small to medium sized veins of deep dermis or the subcutaneous fat tissue are obliterated with organizing thrombosis. The walls show fibrous thickening, sometimes accompanying mononuclear cell infiltrate. Besides subcutaneous veins, thrombosis may also involve the deeper veins.

Sweet's Syndrome-Like Lesions

There is dense, diffuse, or patchy neutrophilic infiltration within the dermis, sometimes extending to the subdermis. In later stages, this neutrophilic infiltration can be replaced by lymphohistiocytic infiltration. The Sweet syndrome-like neutrophilic dermatosis is considered as a neutrophilic vascular reaction not infrequently encountered in BD [30].

Pathergy Reaction (See Also Chap. 4)

In response to a needle-prick, dermal inflammation, composed of lymphocytes, neutrophils, eosinophils, mainly localized around the vessels, are detected starting after 12 h, becoming denser at 24 h [31]. Edema and leukocytoclasia are seen in most cases. Intraepidermal pustules develop, correlated with the clinical pathergy response. There is debate whether vascular changes are primary or secondary in the formation of the pathergy reaction [31, 32].

Haim and Gilhar reported an increase in the number of mast cells in pathergy lesions, however, this finding was not confirmed by others [18, 31, 32].

Ocular Involvement

The most common ocular symptom is a panuveitis, and the presence of retinovascular lesions, especially retinal vasculitis, involving the venous system [33]. Due to retinal vasculitis, hemorrhagic infarction of the retina that may lead to blindness and exudation, also, hemorrhages into the vitreus are common. Venous thrombosis can be seen. As a rare manifestation of BD, conjunctival ulcerations may occur. The histopathologic examination of these ulcers reveal intraepithelial and perivascular infiltration with neutrophils, lymphocytes, plasma cells and histiocytes in conjunctiva [34, 35]. In the central areas, neutrophils were reported to be prominent [35]. The infiltrating lymphocytes are mainly T-cells [35].

Cardiovascular Manifestations

BD is a multisystemic disease affecting vessels of all sizes, ranging from great blood vessels to capillaries. Involvement of great vessels is referred to as vasculo-Behçet's Disease (vBD). The lesions of vBD range from arterial occlusions and aneurysms to superficial thrombophlebitis and occlusion of the superior and inferior vena cavae [36]. Other than visceral organ vessel involvement, the most common systemic vessel involvement of BD is listed in Table 13.1 [37].

With aortic disease, there is irregular fibrous thickening in all layers and focal aneurysmal dilatation [38]. Aneurysm formation most commonly involves the abdominal aorta but also occurs in the aortic arch and the other large vessels [39]. Aneurysms usually have fusiform or saccular shape. The aneurysms are usually filled with a thick thrombus showing a lamellar structure.

With the naked eye, the intimal surface of the entire aorta is usually rough and wrinkled indicating scattered aortitis (Fig. 13.3) [40]. There is loss or interruption of the medial elastic fibers (Fig. 13.4) along with perivascular lymphocytic infiltra-

Table 13.1 Vascular involvement in Behçet's disease (modified from Ref. 37)

Arterial involvement
  Systemic arterial vasculitis
  Aneurysms/ pseudo aneurysms
  Stenosis
  Occlusions
Venous involvement
  Venous occlusion
  Superficial venous thrombosis
  Deep venous thrombosis
  Vena cava thrombosis
  Varices

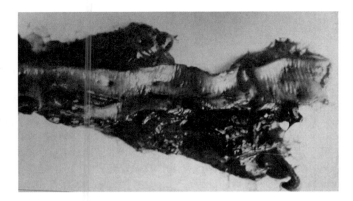

Fig. 13.3 Gross aspect of wrinkled areas on the intimal surface of chronic aortic involvement in vasculo-Behçet's disease

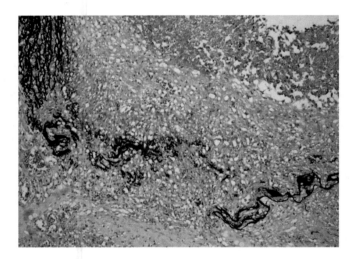

Fig. 13.4 Fragmentation and splitting of elastic fibers in the aneurysm wall (HE×100)

tion with the proliferation of the vasa vasorum. In active aortitis, the cellular infiltrate is predominantly composed of neutrophils, lymphocytes and plasma cells, admixed with histiocytes and eosinophils.

A granulomatous type of vasculitis which is histologically indistinguishable from Takayasu's aortitis can occur particularly in childhood BD, with a grave prognosis [40]. Fibrous thickening of the adventitia and the proliferation of the vaso vasorum accompany chronic large vessel involvement (Fig. 13.5). Occlusion and stenoses frequently are seen in the medium and smaller arteries where the changes in the vasa vasorum are not paramount [41].

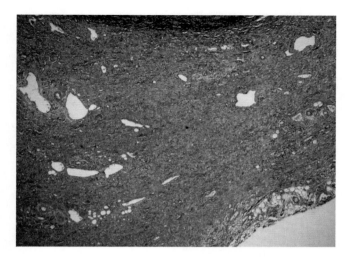

Fig. 13.5   Fibrous thickening of the adventitia and the proliferation of the vaso vasorum (EVG×100)

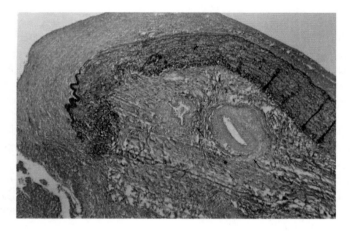

Fig. 13.6   Total loss of elastic fibers in pseudoaneurysm in aorta (*left side of the figure*). Note the myointimal thickening in the vaso vasorum wall (EVG×100)

Other arterial lesions may involve vessels of various sizes, including pulmonary, cerebral, carotid, subclavian, brachial, ulnar, renal, iliac, femoral and popliteal arteries, and arterioles. The pathogenesis of arterial aneurysms is thought to be obliterative endarteritis of vaso vasorum, resulting in dilatation and aneurysm or pseudoaneursym formation (Fig. 13.6) [42, 43]. When the vessel is not thrombosed, the severe inflammation leads to weakening of the arterial wall. This is the mechanism behind the pseudoanuerysms [41].

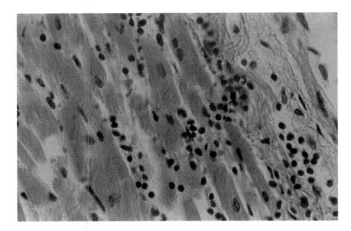

Fig. 13.7 Lymphocytic infiltration among the myocardial muscle fibers in myocardial involvement of BD (=myocarditis) (HE×200)

The luminal obstruction by organized thrombi is the main pathological feature in venous occlusions. The pathogenesis of the thrombotic tendency is unclear (see Chap. 14). Another underlying pathological change in some lesions of BD is a vasculitis involving veins, venules, capillaries, and arterioles. Mostly, it is seen as a leukocytoclastic vasculitis, due to the invasion of the vessel wall by neutrophils, fibrinoid necrosis, leukocytoclasis, endothelial swelling, and extravasation of erythrocytes. Less commonly, a lymphocytic vasculitis can be seen [44]. Cardiomegaly can occasionally be seen along with endocarditis, pericardial effusion, myocardial fibrosis, and aortic valve disease [39]. The second most common manifestation of cardiac involvement is pericarditis [45]. Myocarditis can also be seen with an inflammatory cell infiltrate of predominantly lymphocytes, plasma cells, histiocytes, and small number eosinophils (Fig. 13.7) [46, 47]. This can result in cardiomegaly and myocardial fibrosis. Right ventricular thrombi can be found in patient with vBD and is often associated with pulmonary artery aneurysms (PAAs) [37]. Endomyocardial fibrosis has been reported rarely [48]. Myocardial infarction due to thrombus or vasculitis of the coronary arteries is also another rare presentation of cardiac disease [49].

Pulmonary Manifestations (See Also Chap. 7)

The pulmonary artery is the second most common site of arterial involvement in BD after the aorta while the most frequent pathology in the lung is the (PAA) [50]. BD also is the most common cause of PAA [51]. PAAs are located most frequently in the right lower lobar arteries, followed by the right and the left main pulmonary

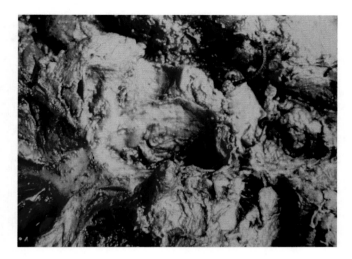

Fig. 13.8 Gross aspect of saccular type of aneurysm in one of the pulmonary arteries of the left lower lobe

arteries [50, 51]. Aneurysms in BD are fusiform or saccular (Fig. 13.8), commonly multiple and bilateral. Their size may reach up to 7 cms [52].

Pathologically, the basic lesion is a lymphocytic and necrotizing vasculitis involving all sizes of pulmonary arteries, veins, and septal capillaries [53]. Pulmonary arteries affected, range from the lobar and segmental branches down to the arterioles [53, 54]. Inflammatory cell infiltration in and around the vessel wall consists mostly of mononuclear inflammatory cells, predominantly lymphocytes. It is transmural in smaller vessels, and subintimal in the large muscular arteries [55]. The large sized vessel involvement is mainly seen in association with vasculitis of the vasa vasorum [53–55]. Some cases show neovascularization of vasa vasorum. The involvement of the vasa vasorum leads to the destruction and loss of elastic fibers and of smooth muscle cells in the media layer or to transmural necrosis ending in formation of true aneurysms. There is fragmentation and splitting of elastic fibers in media initially. Peculiar newly formed collateral vessels lacking elastic lamellae and smooth muscle metaplasia can be seen between the arterioles [53]. Inflammatory thrombotic occlusion is one frequent outcome of the aneurysm (Fig. 13.9). Some of the pulmonary aneurysms can rupture to adjacent bronchus and cause major hemorrhage (Fig. 13.10).

On the basis of these pathological observations, the pathogenesis of PAA is thought to be a chronic ischemic process due to endarteritis obliterans of small vessels, resulting in dilatation and aneurysm or pseudoaneurysm formation and perforation through the bronchial wall [53–55]. It is not uncommon to see aneurysms and pseudoaneurysms side by side in BD [54]. PAA formation seems to be a slowly developing pathology at least in some patients. Striking periadventitial fibrosis develops and is believed to be related to the repetitive vascular inflammatory insults [53, 56].

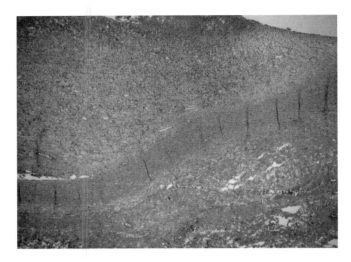

Fig. 13.9 Inflammatory occlusive thrombus formation in lumina of an aneurysm in a pulmonary artery (HE×100)

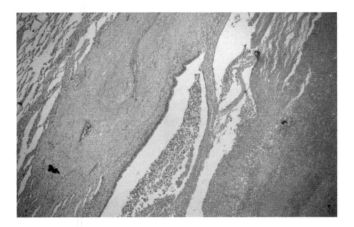

Fig. 13.10 Rupture of the pulmonary artery aneurysm through a bronchus (HE×40)

The weakening and loss of integrity of the vascular layers also cause dissection of the vessel wall alongside the occlusion of the vessel lumen [56]. It is not known why PAAs are often multiple and bilateral whereas peripheral aneurysms are usually single [36]. Thrombosis of the pulmonary arteries in BD is often due to local thrombus formation rather than pulmonary emboli [52]. Thrombotic occlusion and recanalization can be seen not only inside the PAA, but also in some medium and small size arteries (Fig. 13.11).

In addition to PAA, various peripheral pulmonary pathologies are common in BD. The most frequent parenchymal lesions that can be seen on CT, are subpleural

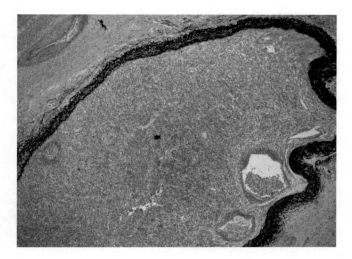

Fig. 13.11 Recanalization in an occlusive thrombus in a pulmonary artery (EVG×100)

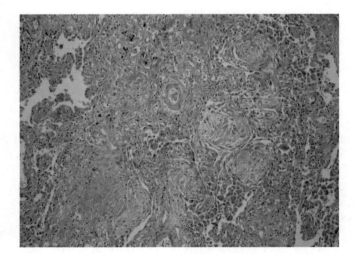

Fig. 13.12 Organizing pneumonia pattern in lung of BD (HE×100)

alveolar infiltrates and wedge-shaped or ill-defined rounded areas of increased opacity, peripheral mosaicism, resulting from focal air trapping [57, 58]. Pathological examination of these lesions shows various histopathological changes such as pulmonary infarcts, pulmonary recurrent pneumonia, bronchitis, fibrosis, and emphysema [39, 57, 59]. These nodular opacities represent hemorrhages, atelectasis, cryptogenic organizing pneumonia (Fig. 13.12), or eosinophilic pneumonia [59, 60]. Some of the nodular opacities can cavitate, and particularly then, it is difficult to differentiate them from lung infections [61, 62]. Pneumonias in BD can be the result of inflammation of pulmonary parenchymal vessels or may occur secondary to immunosuppressive therapy [63, 64].

Vasculitis of the pleura may result in the formation of pleural nodules, which are often difficult to differentiate from parenchymal subpleural lesions. Pleural effusion may be attributed to pulmonary infarction, vasculitis of the pleura, or superior vena cava thrombosis [58].

Neurologic Involvement (See Also Chap. 6)

The first full description of autopsy findings in a patient with neuro Behçet's disease (NB) was reported by Berlin in 1944 [65]. Almost all we know about the pathology of NB is still based on reports of autopsy cases [39, 66–70].

Pathologically, CNS manifestation of BD can be categorized into two main groups (1) Parenchymal CNS involvement (NB), which includes brainstem involvement, hemispheral manifestations, spinal cord lesions, and encephalitic presentations, (2) Nonparenchymal CNS involvement (neuro-vasculo-BD), which includes dural sinus thrombosis, arterial occlusion, and arterial aneurysms [70–72] (see Chap. 6).

Parenchymal CNS Involvement

Parenchymal involvement of CNS is a meningoencephalitis of various kinds.

Many of the pathological changes, as discussed below do not seem to be the result of a true necrotizing cerebral vasculitis. On the other hand, a true vasculitis can also be seen as in Fig. 13.13.

Pathological changes are seen mainly in the midbrain, pons, and medulla. The prominent gross pathological change in most of chronic NB is the atrophy of basal pons, which sometimes goes together with the formation of small cysts. There can be fibrous thickening of the meninges. Marked atrophy of the cerebrum with a prominent enlargement of ventricles has been reported in severe cases [73]. Focal softening and discoloration of the brain tissues is a macroscopic feature of subacute NB [67, 74, 75]. There is perivascular (mainly perivenular or pericapillary) infiltration of lymphocytes/plasma cells and slight glial scarring. A mild myelin breakdown and nerve cell degeneration can be seen. Perivascular inflammatory cell infiltration consists of histiocytes and some microglia as well as lymphocytes and plasma cells. Some gross necrotic foci are characterized by micro-abscess formation histologically [74]. Hiroshi et al. suggested that some findings in brain lesions are closely related to this abscesses formation [75]. They illustrated scattered foci of abscesses in cerebrum and brain stem, where numerous neutrophils were found. In the surrounding micro-abscesses areas, lymphocytic, histiocytic, and leukocytic

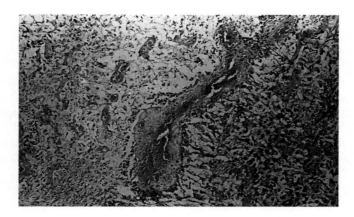

Fig. 13.13 Leukocytoclastic vasculitis in the wall of a medium-sized vessel in the brain paren-chyme. Note the gemistocyte proliferation around the vessel (HE×100)

infiltration was observed, predominantly in the perivascular regions [74]. In chronic cases of NB, histopathology is consistent with an isomorphic gliosis [70]. Diffuse myelin pallor can be seen in the entire white matter in mildly involved cases. It seems to result from severe brain edema, and not from demyelinization.

Another histopathologic finding of chronic NB is the small necrotic foci, characterized with foamy cells, few glial cells and lymphocytic infiltration without perivascular inflammation. This is called encephalomyelopathy [76]. These paren-chymal manifestations of chronic NB are called as secondary demyelination, neuronal loss and gliosis of the recent literature [71, 77]. Arai et al. proposed that it is possible that perivascular inflammation induces ischemia, resulting in destruction of the brain tissue and vessels, demyelination and gliosis [77]. The histological changes can also be seen in the optic nerves. In the bilaterally pseudohypertrophic inferior olivary nuclei, many neuronal cells show vacuolar degeneration with some gliosis [77]. Finally solitary cerebral abscess is very rare.

Nonparenchymal CNS Involvement (Neuro-Vasculo-BD (NvB))

In most of the NvB cases, the vascular pathology is venous [71, 72, 78]. In one-third of NvB patients, cerebral venous sinus thrombosis or thrombophilebitis have been reported [79]. Cerebral venous thrombosis can also cause bilateral subdural effusions [80]. Intracranial cerebral artery stenosis or occlusion is very rare [81, 82]. On the other hand, bilateral internal carotid artery occlusion, verte-bral artery occlusion, and intracranial arteritis, as well as aneurysms have been reported [78, 81, 83, 84]. Most of the cerebral aneurysms in NvB are located in the supratentorial region [74].

Intracranial hemorrhage may rarely occur and presents within ischemic lesions [83]. A rare presentation of NB is the mass lesion that mimics a brain tumor clinically and radiologically. In 1993, Gery et al. described a patient with tumor-like manifestations of NB [85]. Yoshimura et al. pointed out that histopathologically there was necrosis with macrophage and lymphocyte infiltration, together with a small amount glial proliferation, but no perivascular inflammation in this type of tumor-like mass lesion [86]. In such lesions, necrotic areas with perivascular lympho-plasmocytic inflammation and gliosis were reported by different observers [87].

Involvement of the choroid plexus, extensively studied in some other vasculitides, like systemic lupus [88, 89], to our knowledge, has not formally been looked at in BD.

Gastrointestinal Manifestations

The whole alimentary canal from mouth to anus may be involved in patients with BD. Except the oral cavity which is by far the most frequently involved area, the order of frequency can be listed as ileum, colon, other parts of the small intestine, stomach, esophagus, and pharynx [90]. The pathological features of oral apthae have already been described above.

Pharyngeal Involvement

Major lesions are deep, extensive ulcers and/or stenosis which can give pain and difficulty in swallowing in the pharynx [91, 92].

Ulcers are characterized by necrosis of the mucosa and submucosa, and extensive vasculitis in the base of these ulcers may be found [92]. A localized myositis has also been noted [93].

Esophageal and Gastric Involvement

Both are rare in patients with BD.

Single or multiple aphthous ulcers, perforated ulcers, diffuse esophagitis, and severe esophageal stenosis have been described [94, 95]. The most common lesions are the aphthous ulcers in the stomach and duodenum. Punched out ulcers can also be detected. Pyloric stenosis which is a consequence of edematous hypertrophy of the pylorus may occur [96]. A unique study from China proposed that gastroduodenal ulcers were a common manifestation among the Chinese patients [97].

Histopathologic features are usually nonspecific, and similar to peptic and Helicobacter associated gastric and duodenal diseases. Active and chronic nonspecific inflammatory cell infiltration may occur in the mucosa. The experience about the histological features of the gastric and duodenal BD in the surgically resected material is very scanty.

The vasculitis affecting the vessels adjacent the duodenal wall may rupture into the bowel lumen and may cause fatal gastrointestinal bleeding [98].

Intestinal Involvement

Two important generalizations can be made about intestinal involvement, a major cause of morbidity and mortality especially among the patients reported from the Far East, in BD. (1) Intestinal BD is essentially an ischemic bowel disease caused by vasculitis of mesenteric vessels, of the arteries or veins; in the gut wall or in the extramural branches of the mesenteric vessels, (2) Pathology of the said involvement is, in many patients, identical to that found in Crohn's disease (CD).

The whole spectrum of the ischemic bowel diseases caused by mesenteric vascular pathologies can also be seen in patients with BD [90, 99–101].Vasculo-BD affecting aorta, celiac axis, superior and inferior mesenteric arteries, and veins may cause intestinal manifestation [102–105]. Indeed, all vascular pathologies described within the context of BD that affect mesenteric arterial and venous branches of various sizes can also result in intestinal BD [106]. The intestinal manifestations vary depending on the vessel type; the type of vascular pathology and severity and extensiveness of the vascular pathology.

Transient, mild, or moderate degrees of bowel ischemia resulting in acute ischemic enteritis and/or colitis may heal spontaneously. Hyper acute, transmural bowel ischemia generally causes bowel infarction. On the other hand, continuous and permanent ischemia that is over 1 month duration is followed by stricturing ischemia or chronic nonresolving ischemia in the bowel [107, 108].

Stricturing ischemia mimicking CD in both the small and large bowel; and chronic nonresolving ischemia mimicking both CD and ulcerative colitis (UC) in the large bowel are well known [109–114].

Similarities between CD and BD are also well established. The clinical manifestations [115–117], laboratory findings [118–120], radiological findings [121], and pathological findings [122–128] resemble each other.

On the other hand, if the nonresolving chronic mesenteric ischemia occurs in the large bowel in a patient with BD, the clinicopathological picture may mimic ulcerative colitis more as it also occurs in chronic ischemic colitis due to other reasons, where the pathology is similar [129, 130].

The main macroscopic lesion of the intestinal BD is ulceration. Many different types of ulcers have been described, the most common being the aphthous ulcer (Fig. 13.14). Other types are punched out ulcers, volcano-type ulcers, geographic and linear ulcers as well as ulcers of indeterminate appearance. All these lesions may be found in the same patient (Fig. 13.15). Aphthous ulcers are shallow and a few millimeters in diameter with partially irregular borders. Punched out ulcers

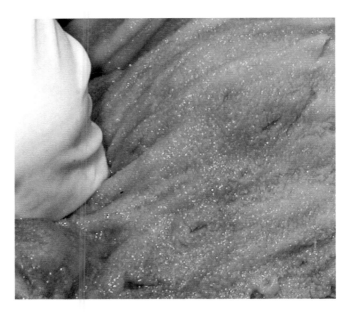

Fig. 13.14 Aphthous ulcers in the small bowel

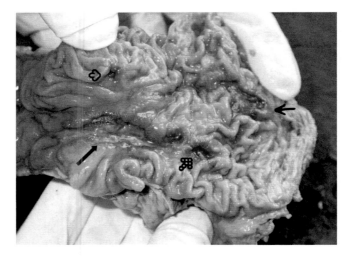

Fig. 13.15 Punch-out ulcer (*blank arrow*), volcano-type ulcer (*dotted arrow*), discrete ulcer (*thin arrow*), and geographic ulcer (*rectangular arrow*)

are a few centimeters in diameter, sharply demarcated, and the depth may vary, but are usually confined to the bowel wall. Volcano-type ulcers are deep oval ulcers with marginal elevation. Their sizes vary and usually are up to one centimeter. They may reach the subserosa or serosal surface. Discrete ulcers may be shallow or very deep.

Geographic ulcers are the largest kind ulcer described in intestinal BD. Perforation and penetration may occur in deep ulcers. Synchronic and/or metachronic multiple bowel perforations are characteristics of intestinal BD. In addition to the linear ulcers, the cobble-stoning, fissures and thickening of the bowel wall, and pseudopolyps, which are the features of CD, can also be seen in intestinal BD. The distribution of these lesions may be local or diffuse [122, 124, 125, 127, 131–133]. Lee et al. have classified the intestinal BD according to the distribution patterns of the lesions such as focal single, focal multiple, segmental, and diffuse [134]. The most frequently involved area is the ileum. Vasa recta are mesenteric vessels between the arquad arcade and the bowel wall. Vasa recta have two branches: vasa longa (long branch) and vasa brava (short branch) [135]. Anthony et al. have shown that short branches of the vasa recta supply the mesenteric margins of the bowel wall, and in the ileum these short vessels are end arteries [136]. This may explain why ileum is the most frequently involved region in intestinal BD characterized by mesenteric vascular pathologies.

Histopathologically, all types of ulcers show nonspecific features. The microscopical variations are directly dependent on the depth, age, and activity of the ulcers. The base of the ulcer is composed of fibrinopurulent exudates and necrotic debris independent of the depth of the ulcer in earlier lesions. Fibrous tissue develops at the base of the chronic ulcer. In most chronic cases, transmural fibrosis occurs. In case of ulcer perforation, the perforated site is characterized by mural necrosis and inflammatory exudation from bowel lumen to serosal surface.

The mucosa adjacent to the chronic ulcer may have signs of chronic enteritis and colitis. Pyloric metaplasia is a common finding, especially in the small intestine. The vasculitic changes, recent and organizing thrombus in the small vessels (small arteries, small veins, and smaller vessels such as arteriole, venule, and capillaries) that are placed immediately adjacent to ulcer base are usually secondary changes due to surrounding fibroinflammatory process. This may cause a false diagnosis of primary vasculitis [122]. Different stages of vasculitis and involvement of both intramural and extramural vessels may be seen in the same specimen (Fig. 13.16). The presence of different stages of the vasculitis and the occurrence of both intramural and extramural vessel pathologies support the diagnosis of a true vasculitis (Fig. 13.17). Arterial involvement associated with venous involvement has also been described in BD [137, 138]. This association may also be seen in mesenteric vessels in intestinal BD (Fig. 13.18).

As emphasized before, intestinal BD may exhibit all the histopathologic features of the CD. Infiltration of Crohn's-like lymphoid follicles throughout the whole thickness of the bowel wall and fibrous obliteration of the submucosa, neuronal hyperplasia, and lymphangiectasia may be seen in patients with intestinal BD. The mucosa of the large bowel may appear entirely normal. The unique striking finding in the mucosa is dense eosinophil infiltration in such cases (Fig. 13.19). Eosinophil activation in the intestinal mucosa occurs in many intestinal diseases including inflammatory bowel disease and NSAID-induced enteropathy [139–142]. This feature creates additional difficulty in the process of differential diagnosis among intestinal BD, NSAID effect, and Crohn's disease, especially in microscopic investigation of the endoscopic biopsy.

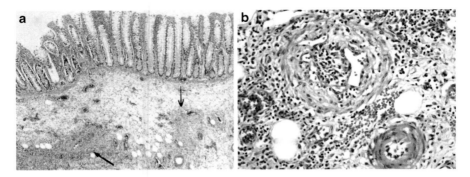

Fig. 13.16 (**a**) Beginning of organization of the thrombus in the submucosal artery with lympho-cytic vasculitis (*rectangular arrow*), complete occlusion with organizing thrombus in the other submucosal vessel (*vertical arrow*). There are not any dense chronic inflammation and fibrosis around the vessels in the submucosa (HE×100). (**b**) The small sized artery is occluded with orga-nizing thrombus in the mesenteric fat tissue outside the bowel wall (the same patient in Fig. 16a) (HE×200)

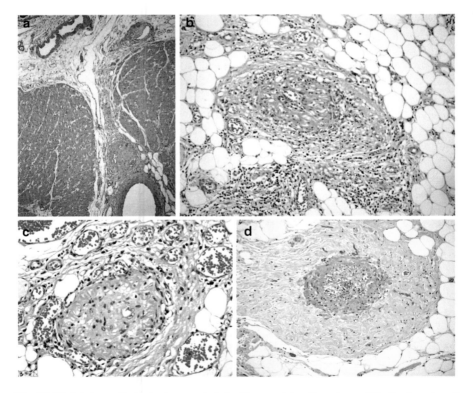

Fig. 13.17 (**a**) A small sized artery occluded with organizing thrombus within the bowel wall (HE×100). (**b–d**) Healing vasculitis and organization of thrombi in different stages in small sized extramural arteries in different locations (the same patient in Fig. 17a) (HE×200)

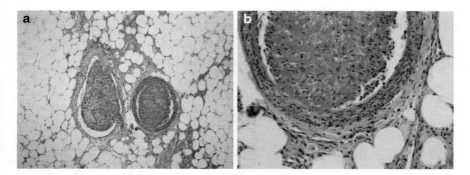

Fig. 13.18 (**a**) Leukocytoclastic vasculitis of the mesenteric artery in BD. Intermedium sized extramural artery with leukocytoclastic vasculitis is occluded with recent thrombus. The vein adjacent to the artery is also occluded with recent thrombus, but vein is not inflamed (HE×100). (**b**) High magnification of the arterial wall in Fig. 18a (HE×400)

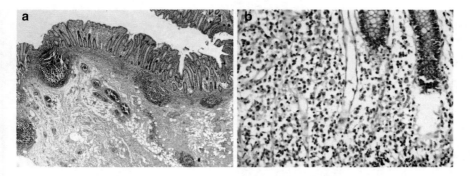

Fig. 13.19 (**a**) Colitis in BD. Architecture of the crypts are normal, there is no goblet cell depletion. Lymphoid hyperplasia and lymphoid follicles are present in the submucosa (HE×40). (**b**) Dense eosinophilic infiltration is striking in the lamina propria (the same patient in Fig. 19a) (HE×400)

Even though less common than seen in CD (~10%), granuloma formation is also seen in intestinal BD [123–127]. Foreign-body granuloma, due to the leakage of luminal material through the bowel wall may occur.

If a large mesenteric vessel has vasculitis and/or aneurysm, it may rupture into the bowel wall and may cause massive bleeding [143]. The microscopic demonstration of the vessel lumen opening into the bowel lumen may be possible in the resected bowel specimen (Fig. 13.20). Gangrenous intestinal manifestations usually develop in the presence of vasculo-BD [102, 144]. Transmural infarction followed by related complications may develop.

Toxic megacolon is characterized by transmural inflammation [145].

In intestinal BD, the erosions in the mucosa, overlying mucosal lymphoid follicles have been reported as early histopathological changes [146]. However, such findings are also true for CD [147]. The findings in endoscopic biopsy in intestinal BD are very similar to CD. The signs of the chronic ileitis such as pyloric metaplasia in the

Fig. 13.20 Ileal artery (with arteritis and organizing thrombus) is ruptured into the bowel lumen (*black dot*) (HE×40)

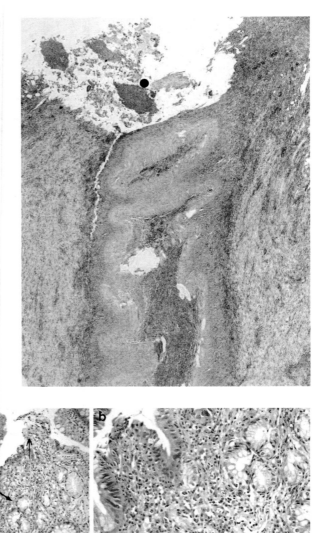

Fig. 13.21 (**a**) Chronic ileitis in BD. Superficial, minute erosion (*thin arrow*), extensive pyloric metaplasia (*rectangular arrows*). Degenerative changes in both of the surface epithelium and villi (HE×200). (**b**) Prominent eosinophil infiltration together with other inflammatory cells in the lamina propria (the same patient in Fig. 21a) (HE×400)

ileal biopsy may suggest the diagnosis of intestinal BD (Fig. 13.21). Mucosal architecture is protected in general [148]. The occurrence of the granuloma in the mucosal biopsy is very rare [123]. It is possible to find the vasculitis in mucosal biopsies. To detect the vasculitis, serial sections of the entire biopsy is recommended [149].

References

1. Jung JY, Kim DY, Bang D (2008) Leg ulcers in Behçet's disease. Br J Dermatol 158:178–179
2. Lee ES, Bang D, Lee S (1997) Dermatologic manifestation of Behçet's disease. Yonsei Med J 38:380–389
3. Cantini F, Salvarani C, Niccoli L et al (1998) Behçet's disease with unusual cutaneous lesions. J Rheumatol 25:2469–2472
4. Bilic M, Mutasim DF (2001) Neutrophilic eccrine hidradenitis in a patient with Behçet's disease. Cutis 68:107–111
5. Nijsten TE, Meuleman L, Lambert J (2002) Chronic pruritic neutrophilic eccrine hidradenitis in a patient with Behçet's disease. Br J Dermatol 147:797–800
6. Mercader-Garcia P, Vilata-Corell JJ, Pardo-Sanchez J et al (2003) Neutrophilic eccrine hidradenitis in a patient with Behçet's disease. Acta Derm Venereol 83:395–396
7. Lee SH, Chung KY, Lee WS et al (1989) Behçet's syndrome associated with bullous necrotizing vasculitis. J Am Acad Dermatol 21:327–330
8. Louthrenoo W, Kasitanon N, Mahanuphab P et al (2003) Kaposi's sarcoma in rheumatic diseases. Semin Arthritis Rheum 32:326–333
9. Kotter I, Aepinus C, Graepler F et al (2001) HHV8 associated Kaposi's sarcoma during triple immunosuppressive treatment with cyclosporin A, azathioprine, and prednisolone for ocular Behçet's disease and complete remission of both disorders with interferon alpha. Ann Rheum Dis 60:83–86
10. Chen KR, Kawahara Y, Miyakawa S et al (1997) Cutaneous vasculitis in Behçet's disease: a clinical and histopathologic study of 20 patients. J Am Acad Dermatol 36:689–696
11. Nazzaro P (1966) Cutaneous manifestations of Behçet's disease. Clinical and histopathological findings. In: Monacelli M, Nazzaro P (eds) International symposium on Behçet's disease, Rome. Karger, Basel, pp 15–41
12. Chun SI, Su WP, Lee S (1990) Histopathologic study of cutaneous lesions in Behçet's syndrome. J Dermatol 17:333–341
13. Gao C (1990) [Clinical pathological analysis of recurrent oral ulcer and Behçet's syndrome]. Zhonghua Kou Qiang Yi Xue Za Zhi 25:82–85, 125
14. Kose O, Stewart J, Waseem A et al (2008) Expression of cytokeratins, adhesion and activation molecules in oral ulcers of Behçet's disease. Clin Exp Dermatol 33:62–69
15. Boyvat A, Heper AO, Kocyigit P et al (2006) Can specific vessel-based papulopustular lesions of Behçet's disease be differentiated from nonspecific follicular-based lesions clinically? Int J Dermatol 45:814–818
16. Jorizzo JL, Abernethy JL, White WL et al (1995) Mucocutaneous criteria for the diagnosis of Behçet's disease: an analysis of clinicopathologic data from multiple international centers. J Am Acad Dermatol 32:968–976
17. Jorizzo JL, Hudson RD, Schmalstieg FC et al (1984) Behçet's syndrome: immune regulation, circulating immune complexes, neutrophil migration, and colchicine therapy. J Am Acad Dermatol 10:205–214
18. Gilhar A, Winterstein G, Turani H et al (1989) Skin hyperreactivity response (pathergy) in Behçet's disease. J Am Acad Dermatol 21:547–552
19. Ilknur T, Pabuccuoglu U, Akin C, Lebe B, Gunes AT (2006) Histopathologic and direct immunofluorescence findings of the papulopustular lesions in Behçet's disease. Eur J Dermatol 16:146–50
20. Ergun T, Gurbuz O, Dogusoy G et al (1998) Histopathologic features of the spontaneous pustular lesions of Behçet's syndrome. Int J Dermatol 37:194–196
21. Alpsoy E, Uzun S, Akman A et al (2003) Histological and immunofluorescence findings of non-follicular papulopustular lesions in patients with Behçet's disease. J Eur Acad Dermatol Venereol 17:521–524
22. Demirkesen C, Tuzuner N, Mat C et al (2001) Clinicopathologic evaluation of nodular cutaneous lesions of Behçet's syndrome. Am J Clin Pathol 116:341–346

23. Kim B, LeBoit PE (2000) Histopathologic features of erythema nodosum-like lesions in Behçet's disease: a comparison with erythema nodosum focusing on the role of vasculitis. Am J Dermatopathol 22:379–390
24. Chun SI, Su WP, Lee S et al (1989) Erythema nodosum-like lesions in Behçet's syndrome: a histopathologic study of 30 cases. J Cutan Pathol 16:259–265
25. Mat C, Demirkesen C, Melikoglu M, Yazici H (2006) Behçet's syndrome. In: Sarzi-Puttini P, Doria A, Girolomoni G, Kuhn A (eds) The skin in systemic autoimmune diseases, Vol 5, Handbook of systemic autoimmune diseases. Elsevier, Amsterdam-Boston-London-New York-Oxford-Paris-Tokyo, pp 186–205
26. Senturk T, Aydintug O, Kuzu I et al (1998) Adhesion molecule expression in erythema nodosum-like lesions in Behçet's disease. A histopathological and immunohistochemical study. Rheumatol Int 18:51–57
27. Uchio E, Matsumoto T, Tanaka SI et al (1999) Soluble intercellular adhesion molecule-1 (ICAM-1), CD4, CD8 and interleukin-2 receptor in patients with Behçet's disease and Vogt-Koyanagi-Harada's disease. Clin Exp Rheumatol 17:179–184
28. Verity DH, Vaughan RW, Kondeatis E et al (2000) Intercellular adhesion molecule-1 gene polymorphisms in Behçet's disease. Eur J Immunogenet 27:73–76
29. Triolo G, Accardo-Palumbo A, Carbone MC et al (1999) Enhancement of endothelial cell E-selectin expression by sera from patients with active Behçet's disease: moderate correlation with anti-endothelial cell antibodies and serum myeloperoxidase levels. Clin Immunol 91:330–337
30. Magro CM, Crowson AN (1995) Cutaneous manifestations of Behçet's disease. Int J Dermatol 34:159–165
31. Ergun T, Gurbuz O, Harvell J et al (1998) The histopathology of pathergy: a chronologic study of skin hyperreactivity in Behçet's disease. Int J Dermatol 37:929–933
32. Haim S, Sobel JD, Friedman-Birnbaum R et al (1976) Histological and direct immunofluorescence study of cutaneous hyperreactivity in Behçet's disease. Br J Dermatol 95:631–636
33. Kim HB (1997) Ophthalmologic manifestation of Behçet's disease. Yonsei Med J 38:390–394
34. Matsuo T, Itami M, Nakagawa H et al (2002) The incidence and pathology of conjunctival ulceration in Behçet's syndrome. Br J Ophthalmol 86:140–143
35. Zamir E, Bodaghi B, Tugal-Tutkun I et al (2003) Conjunctival ulcers in Behçet's disease. Ophthalmology 110:1137–1141
36. Park JH, Han MC, Bettmann MA (1984) Arterial manifestations of Behçet's disease. AJR Am J Roentgenol 143:821–825
37. Calamia KT, Schirmer M, Melikoglu M (2005) Major vessel involvement in Behçet's disease. Curr Opin Rheumatol 17:1–8
38. Fukuda Y, Watanabe I, Hayashi H et al (1980) Pathological studies on Behçet's disease. Ryumachi 20:268–275
39. Lakhanpal S, Tani K, Lie JT et al (1985) Pathologic features of Behçet's syndrome: a review of Japanese autopsy registry data. Hum Pathol 16:790–795
40. Yazawa S, Ishihara A, Kawasaki S (2001) Fatal thoracic aortic aneurysm in a patient with childhood-onset vasculo-Behçet's disease: an autopsy report. Intern Med 40:1154–1157
41. Ko GY, Byun JY, Choi BG et al (2000) The vascular manifestations of Behçet's disease: angiographic and CT findings. Br J Radiol 73:1270–1274
42. Rosenthal T, Rubenstein Z, Adar R et al (1982) Major vessel arteritis with aortic aneurysm in Behçet's disease. Vasa 11:124–127
43. Gruber HE, Weisman MH (1983) Aortic thrombosis during sigmoidoscopy in Behçet's syndrome. Arch Intern Med 143:343–345
44. Kim B, LeBoit PE (1998) Erythema nodosum-like lesions in Behçet's disease: is vasculitis the main pathological feature (abstract)? J Cutan Pathol 25:500
45. Yakut ZI, Odev K (2007) Pulmonary and cardiac involvement in Behçet's disease: 3 case reports. Clin Appl Thromb Hemost 13:318–322

46. Lie JT (1988) Cardiac and pulmonary manifestations of Behçet's syndrome. Pathol Res Pract 183:347–355
47. Higashihara M, Mori M, Takeuchi A et al (1982) Myocarditis in Behçet's disease-a case report and review of the literature. J Rheumatol 9:630–633
48. Turnbull JR, Tunsch A, Adler YD et al (2003) Cardiac manifestation in four patients with Adamantiades–Behçet's disease. Adv Exp Med Biol 528:423–426
49. Schirmer M, Weidinger F, Sandhofer A et al (2003) Valvular disease and myocardial infarctions in a patient with Behçet's disease. J Clin Rheumatol 9:316–320
50. Erkan F, Gul A, Tasali E (2001) Pulmonary manifestations of Behçet's disease. Thorax 56:572–578
51. Hamuryudan V, Yurdakul S, Moral F et al (1994) Pulmonary arterial aneurysms in Behçet's syndrome: a report of 24 cases. Br J Rheumatol 33:48–51
52. Seyahi E, Melikoğlu M, Akman C et al (2006) Pulmonary vascular involvement in Behçet's syndrome. Clin Exp Rheumatol 24:23 (presented in 12th International conference on Behçet's Disease Lisbon 9–23 September 2006)
53. Slavin RE, de Groot WJ (1981) Pathology of the lung in Behçet's disease. Case report and review of the literature. Am J Surg Pathol 5:779–788
54. Hamuryudan V, Oz B, Tuzun H et al (2004) The menacing pulmonary artery aneurysms of Behçet's syndrome. Clin Exp Rheumatol 22:S1–S3
55. Raz I, Okon E, Chajek-Shaul T (1989) Pulmonary manifestations in Behçet's syndrome. Chest 95:585–589
56. Hamuryudan V, Er T, Seyahi E et al (2004) Pulmonary artery aneurysms in Behçet's syndrome. Am J Med 117:867–870
57. Hiller N, Lieberman S, Chajek-Shaul T et al (2004) Thoracic manifestations of Behçet's disease at CT. Radiographics 24:801–808
58. Tunaci A, Berkmen YM, Gokmen E (1995) Thoracic involvement in Behçet's disease: pathologic, clinical, and imaging features. AJR Am J Roentgenol 164:51–56
59. Nanke Y, Kobashigawa T, Yamada T et al (2007) Cryptogenic organizing pneumonia in two patients with Behçet's disease. Clin Exp Rheumatol 25:S103–S106
60. Gul A, Yilmazbayhan D, Buyukbabani N et al (1999) Organizing pneumonia associated with pulmonary artery aneurysms in Behçet's disease. Rheumatology (Oxford) 38:1285–1289
61. Mogulkoc N, Burgess MI, Bishop PW (2000) Intracardiac thrombus in Behçet's disease: a systematic review. Chest 118:479–487
62. Uzun O, Erkan L, Akpolat I et al (2008) Pulmonary involvement in Behçet's disease. Respiration 75:310–321
63. Petty TL, Scoggin CH, Good JT (1977) Recurrent pneumonia in Behçet's syndrome. Roentgenographic documentation during 13 years. JAMA 238:2529–2530
64. Raychaudhuri SP, Siu S (1999) *Pneumocystis carinii* pneumonia in patients receiving immunosuppressive drugs for dermatological diseases. Br J Dermatol 141:528–530
65. Berlin C (1944) Behçet's syndrome with involvement of central nervous system. Report of a case, with necropsy, of lesions of the mount, genitalia and eyes; review of the literature. Arch Derm Syphilol (Chic) 49:227–233
66. Rubinstein LJ, Urich H (1963) Meningo-encephalitis of Behçet's disease: case report with pathological findings. Brain 86:151–160
67. Kawakita H, Nishimura M, Satoh Y et al (1967) Neurological aspects of Behçet's disease. A case report and clinico-pathological review of the literature in Japan. J Neurol Sci 5:417–439
68. Sugihara H, Muto Y, Tsuchiyama H (1969) Neuro-Behçet's syndrome: report of two autopsy cases. Acta Pathol Jpn 19:95–101
69. Totsuka S, Hattori T, Yazaki M et al (1985) Clinicopathologic studies on neuro-Behçet's disease. Folia Psychiatr Neurol Jpn 39:155–166
70. Hirohata S (2008) Histopathology of central nervous system lesions in Behçet's disease. J Neurol Sci 267:41–47

71. Haghighi AB, Sharifzad HR, Matin S et al (2007) The pathological presentations of neuro-Behçet's disease: a case report and review of the literature. Neurologist 13:209–214
72. Serdaroglu P (1998) Behçet's disease and the nervous system. J Neurol 245:197–205
73. Miyakawa T, Murayama E, Deshimaru M et al (1976) Neuro-Behçet's disease showing severe atrophy of the cerebrum. Acta Neuropathol 34:95–103
74. Ho CL, Deruytter MJ (2005) Manifestations of Neuro-Behçet's disease. Report of two cases and review of the literature. Clin Neurol Neurosurg 107:310–314
75. Hiroshi K, Hiroshi N, Akiharu O (1976) Histopathology of Behçet's disease. Review of the literature with a case report. Acta Pathol Jpn 26:383–386
76. McMenemey W, Lawrence BJ (1957) Encephalomyelopathy in Becket's disease; report of necropsy findings in two cases. Lancet 273:353–358
77. Arai Y, Kohno S, Takahashi Y et al (2006) Autopsy case of neuro-Behçet's disease with multifocal neutrophilic perivascular inflammation. Neuropathology 26:579–585
78. Kocer N, Islak C, Siva A et al (1999) CNS involvement in neuro-Behçet's syndrome: an MR study. AJNR Am J Neuroradiol 20:1015–1024
79. Shimizu T, Ehrlich GE, Inaba G et al (1979) Behçet's disease (Behçet's syndrome). Semin Arthritis Rheum 8:223–260
80. Suzuki N, Takeno M, Inaba G (2003) Bilateral subdural effusion in a patient with neuro-Behçet's disease. Ann Rheum Dis 62:374–375
81. Siva A, Altintas A, Saip S (2004) Behçet's syndrome and the nervous system. Curr Opin Neurol 17:347–357
82. Bienenstock H, Murray EM (1961) Behçet's syndrome: report of a case with extensive neurologic manifestation. N Engl J Med 264:1342–1345
83. Kikuchi S, Niino M, Shinpo K et al (2002) Intracranial hemorrhage in neuro-Behçet's syndrome. Intern Med 41:692–695
84. Nakasu S, Kaneko M, Matsuda M (2001) Cerebral aneurysms associated with Behçet's disease: a case report. J Neurol Neurosurg Psychiatry 70:682–684
85. Geny C, Cesaro P, Heran F et al (1993) Pseudotumoral neuro-Behçet's disease. Surg Neurol 39:374–376
86. Yoshimura J, Toyama M, Sekihara Y et al (2001) Neuro-Behçet's disease mimicking a thalamic tumor. No Shinkei Geka 29:527–531
87. Matsuo K, Yamada K, Nakajima K et al (2005) Neuro-Behçet's disease mimicking brain tumor. AJNR Am J Neuroradiol 26:650–653
88. Rhiannon JJ (2008) Systemic lupus erythematosus involving the nervous system: presentation, pathogenesis, and management. Clin Rev Allergy Immunol 34:356–360
89. Duprez T, Nzeusseu A, Peeters A, Houssiau FA (2001) Selective involvement of the choroid plexus on cerebral magnetic resonance images: a new radiological sign in patients with systemic lupus erythematosus with neurological symptoms. J Rheumatol 28:387–391
90. Ebert EC (2009) Gastrointestinal manifestations of Behçet's disease. Dig Dis Sci 54:201–207
91. Brookes GB (1983) Pharyngeal stenosis in Behçet's syndrome. The first reported case. Arch Otolaryngol 109:338–340
92. Yigit O, Alkan S, Basak T et al (2005) Behçet's disease presenting with a hypopharyngeal ulcer. Eur Arch Otorhinolaryngol 262:151–153
93. Hamza M, Ferjaoui M, Elleuch M et al (1985) Pharyngeal stenosis in a case of Behçet's disease. Ann Otolaryngol Chir Cervicofac 102:465–467
94. Yi S, Cheon JH, Kim JH, Lee SK, Kim TI, Lee YC, Kim WH (2009) The prevalence and clinical characteristics of esophageal involvement in patients with Behçet's disease: a single center experience in Korea. J Korean Med Sci 24:52–56
95. Mori S, Yoshihira A, Kawamura H et al (1983) Esophageal involvement in Behçet's disease. Am J Gastroenterol 78:548–553
96. Ozenc A, Bayraktar Y, Baykal A (1990) Pyloric stenosis with esophageal involvement in Behçet's syndrome. Am J Gastroenterol 85:727–728
97. Ning-Sheng L, Ruay-Sheng L, Kuo-Chih T (2005) High frequency of unusual gastric/duodenal ulcers in patients with Behçet's disease in Taiwan: a possible correlation of MHC molecules with the development of gastric/duodenal ulcers. Clin Rheumatol 24:516–520

98. Good AE, Mutchnick MG, Weatherbee L (1982) Duodenal ulcer, hepatic abscesses, and fatal hemobilia with Behçet's syndrome: a case report. Am J Gastroenterol 77:905–909
99. Cappell M (1998) Intestinal (mesenteric) vasculopathy I. Acute superior mesenteric arteriopathy and venopathy. Gastroenterol Clin North Am 27:783–825
100. Cappell M (1998) (mesenteric) vasculopathy II. Ischemic colitis and chronic mesenteric ischemia. Gastroenterol Clin North Am 27:827–860
101. Ha HK, Lee SH, Rha SE et al (2000) Radiologic features of vasculitis involving the gastrointestinal tract. Radiographics 20:779–794
102. Bayraktar Y, Soylu AR, Balkanci F et al (1998) Arterial thrombosis leading to intestinal infarction in a patient with Behçet's disease associated with protein C deficiency. Am J Gastroenterol 93:2556–2558
103. Hong YK, Yoo WH (2008) Massive gastrointestinal bleeding due to the rupture of arterial aneurysm in Behçet's disease: case report and literature review. Rheumatol Int 28: 1151–1154
104. Chubachi A, Saitoh K, Imai H et al (1993) Case report: intestinal infarction after an aneurysmal occlusion of superior mesenteric artery in a patient with Behçet's disease. Am J Med Sci 306:376–378
105. Mercie P, Constans J, Tissot B et al (1996) Thrombosis of the superior mesenteric artery and Behçet's syndrome. Rev Med Interne 17:470–473
106. Kuzu MA, Ozaslan C, Koksoy C et al (1994) Vascular involvement in Behçet's disease: 8-year audit. World J Surg 18:948–953, discussion 53–54
107. Dixon M (1995) The small intestine. In vascular disorders, abnormalities, ischaemia and vasculitis. In: Whitehead R (ed) Gastrointestinal and oesophageal pathology. Churchill Livingstone, Edinburgh, Hong Kong, London, Madrid, Melbourne and New York., pp 665–686
108. Whitehead R, Gratama S (1995) The large intestine. In vascular disorders, abnormalities, ischaemia and vasculitis. In: Whitehead R (ed) Gastrointestinal and oesophageal pathology. Churchill Livingstone, Edinburgh, Hong Kong, London, Madrid, Melbourne and New York, pp 687–709
109. Fagin R, Straus FH, April E, Kirsner JB (1970) An unusual case of ischemic enteritis mimicking regional enteritis. Gastroenterology 59:917–920
110. Eisenberg R, Montgomery CK, Margulis AR (1979) Colitis in the elderly: ischemic colitis mimicking ulcerative and granulomatous colitis. Am J Roentgenol 133:1113–1118
111. Brandt L, Boley SJ, Mitsudo S (1982) Clinical characteristics and natural history of colitis in the elderly. Am J Gastroenterol 77:382–386
112. Gan S, Urbanski S, Coderre SP, Panaccione R (2004) Isolated visceral small artery fibromuscular hyperplasia-induced ischemic colitis mimicking inflammatory bowel disease. Am J Gastroenterol 99:2058–2062
113. Willeke P, Domagk D, Floer M, Bruwer M, Kreuter M, Gaubitz M, Domschke W, Kucharzik T (2005) Ischaemic colitis mimicking inflammatory bowel disease in a young adult receiving oral anticoagulation. Scand J Gastroenterol 40:878–880
114. Kao P, Vecchio JA, Hyman NH, West AB, Blaszyk H (2005) Idiopathic myointimal hyperplasia of mesenteric veins: a rare mimic of idiopathic inflammatory bowel disease. J Clin Gastroenterol 39:704–708
115. Houman MH, Ben Ghorbel I, B'Chir-Hamzaoui S et al (2001) [Intestinal lymphoma associated with Behçet's disease]. Ann Med Interne (Paris) 152:415–418
116. Koksal AS, Ertugrul I, Disibeyaz S et al (2005) Crohn's and Behçet's disease association presenting with superior vena cava thrombosis. Dig Dis Sci 50:1698–1701
117. Akay N, Boyvat A, Heper AO et al (2006) Behçet's disease-like presentation of bullous pyoderma gangrenosum associated with Crohn's disease. Clin Exp Dermatol 31:384–386
118. Fresko I, Ugurlu S, Ozbakir F et al (2005) Anti-Saccharomyces cerevisiae antibodies (ASCA) in Behçet's syndrome. Clin Exp Rheumatol 23:S67–S70
119. Ahmad T, Zhang L, Gogus F et al (2005) CARD15 polymorphisms in Behçet's disease. Scand J Rheumatol 34:233–237
120. Lois E, Michel V, Hugot JP, Reenaers C, Fontaine F, Delforge M, El Yafi F, Colombel JF, Belaiche J (2003) Early development of stricturing or penetrating pattern in Crohn's disease

is influenced by disease location, number of flares, and smoking but not by NOD2/CARD15 genotype. Gut 52:552–557

121. Korman U, Cantasdemir M, Kurugoglu S et al (2003) Enteroclysis findings of intestinal Behçet's disease: a comparative study with Crohn disease. Abdom Imaging 28:308–312

122. Kasahara Y, Tanaka S, Nishino M et al (1981) Intestinal involvement in Behçet's disease: review of 136 surgical cases in the Japanese literature. Dis Colon Rectum 24:103–106

123. Tolia V, Abdullah A, Thirumoorthi MC et al (1989) A case of Behçet's disease with intestinal involvement due to Crohn's disease. Am J Gastroenterol 84:322–325

124. Sayek I, Aran O, Uzunalimoglu B et al (1991) Intestinal Behçet's disease: surgical experience in seven cases. Hepatogastroenterology 38:81–83

125. Masugi J, Matsui T, Fujimori T et al (1994) A case of Behçet's disease with multiple longitudinal ulcers all over the colon. Am J Gastroenterol 89:778–780

126. Houman H, Ben Dahmen F, Ben Ghorbel I et al (2001) [Behçet's disease associated with Crohn's disease]. Ann Med Interne (Paris) 152:480–482

127. Naganuma M, Iwao Y, Kashiwagi K et al (2002) A case of Behçet's disease accompanied by colitis with longitudinal ulcers and granuloma. J Gastroenterol Hepatol 17:105–108

128. Kim ES, Chung WC, Lee KM et al (2007) A case of intestinal Behçet's disease similar to Crohn's colitis. J Korean Med Sci 22:918–922

129. Jarrahnejad P, Gadepalli S, Zurkovsky E et al (2006) Behçet's disease: a rare cause of lower gastrointestinal bleeding. Int J Colorectal Dis 21:856–858

130. Kobashigawa T, Okamoto H, Kato J et al (2004) Ulcerative colitis followed by the development of Behçet's disease. Intern Med 43:243–247

131. Kim JS, Lim SH, Choi IJ et al (2000) Prediction of the clinical course of Behçet's colitis according to macroscopic classification by colonoscopy. Endoscopy 32:635–640

132. Dowling CM, Hill AD, Malone C et al (2008) Colonic perforation in Behçet's syndrome. World J Gastroenterol 14:6578–6580

133. Chou SJ, Chen VT, Jan HC et al (2007) Intestinal perforations in Behçet's disease. J Gastrointest Surg 11:508–514

134. Lee SK, Kim BK, Kim TI et al (2009) Differential diagnosis of intestinal Behçet's disease and Crohn's disease by colonoscopic findings. Endoscopy 41:9–16

135. Moore K (1992) Clinically oriented anatomy, 3rd edn. Williams and Wilkins, Baltimore, Hong Kong, London, Munich, Philadelphia, Sydney, Tokyo, pp 181–182

136. Anthony A, Dhillon AP, Pounder RE, Wakefield AJ (1997) Ulceration of the ileum in Crohn's disease: correlation with vascular anatomy. J Clin Pathol 50:1013–1017

137. Matsumoto T, Uekusa T, Fukuda Y (1991) Vasculo-Behçet's disease: a pathologic study of eight cases. Hum Pathol 22:45–51

138. Kabbaj N, Benjelloun G, Gueddari FZ et al (1993) [Vascular involvements in Behçet's disease. Based on 40 patient records]. J Radiol 74:649–656

139. Haeberle M, Griffen WO Jr (1972) Eosinophilia and regional enteritis. A possible diagnostic aid. Am J Dig Dis 17:200–204

140. Levy A, Yamazaki K, Van Keulen VP, Burgart LJ, Sandborn WJ, Phillips SF, Kephart GM, Gleich GJ, Leiferman KM (2001) Increased eosinophil infiltration and degranulation in colonic tissue from patients with collagenous colitis. Am J Gastroenterol 96:1522–1528

141. Metwai A, Blum AM, Ferraris L, Klein JS, Claudio F, Weinstock JV (1994) Eosinophils within the healthy or inflamed human intestine produce substance P and vasoactive intestinal peptide. J Neuroimmunol 52:69–78

142. Rothenber M, Mishra A, Brandt EB, Hogan SP (2001) Gastrointestinal eosinophils. Immunol Rev 179:139–155

143. Kim SU, Cheon JH, Lim JS et al (2007) Massive gastrointestinal bleeding due to aneurysmal rupture of ileo-colic artery in a patient with Behçet's disease. Korean J Gastroenterol 49:400–404

144. Turanlı M, Senol M, Koyunca A, Aydın C, Arici S (2003) Sigmoid colon perforation as an unusual complication of Behçet's syndrome: report of a case. Surg Today 33:383–386

145. Roenspies U, Saegesser F (1975) Behçet's disease and toxic megacolon. Schweiz Med Wochenschr 105:199–204
146. Takada Y, Fujita Y, Igarashi M et al (1997) Intestinal Behçet's disease – pathognomonic changes in intramucosal lymphoid tissues and effect of a "rest cure" on intestinal lesions. J Gastroenterol 32:598–604
147. Sankey E, Dhillon AP, Anthony A, Wakefield AJ, Sim R, More L, Hudson M, Sawyerr AM, Pounder RE (1993) Early mucosal changes in Crohn's disease. Gut 34:375–381
148. Yurdakul S, Tuzuner N, Yurdakul I et al (1996) Gastrointestinal involvement in Behçet's syndrome: a controlled study. Ann Rheum Dis 55:208–210
149. Tribe C, Scott DGI, Bacon PA (1981) Rectal biopsy in the diagnosis of systemic vasculitis. J Clin Pathol 34:843–850

Chapter 14
Disease Mechanisms

Haner Direskeneli and Güher Saruhan-Direskeneli

Keywords Anti cardiolipin antibodies • Anti endothelial cell antibodies (AECA) • Apoptosis • Autoimmunity • Autoinflammation • B cells • Behcetogenic epitope • BES-1 gene derived peptides • CD4+ T cells • CD8+ cytotoxic T cells • Chemotaxis • CXCL-8 • Dendritic cells • Factor V Leiden • Fibrinolysis • Heat shock proteins • Heme oxygenase-1 • Herpes simplex virus • HLA-B27 • HLA-B51 • HLA-B51 transgenic mice • IFN-γ • IL-17 • IL-2 • Infectious etiology • Innate and adaptive immunity • Mannose binding lectin • MEFV • Microbial flora • Molecular mimicry • Neutrophil activation • NK cells • Pathogenesis • Perforin • Prothrombin mutations • Pyrin • Regulatory T cells • Retinal S antigen • Streptococci • Superoxide production • T cells • Th1 response • Th17 cells • Th2 response • Tissue plasminogen activator • Toll-like receptors • α-Enolase • γδ T-cells

Introduction

Behçet's disease (BD) is a systemic inflammatory disorder with a diverse spectrum of clinical manifestations including mucocutaneous, ocular, vascular, gastro-intestinal, musculoskeletal, and central nervous system involvement (1, 2). A complex genetic background leading to a pro-inflammatory, innate-immune system derived activation perpetuated by adaptive immune responses against environmental and auto-antigens is accepted as the main pathogenic mechanism in BD (3).

H. Direskeneli (✉)
Department of Rheumatology, Marmara University Medical Faculty, Istanbul, Turkey
e-mail: direskeneli@superonline.com

Infectious Etiology

Microbial infection has been implicated in the development of BD since its initial description in 1937. Four principal hypotheses have been suggested: (1) bacterial, with streptococci in the foreground, (2) viral, (3) indirectly via heat shock proteins (HSP), and (4) cross-reactive or molecular mimicry etiologies (4).

As BD starts mostly from the oral mucosal surface (oral apthae as the first manifestation in 70% of the patients), oral microbial flora has long been implicated in BD pathogenesis (5). Oral manifestations are increased after dental manipulations, and an increased skin hypersensitivity to streptococcal antigens has been reported (6–8). Oral hygiene is impaired and is associated with a more severe disease course (9). Oral streptococcal colonization is increased with the dominance of atypical streptococci (10). Recent reports of beneficial antibacterial therapy, which improves oral health (11), also support a role for abnormal oral flora in pathogenesis. On the other hand, long-term, prospective studies are yet to be conducted.

There have been several studies showing an immune hyperreactivity to streptococci (12, 13). E. coli and S. aureus also activate BD lymphocytes to release increased amounts of IFN-γ and IL-6 (13). Recently, streptococcus-related BES-1 gene derived peptides, which are homologous to human-heat-shock protein 60 (HSP60) and retinal protein Brn3b are found to stimulate peripheral blood mononuclear cells (PBMCs) of BD patients producing Th1 type cytokines (7). Behçet's T lymphocytes secrete IFN-γ in response to lower (1–10 pg/ml) doses of staphylococcal superantigens SEB and SEC1 compared to controls, pointing to a general, rather than a specific molecule/organism-related, "T cell hyperreactivity" of BD lymphocytes (14).

Another site of infection in BD is the pustular skin lesion, which has been shown to be not sterile (15). A variety of organisms such as S. aureus, Propionibacterium acnes, and coagulase negative staphylococci as well as gram-negative microorganisms such as E. coli and prevotella species are cultured from BD lesions. It has been suggested that the mere presence and persistence of these bacteria might be more important in pathogenesis than the presence of a particular species.

Herpes Simplex Virus

A viral etiology for BD has first been postulated by H. Behçet's in 1937. Later viral particles were claimed to be isolated from bodily fluids (16). Viral infections such as herpes simplex (HSV), varicella zoster, human cytomegalovirus, Epstein-Barr, human herpes virus 6 (HHV-6), and HHV-7 viruses have all been proposed as etiological factors (17).

Serum anti-HSV-1 antibodies are found in a higher proportion of BD patients compared to controls, and an increased cytotoxic T cell activity against HSV-1 has been reported (18, 19). Although anti-HSV treatment in BD has not been successful (20), antiviral therapy has been shown to be beneficial in the animal models, showing possibly their limited resemblance to human disease (21, 22).

Innate Immunity

Neutrophil Activation

As typical BD lesions such as pustular folliculitis, pathergy reactions, and hypopyon have significant neutrophil infiltrates, neutrophil functions and activation status, pivotal in innate immune response, have been extensively investigated (2). Conflicting reports of increased, normal or decreased superoxide production, phagocytosis, chemotaxis and neutrophil-endothelial adhesion in BD are available. This might reflect differing clinical activity, the discordance between "in vitro" and "in vivo" state of affairs, drug effects, or general methodological problems in investigating neutrophils (23–28). We reported decreased fMLP-stimulated superoxide production in BD and in patients with sepsis. Subsequent re-stimulation of prestimulated BD neutrophils produced impaired increase of superoxide production, implying a state of "in vivo" neutrophil preactivation (29). An in vivo "primed" state of neutrophils with a dual signaling system for activating neutrophil oxidase had previously been suggested (30). Agents such as fMLP or cytokines such as tumor necrosis factor-alpha (TNFα) and granulocyte-monocyte colony-stimulating factor (GM-CSF) have been shown to prime neutrophils in vivo without full activation, which might be the case in BD with its pro-inflammatory cytokine milieu. In HLA-B51 transgenic mice, a presumed model for BD, the only observed abnormality was increased superoxide release in response to fMLP (26). High superoxide responses were also present in HLA-B51$^+$ patients and healthy controls in the same study, but these observations could not be reproduced (29).

Expression of some surface molecules has also found to be increased on neutrophils (29, 31, 32). CXCR-2 expression on neutrophils was shown to be upregulated during the relapsing phase of ocular BD (33). In line with this increased activation, life-span of neutrophils is prolonged in tissue infiltrates. Apoptosis of neutrophils is decreased in the remission and restored in the active phase of uveitis. This might be due to apoptotic cell death, in part via Fas–Fas ligand interaction (34). Similarly, neutrophil apoptosis is found to be decreased and associated with males (35), the gender with generally more severe disease.

γδ T Cells in BD

γδ T cells represent a minor T cell population (1–10% of peripheral blood (PB) T-cells) that express T cell receptors (TCRs) comprising γ and δ heterodimer (36). Vγ9δ2$^+$ T cells, a major subset of γδ T cells in the PB, recognize nonpeptide antigens produced by bacteria. γδ T cells have important roles in innate immunity as a *"first line of defense"* against microorganisms, surveillance against tumors and possibly in modulating auto-immune responses. PB γδ T cells have been observed to be elevated in most studies in BD (29, 37–40), with a polyclonal rather than oligoclonal activation (41). This may indicate that during repeated inflammation, γδ T cells are responding to a wide variety of antigenic stimuli with consequent expansion of γδ T cells expressing various Vγ and Vδ chains.

γδ T cells have been reported to be associated with active BD with higher expressions of CD29, CD69 and production of interferon-γ (IFN-γ) and (TNF-α) (37–39). Significantly greater proportions of the Vδ1+ and Vδ2+ γδ T-cell subsets are activated in patients with active BD and the balance of activation between these subsets favor Vδ2+ T cells (42). Whereas PB γδ T cells are mainly Vδ2+ in local fluids such as bronchoalveolar lavage and cerebrospinal fluid (CSF), γδ T cells are dominated by Vδ1+ T-cells in the intra-ocular fluid, except a study with elevated Vγ9δ2+ T cells (43). Prominent local γδ T cell presence in active BD lesions where HSP60 expression is upregulated suggest possible HSP-γδ T cell interactions (44). KTH-1 also stimulate γδ T cells in short-term T cell cultures and KTH-1 specific γδ T-cell lines secrete pro-inflammatory mediators such as IL-6, IL-8, and TNF-α (13, 45). In Italian BD patients, Vγ9Vδ2+ T lymphocytes are shown to be expanded and express TNF receptor II and IL-12 receptor β1 in active disease. The level of soluble granzyme A is also elevated in the cell culture supernatants of these Vγ9Vδ2+ T cells (46, 47).

T cells responsive to HSP60-derived peptides were mainly of γδ T cell subset in UK (48), whereas CD4+ T cells are reported from Japan and Turkey (12, 49). Long-term T cell lines expanded with repetitive HSP60-peptide stimulations were also mainly CD4+ (50), and no response to HSP60 is observed in any T-cell line derived from intra-ocular fluid of uveitis patients with BD, whereas nonpeptide prenyl pyrophosphate reactive γδ T cells were present (43). Although no functional data is available, the recognition of MICA alleles upregulated in the epithelium by Vδ1 subset merits further studies as BD is shown to have a genetic association with MICA alleles (51).

NK and Cytotoxic T Cells

In earlier studies, NK cell activity of PB cells of patients in the clinically active stage of BD was observed to be significantly lower than in the inactive stage and controls. This was normalized by addition of IFN-α. In contrast, the actual number of NK cells was markedly increased in active disease (52, 53). Increases of PB NK cells and CD56+ T lymphocytes were also observed (54).

When further analyzed, CD11b+CD27−CD62L− phenotype of CD8brightCD56+ T cells were increased in active Behçet's uveitis. These cells were polarized to produce IFN-γ and contained high amounts of preformed intracellular perforin while exclusively expressing surface FasL upon PI stimulation. This suggests that CD8brightCD56+ T cells in Behçet's uveitis are characterized by cytotoxic effector phenotypes with functional NK receptors and function as strong cytotoxic effectors through both Fas ligand-dependent and perforin-dependent pathways (55).

The association of HLA-B*51 and B*2702 with BD has also pointed to regulatory interactions of NK and T cells through HLA class I binding NK receptors. When different expression patterns of HLA-recognizing receptors on NK or T cells were analyzed, increased expression of CD94, a member of C-type lectin receptor family binding HLA-E, was observed on CD16$^+$CD56$^+$ NK and on CD3$^+$ and CD3$^+$CD56$^+$ T cells in BD. The expression of KIR3DL1 receptor from the polymorphic killer immunoglobulin-like receptor (KIR) family, binding HLA-Bw4 motif on HLA-B*51 and *2702 alleles was not different between the controls and diseased (56).

Autoinflammation and BD

A recently introduced concept for BD is "autoinflammation." Autoinflammatory diseases are described as a group of inherited disorders characterized by episodes of seemingly unprovoked, recurrent inflammatory attacks of innate-nature, mainly mediated by neutrophils (57). In contrast to classical autoimmune disorders, no significant high-titer autoantibodies or antigen-specific T cells are present. The prototype disorder is familial Mediterranean fever (FMF), a disease associated with mutations in the MEFV gene, encoding pyrin/marenostrin protein. MEFV is expressed at high levels in neutrophils, monocytes, and dendritic cells (DC), but not in lymphocytes. Amino-terminal of pyrin binds to another pyrin-domain containing protein called apoptosis-associated speck-like protein (ASC) containing a caspase-recruitment domain (CARD) and might regulate IL-1β processing, NF-κB activation and apoptosis through this interaction. However, both inhibitory and enhancing effects of pyrin have been observed depending on the experimental system (58).

Behçet's disease, with some of its clinical features such as recurrent nonscarring muco-cutaneous lesions and nondeforming arthritis with enhanced pro-inflammatory cytokine responses such as IL-1 and IL-18 (32, 59), has been suggested to be in this spectrum (60). When associations between FMF and BD, two common diseases in the Middle-East, have been investigated in recent studies, MEFV mutations are observed more frequently in BD and associate with a more severe disease and vascular involvement (61, 62).

On the other hand, almost all conditions characterized as autoinflammatory diseases have a monogenic inheritance as is the case for FMF. Furthermore, there are also clinical aspects that differ between the two diseases (63). Childhood onset, paroxysmal attacks of serosal inflammation, and fever typical of autoinflammatory disorders are not characteristic of BD, while panuveitis, extensive vasculitis, hyper-coagulability, and a disease course getting milder in late ages are uncommon among the autoinflammatory diseases. Another crucial difference between FMF and BD is the prolonged inflammatory skin response. Pathergy test, a nonspecific response to skin trauma, is typically observed in BD and in some neutrophilic dermatoses such as pyoderma gangrenosum and Sweet's Syndrome (64). Pathergy reaction is shown to be associated with skin flora, as extensive skin cleansing decreases the positivity of the test (65). Chronologically, in studies of pathergy, mixed neutrophil and T cell infiltrations are observed as early as 4 h, with a peak density in 24–48 h in BD patients' skin biopsies (64, 66). No pathergy skin response is reported in FMF (67), although an erysipel-like skin lesions or rarely cutaneous vasculitis with neutrophil infiltrations are observed. Similar to pathergy test, increased skin responses to urate crystals have also been described in BD, which is not observed in FMF (68, 69). On the other hand, urate-induced superoxide production in neutrophils was found to be dose-dependent and similar in magnitude in both BD and FMF and was even higher in FMF monocytes (69). Why this observation does not translate into an increased skin response in FMF is currently unknown. Urate crystals have recently been shown to activate NALP3 inflammasome, a protein complex of cryopyrin, ASC, and a protein called CARDINAL (CARD-inhibitor of NF-κB activating ligand), causing the activation of caspase-1 complex and leading to the release of IL-1β (70).

Adaptive Immunity in BD

Cellular Immunity

The presence and activation of T cells both in the PB and tissue specimens is observed in BD. A possibly antigen-driven change in blood CD4$^+$ and CD8$^+$ T cell repertoire with oligoclonal T cell receptor Vβ subtype increases are observed (40, 71). However, high individual variability of dominant Vβ subtypes between the patients makes it impossible to implicate a single antigen driving the T cell activation. As in most other auto-immune disorders and vasculitides, Th1 type cytokine profile is predominant in BD. Both CD4$^+$ and CD8$^+$ T cells producing Th1 type pro-inflammatory cytokines IL-2 and IFN-γ are increased in the PB and correlate with disease activity (72, 73). However, low IL-2 expression, restored with IFN-α treatment, is also reported (74). IL-12, which drives Th1 response in naive T cells, is elevated in BD sera, in correlation with Th1 lymphocytes. Tissue studies also point to a Th1 type tissue infiltration in BD, possibly driven with IL-12 and IL-23 highly expressed in intestinal and cutaneous lesions (75–77). Both streptococcal antigens and auto-antigens such as αB-crystallin also drive an IL-12 response in PBMCs of BD patients (78, 79).

Th2 lymphocytes and levels of Th2 cytokines are generally low (80), except as reported in a single study in which high IL-4, IL-10, and IL-13 levels were reported in anti-CD3/anti-CD40 stimulated PBMC cultures (81). A complex cytokine profile with both Th1 and Th2 features is also described in oral biopsies (82). Recently, IL-15, an innate-driving cytokine is also found to be increased in BD sera (83).

Th17 cells represent a new subset of T helper cells which mainly produce IL-17A, IL-17F, IL-22, and TNF-α (84). IL-6 and TGF-β induce the differentiation of Th17 cells from naïve T-cells. Th17 cells are suggested to be involved in organ-specific autoimmunity. There is possibly a functional antagonism between Th17 cells and regulatory T cells (84, 85). Active BD is characterized by high levels of IL-6, IL-10, and IL-17 compared to remission (86). Levels of IL-23 and IFN-γ are also elevated in BD patients with active uveitis (87). However, elevated IL-17 levels have not been confirmed in all studies (88). When specific responses to BD-associated antigens are investigated, S-antigen peptides significantly induced the production of IFN-γ and TNF-α but not IL-2, IL-4, and IL-17 by PBMCs in active BD patients (89).

Regulatory Activity in BD

CD4$^+$CD25$^+$ T regulatory cells, with the potential to regulate effector T cells, were increased in the peripheral circulation of active BD patients (90). Similarly, as a local response, CD25$^{+bright}$, FoxP3-expressing CD4$^+$ T cells are increased in the CSF of BD patients (91). However, decreased percentages of regulatory T cells are also reported in PBMCs of BD before ocular attacks (92). As BD can be said to display an uncontrolled inflammation, Hamzaoui et al. suggested that regulatory T cell activity may be impaired and insufficient in BD (93).

Autoimmunity and B Cell Activity

BD does not have the classical clinical features of autoimmunity such as female dominance and association with other autoimmune diseases such as Sjogren's syndrome (94, 95). A good multisystem animal model of BD is not at hand (see Chap. 16). However, BD has various aspects that deserve to be considered as "*autoimmune*". Although the total B cell number is normal, the B cells express increased levels of activation markers such as CD13, CD33, CD80, and memory marker CD45RO (96). However, the low level of CD5$^+$CD19$^+$ B cells, which produce auto-antibodies, differentiates BD from classical auto-antibody mediated disorders. As the current role of B cells in immune system is not limited to antibody production and also include antigen presentation and cytokine secretion, the activated and memory type B cell profile might modulate T cell activation in BD.

Although classical, systemic-disease associated auto-antibodies such as ANA and rheumatoid factor are not observed, auto-antibodies against cell surface antigens such as antiendothelial cells (AECA) or mucosal antigens have previously been shown to be present in BD (97, 98). Recently, with especially proteomic approaches, various antibodies against specific antigens such as α-enolase, α-tropomyosin, kinectin, selenium-binding protein, esterase-D, and carboxy-terminal subunit of Sip1 have also been shown (99–105). Most of these autoantibodies are demonstrated in uveitis patients, and their role in disease pathogenesis is not yet clear.

For an autoimmune etiology, various T cell related auto-antigens have also been investigated in BD patients. Among the candidate antigens, human HSP60 has been the most extensively studied (106). Four immunodominant epitopes of HSP60 induced T and B cell responses in studies from UK, Japan, and Turkey (48, 49, 107, 108). A Th1 type, proinflammatory cytokine response to HSP60-derived peptide $_{336-51}$ with IFN-γ, IL-12, and TNF-α production is demonstrated. HSP60-peptide $_{336-51}$ also upregulated Txk, a tyrosine kinase expressed in Th1 cells and effected IFN-γ gene transcription (109). HSP60-peptide$_{336-51}$ and α-tropomyosin are both shown to cause uveitis in rats, however, without any other clinical features of BD (99, 110). An oral conjugate of peptide$_{336-51}$ and cholera toxin-B are shown to ameliorate uveitis in the animal model, and a preliminary study with this agent has also been reported in BD patients with uveitis (111).

Another crucial element of autoimmunity is the MHC association. Most classical auto-immune disorders are shown to have an MHC class II association, leading to a disease-associated peptide hypothesis (MHC class II associated presentation of pathogenic epitope to CD4$^+$ Th cells) such as *shared-epitope* in rheumatoid arthritis (RA). However, BD is associated with an MHC class I antigen, HLA-B51 (112, 113) and the best known role of MHC class I antigens such as B51 is the presentation of Class-I associated antigens synthesized within the cell to CD8$^+$ cytotoxic-suppressor T cells. A candidate *"Behcetogenic"* epitope as a hypothetical disease-inducing peptide has been described (114). A HLA-B51-restricted peptide from a MICA antigen has also been shown to activate CD8$^+$ T cells in BD patients with upregulated IFN-γ and cytotoxic responses (115).

Another candidate auto-antigen in BD is the retinal S-antigen (S-Ag) found mainly in retina. As retina is usually considered as an immune-privileged site, immune responses are only observed after uveitis-associated tissue destruction. T cell responses against S-Ag are present in various types of human uveitis including BD (89, 116, 117). Among the immuno-dominant epitopes of S-Ag, a peptide (aa 342-355, PDSAg) is found to share homology with a conserved region of the HLA-B molecules (aa 125-138, B27PD) such as B51 and B27, which are associated to uveitis in BD and spondyloarthropathies (118, 119). As this epitope is presented to and recognized by CD4$^+$ T cells, a model of MHC class I molecules becoming antigenic epitopes themselves is proposed (120). According to this model, HLA-derived peptides are prominent in selecting the repertoire of CD4$^+$ T cell receptors and, as a consequence, in defining susceptibility to some auto-immune diseases. Indeed, a significant portion of small peptides eluted from the surface of various HLA class II molecules are found to be HLA class I originated, including B27PD (121). As T cells recognizing class I antigens are a natural part of our immune repertoire, but possibly tolerized in thymus, a break-down of tolerance might occur after uveal inflammation by cross-reactivity of PDS-Ag and B27PD reactive T cells. Elevated pro-inflammatory cytokine and chemokines in uveitis patients might also enhance HLA class I molecule expression on cell surfaces, increasing their intra-cellular turnover and immune antigen presentation. Development of uveitis in rats by both peptides supports this model (122). T cell responses to these uveitogenic peptides were first shown in German uveitis patients (119) and later confirmed in a larger group of BD patients from Turkey (123). Interestingly, only T cells from patients with posterior uveitis but not from HLA-B51$^+$ BD group without uveitis are responsive to uveitogenic peptides. This suggests that serious uvea destruction and activation of PDS-Ag reactive T cells is required for *cross-reacting* anti-B27PD responses. Increased IL-2 and TNF-α expression was also present after PDSAg and B27PD stimulation of PBMCs. Oral feeding of B27PD derived peptide prevented retinal S-antigen uveitis in the animal model and is being tried in refractory uveitis patients as a method of "*oral tolerance*" treatment (124). Other recently described HLA-B27 related immune mechanisms such as heavy-chain association or bacterial persistence have not yet been studied in BD in association with HLA-B51.

Pathways from Innate to Adaptive Responses

The presence of a prolonged inflammation such as nonspecific (pathergy) or urate-induced skin responses suggests that innate and adaptive pathways are integrated in a complex immune response in BD. A unifying hypothesis for BD requires the explanation of these links between the two main arms of the immune system. One explanation might be an unprovoked, uncontrolled, innate-related inflammation causing an adaptive system activation only as a secondary response, as in autoin-flammatory disorders (60). An overactivated cytokine cascade through IL-1, IL-6, TNF-α and chemokines such as CXCL-8 might activate nonspecific and nonpatho-genic T and B cell responses in BD. As an example, increased CD3$^+$HLA-DR$^+$, CD4$^+$CD69$^+$, CD8$^+$CD25$^+$, and CD8$^+$CD69$^+$ T cells were observed in the PB during FMF attacks with elevated IL-12 and IL-18 that may lead to a Th1 polarization (125, 126). However, these adaptive responses seem not to be pathogenic in FMF, as a typical autoinflammatory disorder with neutrophil infiltrations.

Neutrophils, although accepted as the primary effector cells of inflammation, are usually neglected in their role in later stages of immune activation and response (127). They have the capability to present antigen under inflammatory conditions expressing MHC class II and costimulatory molecules. They generate chemotactic signals such as TNF-α that attract monocytes and dendritic cells and influence macrophages to differentiate to a predominantly pro or antiinflammatory state. IFN-γ and B-lymphocyte stimulator (BLyS, BAFF) are also released by neutrophils and cause proliferation and maturation of T and B cells, respectively. In this context, neutrophil activation, cytokine release, and antigen presentation may link innate immune system to adap-tive responses and, by definition, give a broader role to neutrophils than simply "auto-inflammation" if one takes the latter as a limited inflammatory response with-out an effective adaptive component. In this respect, BD requires a more critical analysis of neutrophil activation, and BD neutrophils may have a different profile compared to the autoinflammatory disorders (29). An intriguing hypothesis might also be the role of a "*persistent infection*" in BD. Cryopyrin-associated inflam-masomes in neutrophils can be activated by bacterial peptidoglycans (PGN), bacterial RNA, and various gram-positive bacterial toxins (127, 128). Pathways of inflam-masome and recently described pattern-recognition receptors (PRRs) such as toll-like receptors (TLRs) intersect as both are sensors of bacterial products. The augmented adaptive responses in BD compared to autoinflammatory disorders can be the result of persistent oral and skin infections discussed above (5).

In addition to adaptive responses to bacterial and mammalian "*cross-reactive*" epitopes of human HSP60, a direct activation of innate immunity through TLRs by HSP60 is also shown (106, 129). HSPs released from necrotic (but not apoptotic) cells are observed to activate DCs (130). HSP60 is also shown to induce DC maturation with increased MHC class II, CD40, CD54 and CD86 expressions, and allogeneic T cell proliferation with a Th1 bias (131). Both human HSP60 and streptococcal extracts are shown to activate BD neutrophils to express TLR-6 (132). As another link between oral diseases, TLRs and HSPs, human T-cell proliferative responses to human HSP60 are increased in patients with periodontal disease and this proliferation can be inhibited with anti-TLR-2 antibodies (133). Monocytes of active BD patients showed higher expressions of TLR-2 and TLR-4, and this observation is linked to low levels of serum 25(OH)D$_3$, which inversely correlated with the expressions of TLRs 2/4. In vitro, vitamin D$_3$ was also found to dose-dependently suppress the protein and mRNA expressions of TLR-2 and TLR-4 (134). In another study, heme oxygenase (HO)-1 (an inducible heme-degrading enzyme that is induced by various stresses) suppressing inflammatory responses, is shown to be decreased in PBMCs of active BD patients. HO-1 expression is associated with increased HSP60 and TLR-4 expressions (135).

As neutrophils arrive very early to initiate inflammation in tissues and with a very short life span (127), clearance of apoptotic material by complement system proteins such as mannose-binding lectin (MBL), surfactant protein-A, and SP-D is critical in suppressing inflammation. An adaptive response related to neutrophils in BD may be promoted by aberrant phagocytosis of apoptotic neutrophils by DCs, as shown in ANCA-associated vasculitis (136). In this context, serum MBL levels are shown to be decreased in BD patients, and MBL deficiency may prolong the exposure of neutrophil-related antigens to adaptive immune system (137). A lower bacterial clearance due to low MBL levels may also predispose to bacterial infections and a higher prevalence of S. mutans colonization is observed in patients with low MBL levels in BD (138). The function of classical antigen presenting cells is possibly also disturbed in BD (139). Monocytes are activated and BD patients' monocyte culture supernatants cause increased adhesion of normal neutrophils to endothelial cell monolayers in vitro (140). Plasmacytoid dendritic cells (pDC) are observed to be decreased in PBMCs of BD patients with decreased IFN-β levels (141). A normalization of pDCs and the level of IFN-β are also reported in the same study in patients receiving IFN-α.

Another model points to a possible role of T cells for neutrophil activation in BD. Principal source of CXCL-8, the major neutrophil chemoattractant in BD PB, is lymphocytes (142). Recently, skin-derived T cell clones from BD patients have been shown to produce CXCL-8 and GM-CSF, but failed to secrete IFN-γ or IL-5. These cells might represent a particular subset as they differ from both Th1 and Th2 T cells and are associated with a unique, neutrophil-rich sterile inflammation (143). Auto (HSP60, retinal S-antigen) or microbial-derived antigen stimulated T cell lines, mainly of Th1 phenotype, are also demonstrated in other studies with the PB of BD patients (3, 50). However, lower levels of naïve T cells is also reported from BD patients' synovial fluids and may be related to the nonerosive and self-limiting course of BD arthritis compared to RA (144).

γδ T cells are also another important cell subset that links innate and adaptive responses. The γδ T cells have recently been shown to activate DCs and can present antigen. They are also activated under stress conditions by recognizing damaged cells (145). As these cells respond to both streptococci and HSP60-derived peptides in BD, they might participate in tissue destruction and presentation of the self and foreign antigens to adaptive immune cells (106).

Pathogenesis of Vascular Involvement

Vascular involvement in BD is predominantly venous in contrast to what is seen in other systemic vasculitides. However, the rare presence of pulmonary emboli is suggestive of "sticky" thrombi. In histopathological specimens, in addition to thrombi, inflammatory infiltrates in vessel walls point to a vasculitic process (146). Vasculitis is also present, in varying degrees, in the histopathologic specimens of oral and genital ulcers, erythema nodosum-like lesions, epididymitis, enteritis, and central nervous system lesions in BD. Nonlytic antibodies against endothelial cells are commonly present in both vascular and nonvascular BD (97). A 44 kD endothelial antigen is recognized by IgM AECA of BD patients. These antibodies, which mainly target α-enolase (100), increase the expression of ICAM-1 on EC and can activate mitogen-activated protein cascade through the extra-cellular signal regulated kinase (147). Endothelium-dependent brachial artery flow-mediated dilation is also impaired in BD, which is improved by vitamin C treatment and suggests a role for oxidative stress in vascular involvement (148, 149).

Coagulation and Fibrinolytic Pathway Abnormalities

No specific defect in the coagulation cascade has so far been demonstrated (4, 150). However, both coagulation and fibrinolytic pathways seem to be activated with or without thrombosis. Increased levels of thrombin-antithrombin III complex (TAT) and prothrombin fragment 1+2 support intravascular thrombin generation in these patients as a result of the activation of the coagulation cascade (151, 152). Various procoagulant conditions associated with increased risk of thrombosis, such as deficiencies of protein C, protein S and antithrombin III, factor V Leiden and prothrombin 20210A mutations may also contribute to the prothrombotic state of BD. Several-fold increases in the risk of thrombosis have been described in carriers of factor V Leiden and prothrombin gene mutations in patients with BD (153–155). Increased homocystein levels associated with thrombosis has also been reported (149, 156), however, with conflicting results (157, 158). ACL antibodies do not seem to be important in the thrombotic tendency of BD (159). Increased levels of plasmin-a2-antiplasmin complex (PAP) in BD patients possibly indicate an increased fibrinolytic activity. Some studies also revealed defective fibrinolysis, following venous occlusion or after desmopressin infusion, or impaired plasminogen activator binding kinetics (4). Tissue plasminogen activator (t-PA) activity was observed to be decreased, normal or increased in different studies (160, 161). The concentrations of free t-PA, u-PA, and free plasminogen activator inhibitor-1 (PAI-1) were elevated in BD, but the antigen (free and PAI-1 bound) levels of t-PA and u-PA were normal, suggesting a defective t-PA/PAI-1 complex formation (4, 162). The endothelial dysfunction resulting from immune-mediated vasculitis may be an important factor in the thrombotic tendency seen in many patients (146).

Severity and Gender

One currently underexplored area is the gender differences in BD, a condition pronouncedly more severe among males (1). Severe complications such as vascular, CNS, and pulmonary involvement as well as mortality are related to the male gender. However, serum levels of testosterone and oestradiol are not different among the male patients. Sebum excretion rate, which is under androgenic control, is increased in BD, but also in RA, patients (163). Estrogen is shown to protect against endotoxin-induced uveitis (EIU) in Lewis rats. In EIU, cellular infiltration is more marked in male than in female rats, and ovariectomy increases cellular infiltration. Estrogen decreases E-selectin and IL-6 gene expressions through estrogen receptors in vascular endothelium (164). As another mechanism, fMLP-stimulated superoxide generation from neutrophils is decreased in vitro with estrogen incubation (165). Through these mechanisms, estrogens might suppress the pro-inflammatory functions of vascular endothelium and neutrophils, explaining the milder clinical course in females. Alternatively, it was shown that testesteron augments the neutrophil functions, especially in male BD patients (35).

Behçet's Disease or Syndrome: Observations from the Clinic: Different Antigenic Stimuli or Inflammatory Milieu for Different Manifestations?

The term "Behçet's syndrome" has been suggested by Ehrlich et al. due to a different, milder clinical course in Western populations compared to patients with classical course from the "Silk Route" (166). Although not universally agreed upon, this approach might be helpful in elucidating the predisposing genetic and environmental factors. Various manifestations of BD occurring during the disease course unpredict-ably and unlinked to any previous risk factor might be associated with different organ-specific antigens or genetic predispositions. Therapeutic trials provide interesting clues, as the effects of various popular treatments in BD seem to be organ-specific. Colchicine is especially effective for erythema-nodosum (EN) like lesions and arthritis, but has a limited effect on organ involvement. It is not uncommon to see mucocutaneous lesions relapse in patients under immunosuppressive therapy, which prevents ocular attacks. In a double-blind trial, thalidomide was effective for oral and genital ulcers, but caused a significant increase in EN lesions in the first 8 weeks (167). As an explanation for this surprising observation, the authors suggested that "the cause of aphthous ulcers and EN may not have a common putative denominator in BD".

Immune responses to local antigens such as dermal keratins in psoriasis or synovial antigens such as collagen type II in RA have been reported. Similarly, local, organ-specific antigens might be immuno-pathogenic for patient subgroups with muco-cutaneous, ocular, or articular organ involvements in BD. Retinal S-antigen derived PDSAg, with T cell recognition found only in patients with posterior uveitis, is a candidate organ-specific antigen of this type (123). Similarly, presence of anti-HSP60 and αB-crystallin antibodies mainly in parenchyma neuro-Behçet's, but not in pure vascular form, underlines the fact that even within the same organ, immune responses might reflect different clinical subtypes (168, 169). A different inflammatory milieu, associated with different organ manifestations such as elevated matrix metalloproteinase-2 levels associated with aneurysms and IL-6 with parenchymal neuro-Behçet's, is also possible (170–172).

Conclusions

Both innate and adaptive immune systems are activated in BD with a pro-inflammatory and Th1 type of cytokine profile.

An immune response is possibly triggered by two main mechanisms. According to the "*danger theory*" by P. Matzinger, immune system responds to the alarm signals of injured host cells, which activate antigen presenting cells (173). "*The pattern-recognition theory*" places the role of the microbial "nonself" as the dominant stimuli for innate immune system, which in turn triggers an adaptive response (174). Human HSP60 can be an example of the first and various microbial antigens such as lipoteichoic acid of the second type of stimuli for innate and possibly adaptive immune responses in BD pathogenesis. However, these theories are not mutually exclusive. A recent report shows that whether neutrophil apoptosis is due to infection or nonspecific TLR-signaling determines further T regulatory or Th17 pathway activation (175).

In this context, it might be too simplistic to describe BD as either an autoimmune or an autoinflammatory disease. A new category (first suggested for spondyloarthropathies by McGonagle et al.) should possibly be defined for diseases such as BD, which are unlikely to be classical autoantigen-derived autoimmune diseases (176). An infectious agent is possibly required to trigger the inflammation in BD. It might then be linked to a specific, primary innate, immune abnormality (with a genetic mutation effecting an adhesion molecule or a pro-inflammatory cytokine), which predisposes to early or more intense neutrophil and T cell responses. Alternatively, a broad intra-cellular signaling abnormality of a transcription factor, which lowers the threshold of inflammatory responses to external stimuli, as proposed for FMF with decreased pyrine expression of neutrophils, might be present (*hyperreactivity model*).

However, unlike classical autoinflammatory disorders, an adaptive response is also sustained through bacterial persistence or autoantigen-activated dendritic, T or B cells. Clarification of these mechanisms might help to elucidate how both antimicrobial and immunosuppressant therapies seem to be effective in BD and might pave the way for more specific immune interventions.

References

1. Yazici H, Fresko I, Yurdakul S (2007) Behçet's syndrome: disease manifestations, management, and advances in treatment. Nat Clin Pract Rheumatol 3(3):148–155
2. Sakane T, Takeno M, Suzuki N, Inaba G (1999) Behçet's disease. N Engl J Med 341(17): 1284–1291
3. Direskeneli H (2001) Behçet's disease: infectious aetiology, new autoantigens, and HLA-B51. Ann Rheum Dis 60(11):996–1002
4. Zierhut M, Mizuki N, Ohno S, Inoko H, Gul A, Onoe K et al (2003) Immunology and functional genomics of Behçet's disease. Cell Mol Life Sci 60(9):1903–1922
5. Mumcu G, Inanc N, Yavuz S, Direskeneli H (2007) The role of infectious agents in the pathogenesis, clinical manifestations and treatment strategies in Behçet's disease. Clin Exp Rheumatol 25(4 Suppl 45):S27–S33
6. Verity DH, Wallace GR, Vaughan RW, Stanford MR (2003) Behçet's disease: from Hippocrates to the third millennium. Br J Ophthalmol 87(9):1175–1183
7. Kaneko F, Oyama N, Yanagihori H, Isogai E, Yokota K, Oguma K (2008) The role of streptococcal hypersensitivity in the pathogenesis of Behçet's disease. Eur J Dermatol 18(5):489–498
8. The Behçet's Disease Research Committee of Japan (1989) Skin hypersensitivity to streptococcal antigens and the induction of systemic symptoms by the antigens in Behçet's disease – a multicenter study. J Rheumatol 16(4):506–511
9. Mumcu G, Ergun T, Inanc N, Fresko I, Atalay T, Hayran O et al (2004) Oral health is impaired in Behçet's disease and is associated with disease severity. Rheumatology (Oxford) 43(8):1028–1033
10. Isogai E, Ohno S, Kotake S, Isogai H, Tsurumizu T, Fujii N et al (1990) Chemiluminescence of neutrophils from patients with Behçet's disease and its correlation with an increased proportion of uncommon serotypes of *Streptococcus sanguis* in the oral flora. Arch Oral Biol 35(1):43–48
11. Karacayli U, Mumcu G, Simsek I, Pay S, Kose O, Erdem H et al (2009) The close association between dental and periodontal treatments and oral ulcer course in Behçet's disease: a prospective clinical study. J Oral Pathol Med 38(5):410–415
12. Kibaroglu A, Eksioglu-Demiralp E, Akoglu T, Direskeneli H (2004) T and NK cell subset changes with microbial extracts and human HSP60-derived peptides in Behçet's disease. Clin Exp Rheumatol 22(4 Suppl 34):S59–S63
13. Hirohata S, Oka H, Mizushima Y (1992) Streptococcal-related antigens stimulate production of IL6 and interferon-gamma by T cells from patients with Behçet's disease. Cell Immunol 140(2):410–419
14. Hirohata S, Hashimoto T (1998) Abnormal T cells responses to bacterial antigens in patients with Behçet's disease. Clin Exp Immunol 112:317–324
15. Hatemi G, Bahar H, Uysal S, Mat C, Gogus F, Masatlioglu S et al (2004) The pustular skin lesions in Behçet's syndrome are not sterile. Ann Rheum Dis 63(11):1450–1452
16. Sezer FN (1953) The isolation of a virus as the cause of Behçet's diseases. Am J Ophthalmol 36(3):301–315
17. Lee S, Bang D, Cho YH, Lee ES, Sohn S (1996) Polymerase chain reaction reveals herpes simplex virus DNA in saliva of patients with Behçet's disease. Arch Dermatol Res 288(4): 179–183

18. Hamzaoui K, Ayed K, Slim A, Hamza M, Touraine J (1990) Natural killer cell activity, interferon-gamma and antibodies to herpes viruses in patients with Behçet's disease. Clin Exp Immunol 79(1):28–34
19. Hamza M, Elleuch M, Slim A, Hamzaoui K, Ayed K (1990) Antibodies to herpes simplex virus in patients with Behçet's disease. Clin Rheumatol 9(4):498–500
20. Davies UM, Palmer RG, Denman AM (1988) Treatment with acyclovir does not affect orogenital ulcers in Behçet's syndrome: a randomized double-blind trial. Br J Rheumatol 27(4):300–302
21. Sohn S, Bang D, Lee ES, Kwon HJ, Lee SI, Lee S (2001) Experimental studies on the antiviral agent famciclovir in Behçet's disease symptoms in ICR mice. Br J Dermatol 145(5):799–804
22. Sohn S, Lutz M, Kwon HJ, Konwalinka G, Lee S, Schirmer M (2004) Therapeutic effects of gemcitabine on cutaneous manifestations in an Adamantiades–Behçet's disease-like mouse model. Exp Dermatol 13(10):630–634
23. Mege JL, Dilsen N, Sanguedolce V, Gul A, Bongrand P, Roux H et al (1993) Overproduction of monocyte derived tumor necrosis factor alpha, interleukin (IL) 6, IL-8 and increased neutrophil superoxide generation in Behçet's disease. A comparative study with familial Mediterranean fever and healthy subjects. J Rheumatol 20(9):1544–1549
24. Pronai L, Ichikawa Y, Nakazawa H, Arimori S (1991) Enhanced superoxide generation and the decreased superoxide scavenging activity of peripheral blood leukocytes in Behçet's disease – effects of colchicine. Clin Exp Rheumatol 9(3):227–233
25. Carletto A, Pacor ML, Biasi D, Caramaschi P, Zeminian S, Bellavite P et al (1997) Changes of neutrophil migration without modification of in vitro metabolism and adhesion in Behçet's disease. J Rheumatol 24(7):1332–1336
26. Takeno M, Kaiyone A, Yamashita N, Takiguchi M, Mizushima Y, Kaneoka H et al (1995) Excessive function of peripheral blood neutrophils from patients with Behçet's disease and from HLA-B51 transgenic mice. Arthritis Rheum 38:426–433
27. Tuzun B, Tuzun Y, Yurdakul S, Hamuryudan V, Yazici H, Ozyazgan Y (1999) Neutrophil chemotaxis in Behçet's syndrome. Ann Rheum Dis 58(10):658
28. Sahin S, Akoglu T, Direskeneli H, Sen LS, Lawrence R (1996) Neutrophil adhesion to endothelial cells and factors affecting adhesion in patients with Behçet's disease. Ann Rheum Dis 55(2):128–133
29. Eksioglu-Demiralp E, Direskeneli H, Kibaroglu A, Yavuz S, Ergun T, Akoglu T (2001) Neutrophil activation in Behçet's disease. Clin Exp Rheumatol 19(5 Suppl 24):S19–S24
30. Hallett MB, Lloyds D (1995) Neutrophil priming: the cellular signals that say 'amber' but not 'green'. Immunol Today 16(6):264–268
31. Ureten K, Ertenli I, Ozturk MA, Kiraz S, Onat AM, Tuncer M et al (2005) Neutrophil CD64 expression in Behçet's disease. J Rheumatol 32(5):849–852
32. Pay S, Musabak U, Simsek I, Pekel A, Erdem H, Dinc A et al (2006) Expression of CXCR-1 and CXCR-2 chemokine receptors on synovial neutrophils in inflammatory arthritides: does persistent or increasing expression of CXCR-2 contribute to the chronic inflammation or erosive changes? Joint Bone Spine 73(6):691–696
33. Qiao H, Sonoda KH, Ariyama A, Kuratomi Y, Kawano Y, Ishibashi T (2005) CXCR2 Expression on neutrophils is upregulated during the relapsing phase of ocular Behçet disease. Curr Eye Res 30(3):195–203
34. Fujimori K, Oh-i K, Takeuchi M, Yamakawa N, Hattori T, Kezuka T et al (2008) Circulating neutrophils in Behçet's disease is resistant for apoptotic cell death in the remission phase of uveitis. Graefes Arch Clin Exp Ophthalmol 246(2):285–290
35. Yavuz S, Ozilhan G, Elbir Y, Tolunay A, Eksioglu-Demiralp E, Direskeneli H (2007) Activation of neutrophils by testosterone in Behçet's disease. Clin Exp Rheumatol 25(4 Suppl 45): S46–S51
36. Chen ZW, Letvin NL (2003) Adaptive immune response of Vgamma2Vdelta2 T cells: a new paradigm. Trends Immunol 24(4):213–219
37. Hamzaoui K, Hamzaoui A, Hentati F, Kahan A, Ayed K, Chabbou A et al (1994) Phenotype and functional profile of T cell expressing gamma delta receptor from patients with active Behçet's disease. J Rheumatol 21:2301–2306

38. Freysdottir J, Lau S, Fortune F (1999) Gammadelta T cells in Behçet's disease (BD) and recurrent aphthous stomatitis (RAS). Clin Exp Immunol 118:451–457
39. Bank I, Duvdevani M, Livneh A (2003) Expansion of [gamma][delta] T-cells in Behçet's disease: role of disease activity and microbial flora in oral ulcers. J Lab Clin Med 141(1):33–40
40. Direskeneli H, Eksioglu-Demiralp E, Kibaroglu A, Yavuz S, Ergun T, Akoglu T (1999) Oligoclonal T cell expansions in patients with Behçet's disease. Clin Exp Immunol 117(1): 166–170
41. Freysdottir J, Hussain L, Farmer I, Lau S-H, Fortune F (2006) Diversity of gammadelta T cells in patients with Behçet's disease is indicative of polyclonal activation. Oral Dis 12(3): 271–277
42. Yasuoka H, Yamaguchi Y, Mizuki N, Nishida T, Kawakami Y, Kuwana M (2008) Preferential activation of circulating CD8+ and gammadelta T cells in patients with active Behçet's disease and HLA-B51. Clin Exp Rheumatol 26(4 Suppl 50):S59–S63
43. Verjans G, van Hagen PM, van der Kooi A, Osterhaus AD, Baarsma GS (2002) V[gamma]9V[delta]2 T cells recovered from eyes of patients with Behçet's disease recognize non-peptide prenyl pyrophosphate antigens. J Neuroimmunol 130(1-2):46–54
44. Ergun T, Ince U, Eksioglu-Demiralp E, Direskeneli H, Gurbuz O, Gurses L et al (2001) HSP 60 expression in mucocutaneous lesions of Behçet's disease. J Am Acad Dermatol 45(6): 904–909
45. Mochizuki N, Suzuki N, Takeno M, Nagafuchi H, Harada T, Kaneoka H, Yamashita N, Hirayama K, Nakajima T, Mizushima Y et al (1994) Fine antigen specificity of human gamma delta T cell lines established by repetitive stimulation with a serotype (KTH-1) of a gram-positive bacterium, *Streptococcus sanguis*. Eur J Immunol 24:1536–43
46. Triolo G, Accardo-Palumbo A, Dieli F, Ciccia F, Ferrante A, Giardina E et al (2003) Vgamma9/Vdelta2 T lymphocytes in Italian patients with Behçet's disease: evidence for expansion, and tumour necrosis factor receptor II and interleukin-12 receptor beta1 expression in active disease. Arthritis Res Ther 5(5):R262–R268
47. Accardo-Palumbo AFA, Cadelo M, Ciccia F, Parrinello G, Lipari L, Giardina AR, Riili M, Giardina E, Dieli F, Triolo G (2004) The level of soluble Granzyme A is elevated in the plasma and in the Vgamma9/Vdelta2 T cell culture supernatants of patients with active Behçet's disease. Clin Exp Rheumatol 22(4 Suppl 34):S45–S49
48. Hasan A, Fortune F, Wilson A, Warr K, Shinnick T, Mizushima Y et al (1996) Role of gamma delta T cells in pathogenesis and diagnosis of Behçet's disease. Lancet 347(9004):789–794
49. Kaneko S, Suzuki N, Yamashita N, Nagafuchi H, Nakajima T, Wakisaka S et al (1997) Characterization of T cells specific for an epitope of human 60-kD heat shock protein (hsp) in patients with Behçet's disease (BD) in Japan. Clin Exp Immunol 108(2):204–212
50. Saruhan-Direskeneli G, Celet B, Eksioglu-Demiralp E, Direskeneli H (2001) Human HSP 60 peptide responsive T cell lines are similarly present in both Behçet's disease patients and healthy controls. Immunol Lett 79(3):203–208
51. Mizuki N, Ota M, Kimura M, Ohno S, Ando H, Katsuyama Y et al (1997) Triplet repeat polymorphism in the transmembrane region of the MICA gene: a strong association of six GCT repetitions with Behçet's disease. Proc Natl Acad Sci U S A 94(4):1298–1303
52. Kaneko F, Takahashi Y, Muramatsu R, Adachi K, Miura Y, Nakane A et al (1985) Natural killer cell numbers and function in peripheral lymphoid cells in Behçet's disease. Br J Dermatol 113(3):313–318
53. Hamzaoui K, Ayed K, Hamza M, Touraine JL (1988) Natural killer cells in Behçet's disease. Clin Exp Immunol 71(1):126–131
54. Suzuki Y, Hoshi K, Matsuda T, Mizushima Y (1992) Increased peripheral blood gamma delta+T cells and natural killer cells in Behçet's disease. J Rheumatol 19(4):588–592
55. Ahn JK, Chung H, Lee DS, Yu YS, Yu HG (2005) CD8brightCD56+ T cells are cytotoxic effectors in patients with active Behçet's uveitis. J Immunol 175(9):6133–6142
56. Saruhan-Direskeneli G, Uyar FA, Cefle A, Onder SC, Eksioglu-Demiralp E, Kamali S et al (2004) Expression of KIR and C-type lectin receptors in Behçet's disease. Rheumatology (Oxford) 43(4):423–427

57. Stojanov S, Kastner DL (2005) Familial autoinflammatory diseases: genetics, pathogenesis and treatment. Curr Opin Rheumatol 17(5):586–599
58. Ting JP, Kastner DL, Hoffman HM (2006) CATERPILLERs, pyrin and hereditary immunological disorders. Nat Rev Immunol 6(3):183–195
59. Musabak U, Pay S, Erdem H, Simsek I, Pekel A, Dinc A et al (2006) Serum interleukin-18 levels in patients with Behçet's disease. Is its expression associated with disease activity or clinical presentations? Rheumatol Int 26(6):545–550
60. Gul A (2005) Behet's disease as an autoinflammatory disorder. Curr Drug Targets Inflamm Allergy 4(1):81–83
61. Atagunduz P, Ergun T, Direskeneli H (2003) MEFV mutations are increased in Behçet's disease (BD) and are associated with vascular involvement. Clin Exp Rheumatol 21(4 Suppl 30):S35–S37
62. Rabinovich E, Shinar Y, Leiba M, Ehrenfeld M, Langevitz P, Livneh A (2007) Common FMF alleles may predispose to development of Behçet's disease with increased risk for venous thrombosis. Scand J Rheumatol 36(1):48–52
63. Yazici H, Fresko I (2005) Behçet's disease and other autoinflammatory conditions: what's in a name? Clin Exp Rheumatol 23(4 Suppl 38):S1–S2
64. Ergun T, Gurbuz O, Harvell J, Jorizzo J, White W (1998) The histopathology of pathergy: a chronologic study of skin hyperreactivity in Behçet's disease. Int J Dermatol 37(12):929–933
65. Fresko I, Yazici H, Bayramicli M, Yurdakul S, Mat C (1993) Effect of surgical cleaning of the skin on the pathergy phenomenon in Behçet's syndrome. Ann Rheum Dis 52(8): 619–620
66. Melikoglu M, Uysal S, Krueger JG, Kaplan G, Gogus F, Yazici H et al (2006) Characterization of the divergent wound-healing responses occurring in the pathergy reaction and normal healthy volunteers. J Immunol 177(9):6415–6421
67. Tunc R, Uluhan A, Melikoglu M, Ozyazgan Y, Ozdogan H, Yazici H (2001) A reassessment of the International Study Group criteria for the diagnosis (classification) of Behçet's syndrome. Clin Exp Rheumatol 19(5 Suppl 24):S45–S47
68. Cakir N, Yazici H, Chamberlain MA, Barnes CG, Yurdakul S, Atasoy S et al (1991) Response to intradermal injection of monosodium urate crystals in Behçet's syndrome. Ann Rheum Dis 50(9):634–636
69. Gogus F, Fresko I, Elbir Y, Eksioglu-Demiralp E, Direskeneli H (2005) Oxidative burst response to monosodium urate crystals in patients with Behçet's syndrome. Clin Exp Rheumatol 23(4 Suppl 38):S81–S85
70. Martinon F, Petrilli V, Mayor A, Tardivel A, Tschopp J (2006) Gout-associated uric acid crystals activate the NALP3 inflammasome. Nature 440(7081):237–241
71. Esin S, Gul A, Hodara V, Jeddi-Tehrani M, Dilsen N, Konice M et al (1997) Peripheral blood T cell expansions in patients with Behçet's disease. Clin Exp Immunol 107(3):520–527
72. Frassanito M, Dammacco R, Cafforio P, Dammacco F (1999) Th1 polarization of the immune response in Behçet's disease. Arthritis Rheum 42:1967–1974
73. Sugi-Ikai N, Nakazawa M, Nakamura S, Ohno S, Minami M (1998) Increased frequencies of interleukin-2 and interferon-gamma-producing T cells in patients with active Behçet's disease. Invest Ophthalmol Vis Sci 39(6):996–1004
74. Amberger M, Groll S, Gunaydin I, Deuter C, Vonthein R, Kotter I (2007) Intracellular cytokine patterns in Behçet's disease in comparison to ankylosing spondylitis – influence of treatment with interferon-alpha2a. Clin Exp Rheumatol 25(4 Suppl 45):S52–S57
75. Imamura Y, Kurokawa MS, Yoshikawa H, Nara K, Takada E, Masuda C et al (2005) Involvement of Th1 cells and heat shock protein 60 in the pathogenesis of intestinal Behçet's disease. Clin Exp Immunol 139(2):371–378
76. Nara K, Kurokawa MS, Chiba S, Yoshikawa H, Tsukikawa S, Matsuda T et al (2008) Involvement of innate immunity in the pathogenesis of intestinal Behçet's disease. Clin Exp Immunol 152(2):245–251
77. Lew W, Chang JY, Jung JY, Bang D (2008) Increased expression of interleukin-23 p19 mRNA in erythema nodosum-like lesions of Behçet's disease. Br J Dermatol 158(3):505–511

78. Yanagihori H, Oyama N, Nakamura K, Mizuki N, Oguma K, Kaneko F (2006) Role of IL-12B promoter polymorphism in Adamantiades–Behçet's disease susceptibility: an involvement of Th1 immunoreactivity against *Streptococcus sanguinis* antigen. J Invest Dermatol 126(7): 1534–1540

79. Kulaber A, Tugal-Tutkun I, Yentur SP, Akman-Demir G, Kaneko F, Gul A et al (2007) Pro-inflammatory cellular immune response in Behçet's disease. Rheumatol Int 27(12):1113–1118

80. Mantas C, Direskeneli H, Eksioglu-Demiralp E, Akoglu T (1999) Serum levels of Th2 cytokines IL-4 and IL-10 in Behçet's disease. J Rheumatol 26(2):510–512

81. Raziuddin S, al-Dalaan A, Bahabri S, Siraj AK, al-Sedairy S (1998) Divergent cytokine production profile in Behçet's disease. Altered Th1/Th2 cell cytokine pattern. J Rheumatol 25(2):329–33

82. Dalghous AM, Freysdottir J, Fortune F (2006) Expression of cytokines, chemokines, and chemokine receptors in oral ulcers of patients with Behçet's disease (BD) and recurrent aphthous stomatitis is Th1-associated, although Th2-association is also observed in patients with BD. Scand J Rheumatol 35(6):472–475

83. Curnow SJ, Pryce K, Modi N, Knight B, Graham EM, Stewart JE et al (2008) Serum cytokine profiles in Behçet's disease: is there a role for IL-15 in pathogenesis? Immunol Lett 121(1):7–12

84. Romagnani S (2008) Human Th17 cells. Arthritis Res Ther 10(2):206

85. Oukka M (2007) Interplay between pathogenic Th17 and regulatory T cells. Ann Rheum Dis 66(Suppl 3):iii87–iii90

86. Hamzaoui K, Hamzaoui A, Guemira F, Bessioud M, Hamza M, Ayed K (2002) Cytokine profile in Behçet's disease patients. Relationship with disease activity. Scand J Rheumatol 31(4):205–210

87. Chi W, Zhu X, Yang P, Liu X, Lin X, Zhou H et al (2008) Upregulated IL-23 and IL-17 in Behçet's patients with active uveitis. Invest Ophthalmol Vis Sci 49(7):3058–3064

88. Saruhan-Direskeneli G, Yentur SP, Akman-Demir G, Isik N, Serdaroglu P (2003) Cytokines and chemokines in neuro-Behçet's disease compared to multiple sclerosis and other neurological diseases. J Neuroimmunol 145(1–2):127–134

89. Zhao C, Yang P, He H, Lin X, Li B, Zhou H et al (2008) S-antigen specific T helper type 1 response is present in Behçet's disease. Mol Vis 14:1456–1464

90. Hamzaoui K, Hamzaoui A, Houman H (2006) CD4+CD25+ regulatory T cells in patients with Behçet's disease. Clin Exp Rheumatol 24(5 Suppl 42):S71–S78

91. Hamzaoui K, Houman H, Hamzaoui A (2007) Regulatory T cells in cerebrospinal fluid from Behçet's disease with neurological manifestations. J Neuroimmunol 187(1–2):201–204

92. Nanke Y, Kotake S, Goto M, Ujihara H, Matsubara M, Kamatani N (2008) Decreased percentages of regulatory T cells in peripheral blood of patients with Behçet's disease before ocular attack: a possible predictive marker of ocular attack. Mod Rheumatol 18(4):354–358

93. Hamzaoui K (2007) Paradoxical high regulatory T cell activity in Behçet's disease. Clin Exp Rheumatol 25(4 Suppl 45):S107–S113

94. Yazici H (1997) The place of Behçet's syndrome among the autoimmune diseases. Int Rev Immunol 14(1):1–10

95. Gunaydin I, Ustundag C, Kaner G, Pazarli H, Yurdakul S, Hamuryudan V et al (1994) The prevalence of Sjogren's syndrome in Behçet's syndrome. J Rheumatol 21(9):1662–1664

96. Eksioglu-Demiralp E, Kibaroglu A, Direskeneli H, Yavuz S, Karsli F, Yurdakul S et al (1999) Phenotypic characteristics of B cells in Behçet's disease: increased activity in B cell subsets. J Rheumatol 26(4):826–832

97. Direskeneli H, Keser G, D'Cruz D, Khamashta MA, Akoglu T, Yazici H et al (1995) Anti-endothelial cell antibodies, endothelial proliferation and von Willebrand factor antigen in Behçet's disease. Clin Rheumatol 14(1):55–61

98. Michelson JB, Chisari FV, Kansu T (1985) Antibodies to oral mucosa in patients with ocular Behçet's disease. Ophthalmology 92(9):1277–1281

99. Mor F, Weinberger A, Cohen IR (2002) Identification of alpha-tropomyosin as a target self-antigen in Behçet's syndrome. Eur J Immunol 32(2):356–365

100. Lee KH, Chung HS, Kim HS, Oh SH, Ha MK, Baik JH et al (2003) Human alpha-enolase from endothelial cells as a target antigen of anti-endothelial cell antibody in Behçet's disease. Arthritis Rheum 48(7):2025–2035
101. Mahesh SP, Li Z, Buggage R, Mor F, Cohen IR, Chew EY et al (2005) Alpha tropomyosin as a self-antigen in patients with Behçet's disease. Clin Exp Immunol 140(2):368–375
102. Lu Y, Ye P, Chen SL, Tan EM, Chan EK (2005) Identification of kinectin as a novel Behçet's disease autoantigen. Arthritis Res Ther 7(5):R1133–R1139
103. Okunuki Y, Usui Y, Kezuka T, Hattori T, Masuko K, Nakamura H et al (2008) Proteomic surveillance of retinal autoantigens in endogenous uveitis: implication of esterase D and brain-type creatine kinase as novel autoantigens. Mol Vis 14:1094–1104
104. Okunuki Y, Usui Y, Takeuchi M, Kezuka T, Hattori T, Masuko K et al (2007) Proteomic surveillance of autoimmunity in Behçet's disease with uveitis: selenium binding protein is a novel autoantigen in Behçet's disease. Exp Eye Res 84(5):823–831
105. Delunardo F, Conti F, Margutti P, Alessandri C, Priori R, Siracusano A et al (2006) Identification and characterization of the carboxy-terminal region of Sip-1, a novel autoantigen in Behçet's disease. Arthritis Res Ther 8(3):R71
106. Direskeneli H, Saruhan-Direskeneli G (2003) The role of heat shock proteins in Behçet's disease. Clin Exp Rheumatol 21(4 Suppl 30):S44–S48
107. Direskeneli H, Eksioglu-Demiralp E, Yavuz S, Ergun T, Shinnick T, Lehner T et al (2000) T cell responses to 60/65 kDa heat shock protein derived peptides in Turkish patients with Behçet's disease. J Rheumatol 27(3):708–713
108. Direskeneli H, Hasan A, Shinnick T, Mizushima R, van der Zee R, Fortune F et al (1996) Recognition of B-cell epitopes of the 65 kDa HSP in Behçet's disease. Scand J Immunol 43(4):464–471
109. Nagafuchi H, Takeno M, Yoshikawa H, Kurokawa MS, Nara K, Takada E et al (2005) Excessive expression of Txk, a member of the Tec family of tyrosine kinases, contributes to excessive Th1 cytokine production by T lymphocytes in patients with Behçet's disease. Clin Exp Immunol 139(2):363–370
110. Hu W, Hasan A, Wilson A, Stanford MR, Li-Yang Y, Todryk S et al (1998) Experimental mucosal induction of uveitis with the 60-kDa heat shock protein-derived peptide 336-351. Eur J Immunol 28(8):2444–2455
111. Stanford M, Whittall T, Bergmeier LA, Lindblad M, Lundin S, Shinnick T et al (2004) Oral tolerization with peptide 336-351 linked to cholera toxin B subunit in preventing relapses of uveitis in Behçet's disease. Clin Exp Immunol 137(1):201–208
112. Ohno S, Asanuma T, Sugiura S, Wakisaka A, Aizawa M, Itakura K (1978) HLA-Bw51 and Behçet's disease. JAMA 240(6):529
113. Gul A, Hajeer AH, Worthington J, Barrett JH, Ollier WE, Silman AJ (2001) Evidence for linkage of the HLA-B locus in Behçet's disease, obtained using the transmission disequilibrium test. Arthritis Rheum 44(1):239–240
114. Falk K, Rotzschke O, Takiguchi M, Gnau V, Stevanovic S, Jung G et al (1995) Peptide motifs of HLA-B51, -B52 and -B78 molecules, and implications for Behçet's disease. Int Immunol 7(2):223–228
115. Yasuoka H, Okazaki Y, Kawakami Y, Hirakata M, Inoko H, Ikeda Y et al (2004) Autoreactive CD8+ cytotoxic T lymphocytes to major histocompatibility complex class I chain-related gene A in patients with Behçet's disease. Arthritis Rheum 50(11):3658–3662
116. Yamamoto J, Minami M, Inaba G, Masuda K, Mochizuki M (1993) Cellular autoimmunity to retinal specific antigens in patients with Behçet's disease. Br J Ophthalmol 77(9):584–9
117. Zhao C, Yang P, He H, Lin X, Du L, Zhou H et al (2009) Retinal S-antigen Th1 cell epitope mapping in patients with Behçet's disease. Graefes Arch Clin Exp Ophthalmol 247(4):555–560
118. Gul A, Uyar FA, Inanc M, Ocal L, Barrett JH, Aral O et al (2002) A weak association of HLA-B*2702 with Behçet's disease. Genes Immun 3(6):368–372
119. Wildner G, Thurau SR (1994) Cross-reactivity between an HLA-B27-derived peptide and a retinal autoantigen peptide: a clue to major histocompatibility complex association with autoimmune disease. Eur J Immunol 24(11):2579–2585

120. Baum H, Davies H, Peakman M (1996) Molecular mimicry in the MHC: hidden clues to autoimmunity? Immunol Today 17(2):64–70
121. Chicz RM, Urban RG, Gorga JC, Vignali DA, Lane WS, Strominger JL (1993) Specificity and promiscuity among naturally processed peptides bound to HLA-DR alleles. J Exp Med 178(1):27–47
122. Wildner G, Diedrichs-Mohring M, Thurau SR (2008) Rat models of autoimmune uveitis. Ophthalmic Res 40(3–4):141–144
123. Kurhan-Yavuz S, Direskeneli H, Bozkurt N, Ozyazgan Y, Bavbek T, Kazokoglu H et al (2000) Anti-MHC autoimmunity in Behçet's disease: T cell responses to an HLA-B-derived peptide cross-reactive with retinal-S antigen in patients with uveitis. Clin Exp Immunol 120(1):162–166
124. Thurau SR, Wildner G (2002) Oral tolerance for treating uveitis – new hope for an old immunological mechanism. Prog Retin Eye Res 21(6):577–589
125. Musabak U, Sengul A, Oktenli C, Pay S, Yesilova Z, Kenar L et al (2004) Does immune activation continue during an attack-free period in familial Mediterranean fever? Clin Exp Immunol 138(3):526–533
126. Simsek I, Pay S, Pekel A, Dinc A, Musabak U, Erdem H et al (2007) Serum proinflammatory cytokines directing T helper 1 polarization in patients with familial Mediterranean fever. Rheumatol Int 27(9):807–811
127. Nathan C (2006) Neutrophils and immunity: challenges and opportunities. Nat Rev Immunol 6(3):173–182
128. Martinon F, Agostini L, Meylan E, Tschopp J (2004) Identification of bacterial muramyl dipeptide as activator of the NALP3/cryopyrin inflammasome. Curr Biol 14(21):1929–1934
129. Vabulas RM, Wagner H, Schild H (2002) Heat shock proteins as ligands of toll-like receptors. Curr Top Microbiol Immunol 270:169–184
130. Basu S, Binder RJ, Suto R, Anderson KM, Srivastava PK (2000) Necrotic but not apoptotic cell death releases heat shock proteins, which deliver a partial maturation signal to dendritic cells and activate the NF-kappa B pathway. Int Immunol 12(11):1539–1546
131. Flohe SB, Bruggemann J, Lendemans S, Nikulina M, Meierhoff G, Flohe S et al (2003) Human heat shock protein 60 induces maturation of dendritic cells versus a Th1-promoting phenotype. J Immunol 170(5):2340–2348
132. Yavuz S, Elbir Y, Tulunay A, Eksioglu-Demiralp E, Direskeneli H (2008) Differential expression of toll-like receptor 6 on granulocytes and monocytes implicates the role of micro-organisms in Behçet's disease etiopathogenesis. Rheumatol Int 28(5):401–406
133. Hasan A, Sadoh D, Palmer R, Foo M, Marber M, Lehner T (2005) The immune responses to human and microbial heat shock proteins in periodontal disease with and without coronary heart disease. Clin Exp Immunol 142(3):585–594
134. Do JE, Kwon SY, Park S, Lee ES (2008) Effects of vitamin D on expression of Toll-like receptors of monocytes from patients with Behçet's disease. Rheumatology (Oxford) 47(6):840–848
135. Kirino Y, Takeno M, Watanabe R, Murakami S, Kobayashi M, Ideguchi H et al (2008) Association of reduced heme oxygenase-1 with excessive Toll-like receptor 4 expression in peripheral blood mononuclear cells in Behçet's disease. Arthritis Res Ther 10(1):R16
136. Harper L, Williams JM, Savage CO (2004) The importance of resolution of inflammation in the pathogenesis of ANCA-associated vasculitis. Biochem Soc Trans 32(Pt 3):502–506
137. Inanc N, Mumcu G, Birtas E, Elbir Y, Yavuz S, Ergun T et al (2005) Serum mannose-binding lectin levels are decreased in Behçet's disease and associated with disease severity. J Rheumatol 32(2):287–291
138. Mumcu G (2009) Association of salivary S. mutans colonization, mannose-binding lectin deficiency and male gender in Behçet's disease. Clin Exp Rheumatol 27(2 Suppl 53):S32–S36
139. Pay S, Simsek I, Erdem H, Dinc A (2007) Immunopathogenesis of Behçet's disease with special emphasize on the possible role of antigen presenting cells. Rheumatol Int 27(5):417–424
140. Sahin S, Lawrence R, Direskeneli H, Hamuryudan V, Yazici H, Akoglu T (1996) Monocyte activity in Behçet's disease. Br J Rheumatol 35(5):424–429

141. Pay S, Simsek I, Erdem H, Pekel A, Musabak U, Sengul A et al (2007) Dendritic cell subsets and type I interferon system in Behçet's disease: does functional abnormality in plasmacytoid dendritic cells contribute to Th1 polarization? Clin Exp Rheumatol 25(4 Suppl 45):S34–S40

142. Mantas C, Direskeneli H, Oz D, Yavuz S, Akoglu T (2000) IL-8 producing cells in patients with Behçet's disease. Clin Exp Rheumatol 18(2):249–251

143. Keller M, Spanou Z, Schaerli P, Britschgi M, Yawalkar N, Seitz M et al (2005) T cell-regulated neutrophilic inflammation in autoinflammatory diseases. J Immunol 175(11): 7678–7686

144. Pay S, Musabak U, Simsek I, Erdem H, Pekel A, Sengul A et al (2007) Synovial lymphoid neogenetic factors in Behçet's synovitis: do they play a role in self-limiting and subacute course of arthritis? Clin Exp Rheumatol 25(4 Suppl 45):S21–S26

145. Munz C, Steinman RM, Fujii S (2005) Dendritic cell maturation by innate lymphocytes: coordinated stimulation of innate and adaptive immunity. J Exp Med 202(2):203–207

146. Melikoglu M, Kural-Seyahi E, Tascilar K, Yazici H (2008) The unique features of vasculitis in Behçet's syndrome. Clin Rev Allergy Immunol 35(1–2):40–46

147. Lee KH, Cho HJ, Kim HS, Lee WJ, Lee S, Bang D (2002) Activation of extracellular signal regulated kinase 1/2 in human dermal microvascular endothelial cells stimulated by anti-endothelial cell antibodies in sera of patients with Behçet's disease. J Dermatol Sci 30(1):63–72

148. Chambers JC, Haskard DO, Kooner JS (2001) Vascular endothelial function and oxidative stress mechanisms in patients with Behçet's syndrome. J Am Coll Cardiol 37(2):517–520

149. Kayikcioglu M, Aksu K, Hasdemir C, Keser G, Turgan N, Kultursay H et al (2006) Endothelial functions in Behçet's disease. Rheumatol Int 26(4):304–308

150. Kiraz S, Ertenli I, Ozturk MA, Haznedaroglu IC, Celik I, Calguneri M (2002) Pathological haemostasis and "prothrombotic state" in Behçet's disease. Thromb Res 105(2):125–133

151. Espinosa G, Font J, Tassies D, Vidaller A, Deulofeu R, Lopez-Soto A et al (2002) Vascular involvement in Behçet's disease: relation with thrombophilic factors, coagulation activation, and thrombomodulin. Am J Med 112(1):37–43

152. Haznedaroglu IC, Ozcebe OI, Ozdemir O, Celik I, Dundar SV, Kirazli S (1996) Impaired haemostatic kinetics and endothelial function in Behçet's disease. J Intern Med 240(4):181–187

153. Gul A, Ozbek U, Ozturk C, Inanc M, Konice M, Ozcelik T (1996) Coagulation factor V gene mutation increases the risk of venous thrombosis in Behçet's disease. Br J Rheumatol 35(11):1178–1180

154. Verity DH, Vaughan RW, Madanat W, Kondeatis E, Zureikat H, Fayyad F et al (1999) Factor V Leiden mutation is associated with ocular involvement in Behçet's disease. Am J Ophthalmol 128(3):352–356

155. Mammo L, Al-Dalaan A, Bahabri SS, Saour JN (1997) Association of factor V Leiden with Behçet's disease. J Rheumatol 24(11):2196–2198

156. Ates A, Aydintug O, Olmez U, Duzgun N, Duman M (2005) Serum homocysteine level is higher in Behçet's disease with vascular involvement. Rheumatol Int 25(1):42–44

157. Ricart JM, Vaya A, Todoli J, Calvo J, Villa P, Estelles A et al (2006) Thrombophilic risk factors and homocysteine levels in Behçet's disease in eastern Spain and their association with thrombotic events. Thromb Haemost 95(4):618–624

158. Feki M, Houman H, Ghannouchi M, Smiti-Khanfir M, Hamzaoui K, El Matri L et al (2004) Hyperhomocysteinaemia is associated with uveitis but not with deep venous thrombosis in Behçet's disease. Clin Chem Lab Med 42(12):1417–23

159. Tokay S, Direskeneli H, Yurdakul S, Akoglu T (2001) Anticardiolipin antibodies in Behçet's disease: a reassessment. Rheumatology (Oxford) 40(2):192–195

160. Hampton KK, Chamberlain MA, Menon DK, Davies JA (1991) Coagulation and fibrinolytic activity in Behçet's disease. Thromb Haemost 66(3):292–294

161. Mishima H, Masuda K, Shimada S, Toki N, Tsushima H, Gocho M (1985) Plasminogen activator activity levels in patients with Behçet's syndrome. Arch Ophthalmol 103(7):935–936

162. Haznedaroglu IC, Celik I, Buyukasik Y, Kosar A, Kirazli S, Dundar SV (1998) Haemostasis, thrombosis, and endothelium in Behçet's disease. Acta Haematol 99(4):236–237

163. Yazici H, Mat C, Deniz S, Iscimen A, Yurdakul S, Tuzun Y et al (1987) Sebum production is increased in Behçet's syndrome and even more so in rheumatoid arthritis. Clin Exp Rheumatol 5(4):371–374

164. Miyamoto N, Mandai M, Suzuma I, Suzuma K, Kobayashi K, Honda Y (1999) Estrogen protects against cellular infiltration by reducing the expressions of E-selectin and IL-6 in endotoxin-induced uveitis. J Immunol 163(1):374–379

165. Buyon JP, Korchak HM, Rutherford LE, Ganguly M, Weissmann G (1984) Female hormones reduce neutrophil responsiveness in vitro. Arthritis Rheum 27(6):623–630

166. Ehrlich GE (1998) Behçet's disease and the emergence of thalidomide. Ann Intern Med 128(6):494–495

167. Hamuryudan V, Mat C, Saip S, Ozyazgan Y, Siva A, Yurdakul S et al (1998) Thalidomide in the treatment of the mucocutaneous lesions of the Behçet's syndrome. A randomized, double-blind, placebo-controlled trial. Ann Intern Med 128(6):443–450

168. Celet B, Akman-Demir G, Serdaroglu P, Yentur SP, Tasci B, van Noort JM et al (2000) Anti-alpha B-crystallin immunoreactivity in inflammatory nervous system diseases. J Neurol 247(12):935–939

169. Tasci B, Direskeneli H, Serdaroglu P, Akman-Demir G, Eraksoy M, Saruhan-Direskeneli G (1998) Humoral immune response to mycobacterial heat shock protein (hsp)65 in the cerebrospinal fluid of neuro-Behçet's patients. Clin Exp Immunol 113(1):100–104

170. Pay S, Abbasov T, Erdem H, Musabak U, Simsek I, Pekel A et al (2007) Serum MMP-2 and MMP-9 in patients with Behçet's disease: do their higher levels correlate to vasculo-Behçet's disease associated with aneurysm formation? Clin Exp Rheumatol 25(4 Suppl 45):S70–S75

171. Hirohata S, Isshi K, Oguchi H, Ohse T, Haraoka H, Takeuchi A et al (1997) Cerebrospinal fluid interleukin-6 in progressive Neuro-Behçet's syndrome. Clin Immunol Immunopathol 82(1):12–17

172. Akman-Demir G, Tuzun E, Icoz S, Yesilot N, Yentur SP, Kurtuncu M et al (2008) Interleukin-6 in neuro-Behçet's disease: association with disease subsets and long-term outcome. Cytokine 44(3):373–376

173. Matzinger P (2002) The danger model: a renewed sense of self. Science 296(5566):301–305

174. Medzhitov R, Janeway CA Jr (2002) Decoding the patterns of self and nonself by the innate immune system. Science 296(5566):298–300

175. Torchinsky MB, Garaude J, Martin AP, Blander JM (2009) Innate immune recognition of infected apoptotic cells directs T(H)17 cell differentiation. Nature 458(7234):78–82

176. McGonagle D, Savic S, McDermott MF (2007) The NLR network and the immunological disease continuum of adaptive and innate immune-mediated inflammation against self. Semin Immunopathol 29(3):303–313

Chapter 15
Genetics of Behçet's Disease

Ahmet Gül and Shigeaki Ohno

Keywords Behçet's disease • Familial aggregation • Sibling recurrence risk ratio (λs) • HLA-B51 • MICA • HLA-A26 • Linkage study • Genomewide association study

Behçet's disease (BD) is a systemic inflammatory disorder of unknown etiology. It is generally accepted as a multifactorial disease with a strong genetic background, and the disease manifestations are considered to be triggered by various environmental factors in genetically susceptible individuals [1, 2].

There are several clues supporting involvement of genetic factors in the pathogenesis of BD, which include familial aggregation, distinct geographic distribution, and its association with the HLA-B51 antigen.

Familial Aggregation

Although majority of BD patients are seen as sporadic cases, increased frequency of BD has long been noted among the relatives [3–16]. Varying frequencies of patients with a positive family history for BD were described in large series of patients, with a tendency for higher figures in the Middle Eastern patients compared to the patients from Asian and European countries [16, 17].

Gül and colleagues analyzed the sibling recurrence risk ratio (λs) for quantifying the familial aggregation in BD [17]. They calculated the sibling recurrence rate as 4.2 by taking into account only the immediately older sibling, or if an older sibling is not available, immediately younger sibling for evaluation. By using the prevalence rates of BD in Turkey, λs value was found to be 11.4–52.5 for BD [17].

A. Gül (✉)
Department of Internal Medicine, Division of Rheumatology, Istanbul
Faculty of Medicine, Istanbul University, Istanbul, Turkey
e-mail: agul@istanbul.edu.tr

Y. Yazıcı and H. Yazıcı (eds.), *Behçet's Syndrome*,
DOI 10.1007/978-1-4419-5641-5_15, © Springer Science+Business Media, LLC 2010

This λs value was considered as strongly supporting the contribution of genetics to the multifactorial pathogenesis of BD.

Familial clustering was more frequently observed among juvenile-onset (<16) BD patients [18, 19]. Molinary and colleagues conducted a segregation analysis using the pedigree data of 106 BD cases. They included "possible" BD patients who had only two of the classical disease manifestations into the analysis, and they found a pattern compatible with autosomal recessive inheritance in pediatric BD subgroup, and no Mendelian pattern in adult-onset patients [19]. This study suggested a genetic heterogeneity with a higher impact of genetic load in juvenile BD cases [19].

Frequency of HLA-B51 was found to be higher in familial patients [11, 12]. However, presence of unaffected siblings with risk alleles also showed the complex nature of the disease indicating the contribution of other genes and/or environmental factors [11, 20]. A comparison of related pairs of patients according to their age at onset also supports involvement of both genetic and environmental factors in the pathogenesis [21, 22].

Another study from Turkey documented clues for genetic anticipation in the form of earlier disease onset in the second generation compared with their affected parents in 15 out of 18 familial cases studied [23]. However, no trinucleotide repeat expansion data are yet available to further support this observation.

No large series of twins concordant or discordant for BD were reported so far [24–26]. Therefore, large series of monozygotic and dizygotic twins are being awaited for heritability analysis to assess the relative contribution of genes and environment to the pathogenesis of BD.

Geographic Distribution

Epidemiology of BD has a distinct feature in terms of its geographic distribution. Prevalence of BD is much higher in an area extending from the Mediterranean basin to Japan, between 30° and 45° latitudes North, which overlaps with the ancient Silk Road [27]. There is no known specific environmental factor common along this route, but shared genetic factors may explain the clustering of BD cases. The frequency of BD-related HLA-B51 allele is higher in the healthy population living along this region, and distribution of HLA-B51 allele is suggested to play a role in the disease clustering [27, 28].

HLA-B51 and Other MHC Associations

BD is strongly associated with a class I major histocompatibility complex (MHC) allele, HLA-B51. This association was first reported in Japanese BD patients [28–30]. Association of HLA-B51 with BD was later confirmed in other ethnic groups, including those in which BD is seen very rarely [1, 2, 16, 27, 31–34].

No disease specific differences were observed in the sequence of HLA-B51 alleles between BD patients and healthy controls, neither in the coding region nor in the regulatory sequences [35, 36]. HLA-B51 is a split antigen of HLA-B5, and the other split antigen HLA-B52 has not been associated with BD despite some exceptional reports [37, 38]. HLA-B51 differs from HLA-B52 only by two amino-acids in the α1 helix. Asparagine and phenylalanine at positions 63 and 67 of the HLA-B51 molecule are replaced with glutamic acid and serine in the HLA-B52 at the same positions [39]. These two aminoacids are located at the B pocket of the antigen binding groove (Fig. 15.1). HLA-B51 allele can bind peptides with eight or nine aminoacids and a hydrophobic C-terminus [40]. Later studies suggested that B pocket can be occupied by small aminoacids alanine and proline, and changes in the B pocket can affect the motif of the peptides that can bind to HLA molecule [41]. Isoleucine and valine were identified as dominant anchor residues in the C-terminus of the refined peptide motif which binds to relatively small F pocket, and aminoacids making the F pocket are conserved in all HLA-B51 alleles [41].

HLA-B51 allele has 73 different subtypes (HLA-B*5101–B*5173), and they all share the same aminoacid sequence at the B pocket of the antigen binding groove except for B*5107 and B*5122. HLA-B*5101 is the dominant subtype of the B51 molecule, and molecular HLA-B51 typing in different ethnic groups suggests that HLA-B51 subtypes in BD patients are not different from those in healthy controls, with HLA-B*5101 and -B*5108 as the main subtypes [42–46].

Molecular typing of HLA-B51 molecules suggests that presentation of certain BD-associated peptides with its specific B and F pocket features might be one of

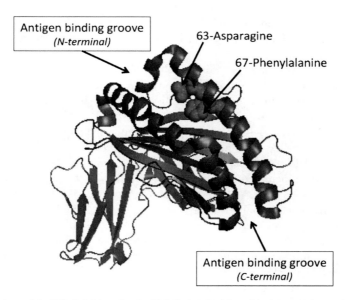

Fig. 15.1 A model of HLA-B51 molecule (1E28) showing the critical asparagine and phenylala-nine at positions 63 and 67 in its antigen binding groove (drawn by PyMOL)

the pathogenic mechanisms behind the susceptibility to BD. So far, only major histocompatibility complex class I chain-related gene A (MICA)-derived nonamer peptide (AAAAAIFVI) was shown to induce T cells in less than one-third of active HLA-B51 positive BD patients compared to none of the healthy controls [47].

HLA-B51, as a class I molecule, also interacts with a group of receptors expressed on natural killer (NK) cells, CD8+ and γδ T cells [48]. The killer immunoglobulin-like receptors (KIR), bind to conserved Bw4 epitopes at residues 77–83 of the α1-helix, which are shared by different allellic groups of HLA class I molecules. Engagement of these receptors can result in selective inhibition of NK or T cell mediated cytotoxicity. A relative predispositional effects analysis, conducted to search for weaker HLA-B associations with BD masked by strong HLA-B51 association, revealed a weak association of HLA-B*2702 with BD, which shares the same Bw4 motif with HLA-B51 [49]. Investigation of HLA-B51 interacting KIR3DL1/DS1 polymorphism documented the association of DL1/DL1 genotype with BD in Bw4-motif positive patients [50]. These preliminary studies support an alternative hypothesis that the pathogenic role of HLA-B51 may also include its interaction with KIR3DL1 molecules expressed on inflammatory cells.

HLA-B51-derived peptides can be presented by HLA class II molecules. HLA class I heavy chain misfolding as well as enhanced expression due to up-regulated immune response increase the possibility of class I-derived peptide presentation. Wildner and Thurau identified a polymorphic HLA-B sequence common in HLA-B27, -B51, and several other HLA-B alleles (B27PD), which shares aminoacid homologies with retinal soluble antigen (S-Ag)-derived peptide [51]. Kurhan-Yavuz and colleagues demonstrated increased T cell response against retinal S-Ag, retinal S-Ag derived peptide, and B27PD peptide in BD patients with posterior uveitis compared with those BD patients without eye disease or patients with non-BD anterior uveitis [52].

HLA-B51 is one of the slow folding MHC molecules [53]. However, there is no data showing the role of HLA-B51 folding problems and unfolded protein response in BD pathogenesis similar to the observations on HLA-B27 in ankylosing spondylitis animal models [54].

There is only one HLA-B*5101 heavy chain transgenic mouse model developed so far in investigating the direct role of HLA-B51 molecules in BD [55]. No manifestation typical for BD was observed in these transgenic animals. HLA-B51 transgenic animals showed an increased neutrophil activity following f-Met-Leu-Phe (fMLP) stimulation compared to HLA-B35 and nontransgenic mice [55]. A similar enhanced neutrophil activity was reported in HLA-B51 positive healthy individuals [11, 55, 56]. Extrapolating from the experience with HLA-B27 animal models, it is still needed to have a high heavy chain copy number transgenic animal models with and without human β2-microglobulin in different strains of mice and rats to explore the role of HLA-B51 in BD [57].

In addition to association studies, analysis of 12 multicase families confirmed the genetic linkage of the HLA-B locus to BD by using the transmission disequilibrium test [58]. Contribution of the HLA-B locus to the overall genetic susceptibility to BD was estimated to be 19% assuming multiplicative interaction between disease susceptibility loci [58]. This result supports the need for studies to look for other susceptibility loci.

Other MHC Associations

Linkage disequilibrium (LD) is high in the MHC, especially in the class I region with larger haplotype blocks [59]. It has long been discussed whether HLA-B51 has a direct role in the BD pathogenesis, or whether this strong association reflects LD with one or more susceptibility genes located close to the HLA-B locus (Fig. 15.2). The tumor necrosis factor (TNF) and lymphotoxin genes, which are located centromeric to HLA-B, were investigated first as possible candidate susceptibility genes. The analysis of the genomic segment between the TNF and HLA-B loci revealed a strong association of MICA gene with BD, which is located 46-kb centromeric to HLA-B [60]. The MICA gene *009 allele and its transmembrane region microsatellite polymorphism A6 allele were found to be significantly increased in BD patients [60–62]. Fine mapping of the region in different ethnic groups revealed HLA-B as the gene providing strongest association with BD, and all other associations including the MICA were resulting from strong LD with HLA-B51 [63]. However, it is still hard to rule out individual contribution of the MICA gene on an HLA-B51 haplotype to the BD susceptibility through its interaction with NK and γδ T cells.

Within the MHC region, no association with class II antigens was observed [64], but HLA-B51-associated LD extends to telomeric part of class I region. Weaker associations with HLA-Cw14, Cw15, and C*16 alleles [65, 66] and a negative association with nonclassical HLA-E*0101 and HLA-G*010101 alleles [67] were reported. Recent studies suggest a second HLA class I region association independent of HLA-B51 [68]. Meguro and colleagues reported the association of HLA-A26 allele and HLA-A*26-F*010101-G*010102 haplotype with BD even in HLA-B51 negative patients in Japan [68]. Association of HLA-A26 allele with BD was also observed in Taiwanese and Greek patients. These observations suggest that contribution of the MHC region to the BD susceptibility includes both HLA-B51 and other classical or nonclassical HLA associations with possible different pathogenic mechanisms.

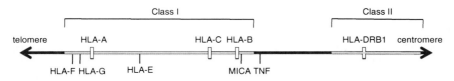

Fig. 15.2 Genetic map of the major histocompatibility complex (MHC) in short arm of chromosome 6 showing the Behçet's disease-associated loci in class I region

Non-HLA Genes and Behçet's Disease

As a complex disease, non-HLA genetic polymorphisms can also contribute to the BD susceptibility. For investigation of these susceptibility genes, a candidate gene approach was frequently preferred by investigators despite no clear evidence for

Table 15.1 List of non-HLA genes reported to be associated with Behçet's disease

Name	Ethnic groups
Cytokines, chemokines and their receptors	
Tumor necrosis factor (TNF)	British Caucasian, Turkish, Korean, Tunisian [69–72]
Interleukin 1 gene cluster	Turkish [73]
Interleukin 6 (IL6)	Korean [74]
Interleukin 8 (IL8/CXCL8)	Korean [75]
Interleukin 10 (IL10)	British Caucasian [76]
Interleukin 12 p40 (IL12B)	Japanese [77]
Interleukin-17F (IL17F)	Korean [78]
Interleukin 18 (IL18)	Korean [79]
Chemokine receptor 5 (CCR5)	Iranian [80]
Other immune response genes	
Natural resistance associated macrophage protein 1 (NRAMP1)	Turkish, Korean [81, 82]
CTLA4	Tunisian, Korean [83, 84]
Mannose binding lectin	Japanese, Korean [85, 86]
Ficolin 2 (FCN2)	Japanese [87]
Small ubiquitin-like modifier 4 (SUMO4)	Chinese [88]
Fc receptor-like 3 gene (FCRL3)	Chinese [89]
CD94/NKG2A	Korean [90]
PTPN22 (negative association)	British Caucasian, Middle Eastern [91]
CD28	Turkish [92]
Pathogen associated molecular pattern receptors	
Toll-like receptor 4 (TLR4)	Japanese, Korean [93, 94]
Autoinflammatory polymorphisms	
Pyrin (MEFV)	Turkish, European, Jewish, Palestinian [95–99]
TNF receptor p55 (TNFRSF1A)	European [100]
Vascular and procoagulant polymorphisms	
Intercellular adhesion molecule-1 (ICAM1)	Palestinian/Jordanian, Italian, Korean, Lebanese [101–104]
Endothelial nitric oxide synthase (eNOS)	Italian, Korean, Turkish, Tunisian [105–108]
Factor V Leiden	Turkish, Arabian [109–111]
Prothrombin	Turkish, Spanish [112, 113]
Manganese superoxide dismutase (SOD)	Japanese [114]
Others	
Cytochrome P450	Turkish, Taiwanese [115, 116]
N-acetyltransferase 2	Turkish [117]

utilizing this method in deciphering the pathogenic mechanisms of BD. Most of these association studies were carried out using small numbers of cases and controls with limited power. The list of non-HLA genes reported to be associated with BD are given in Table 15.1 [69–117]. Among the reported associations, only a few were replicated in different ethnic groups, including polymorphisms in the TNF, MEFV, ICAM1, and eNOS genes. None of these polymorphisms are disease specific, and they are considered to be contributing to a disease-specific inflammatory reaction.

Another approach for investigating complex disease susceptibility genes is screening of whole genome without a priori hypothesis about disease pathogenesis. A genomewide linkage screen using 193 individuals from 28 multicase BD families of Turkish origin with 83 affecteds revealed evidence for linkage to 15 non-HLA chromosomal regions: 1p36, 4p15, 5q12, 5q23, 6q16, 6q25–26, 7p21, 10q24, 12p12–13, 12q13, 16q12, 16q21–23, 17p13, 20q12–13, and Xq26–28 [118]. The linkage peak in the short arm of chromosome 6 (the maximum nonparametric linkage score 3.7) confirmed the strong association of HLA-B locus and also suggested another telomeric susceptibility loci [118, 119]. After the addition of further markers, high maximum nonparametric linkage scores were observed at chromosome 12p12-13 (3.94) and 6q25-26 (3.14).

Linkage studies in families are expected to identify rare, but penetrant genetic variations. However, genomewide association studies (GWAS) in large number of cases and controls can reveal common, but less penetrant polymorphisms affecting the disease susceptibility. A recent GWAS investigated 300 Japanese BD patients and 300 healthy controls with 23,465 microsatellite markers. This study identified six possible genomic regions, including two from the MHC region, one corresponding to HLA-B and the other to HLA-A [68]. Other non-HLA microsatellite markers suggested chromosomal regions 3p12 (D3S0186i), 6q25.1 (536G12Aa), 12p12.1 (D12S0645i), and 22q11.22 (D22S0104im) as possible genomic segments harboring disease susceptibility loci, two of which overlap with the findings of the previous linkage study [68]. Current GWAS approach enables us to analyze thousands of samples using chips for >300,000 single nucleotide polymorphisms in a relatively short time. Results of GWAS from different ethnic groups are eagerly being awaited to clarify the genetics of BD further.

References

1. Gül A (2001) Behçet's disease: an update on the pathogenesis. Clin Exp Rheumatol 19(Suppl 24):S6–S12
2. Zierhut M, Mizuki N, Ohno S et al (2003) Immunology and functional genomics of Behçet's disease. Cell Mol Life Sci 60:1903–1922
3. Fowler TJ, Humpston DJ, Nussey AM, Small M (1968) Behçet's syndrome with neurological manifestations in two sisters. Br Med J 2:473–474
4. Mason RM, Barnes CG (1969) Behçet's syndrome with arthritis. Ann Rheum Dis 28:95–103
5. Fadli ME, Youssef MM (1973) Neuro-Behçet's syndrome in the United Arab Republic. Eur Neurol 9:76–89

6. Chajek T, Fainaru M (1975) Behçet's disease: report of 41 cases and a review of the literature. Medicine (Baltimore) 54:179–196
7. Goolamali SK, Comaish JS, Hassanyeh F (1976) Familial Behçet's syndrome. Br J Dermatol
   95:637–642
8. Nahir M, Scharf Y, Gidoni O et al (1978) HL-A antigens in Behçet's disease. A family study.
   Dermatologica 156:205–208
9. Abdel-Aziz AH, Fairburn EA (1978) Familial Behçet's syndrome. Cutis 21:649–652
10. Dündar SV, Gencalp U, Simsek H (1985) Familial cases of Behçet's disease. Br J Dermatol
    113:319–321
11. Chajek-Shaul T, Pisanty S, Knobler H et al (1987) HLA-B51 may serve as an immunoge-
    netic marker for a subgroup of patients with Behçet's syndrome. Am J Med 83:666–672
12. Akpolat T, Koc Y, Yeniay I et al (1992) Familial Behçet's disease. Eur J Med 1:391–395
13. Villanueva JL, Gonzalez-Dominguez J, Gonzalez-Fernandez R et al (1993) HLA antigen famil-
    ial study in complete Behçet's syndrome affecting three sisters. Ann Rheum Dis 52:155–157
14. Nishiura K, Kotake S, Ichiishi A, Matsuda H (1996) Familial occurrence of Behçet's disease.
    Jpn J Ophthalmol 40:255–259
15. Nishiyama M, Nakae K, Umehara T (2001) A study of familial occurrence of Behçet's
    disease with and without ocular lesions. Jpn J Ophthalmol 45:313–316
16. Fietta P (2005) Behçet's disease: familial clustering and immunogenetics. Clin Exp
    Rheumatol 23(Suppl 38):S96–S105
17. Gül A, Inanc M, Ocal L et al (2000) Familial aggregation of Behçet's disease in Turkey. Ann
    Rheum Dis 59:622–625
18. Treudler R, Orfanos CE, Zouboulis CC (1999) Twenty-eight cases of juvenile-onset
    Adamantiades-Behçet's disease in Germany. Dermatology 199:15–19
19. Koné-Paut I, Geisler I, Wechsler B et al (1999) Familial aggregation in Behçet's disease:
    high frequency in siblings and parents of pediatric probands. J Pediatr 135:89–93
20. Hayasaka S, Kurome H, Noda S (1994) HLA antigens in a Japanese family with Behçet's
    disease. Graefes Arch Clin Exp Ophthalmol 232:589–590
21. Nishiyama M, Nakae K, Kuriyama T et al (2002) A study among related pairs of Japanese
    patients with familial Behçet's disease: group comparisons by interval of disease onsets.
    J Rheumatol 29:743–747
22. Aronsson A, Tegner E (1983) Behçet's syndrome in two brothers. Acta Derm Venereol
    63:73–74
23. Fresko I, Soy M, Hamuryudan V et al (1998) Genetic anticipation in Behçet's syndrome.
    Ann Rheum Dis 57:45–48
24. Hamuryudan V, Yurdakul S, Ozbakir F et al (1991) Monozygotic twins concordant for
    Behçet's syndrome. Arthritis Rheum 34:1071–1072
25. Gül A, Inanç M, Ocal L et al (1997) HLA-B51 negative monozygotic twins discordant for
    Behçet's disease. Br J Rheumatol 36:922–923
26. Kobayashi T, Sudo Y, Okamura S et al (2005) Monozygotic twins concordant for intestinal
    Behçet's disease. J Gastroenterol 40:421–425
27. Verity DH, Marr JE, Ohno S et al (1999) Behçet's disease, the Silk Road and HLA-B51:
    historical and geographical perspectives. Tissue Antigens 54:213–220
28. Ohno S, Ohguchi M, Hirose S et al (1982) Close association of HLA-Bw51 with Behçet's
    disease. Arch Ophthalmol 100:1455–1458
29. Ono S, Aoki K, Sugiura S et al (1973) HL-A5 and Behçet's disease. Lancet 2:1383–1384
30. Ono S, Nakayama E, Sugiura S et al (1975) Specific histocompatibility antigens associated
    with Behçet's disease. Am J Ophthalmol 80:636–641
31. Kilmartin DJ, Finch A, Acheson RW (1997) Primary association of HLA-B51 with Behçet's
    disease in Ireland. Br J Ophthalmol 81:649–653
32. Ambresin A, Tran T, Spertini F, Herbort C (2002) Behçet's disease in Western Switzerland:
    epidemiology and analysis of ocular involvement. Ocul Immunol Inflamm 10:53–63
33. Pipitone N, Boiardi L, Olivieri I et al (2004) Clinical manifestations of Behçet's disease in 137
    Italian patients: results of a multicenter study. Clin Exp Rheumatol 22(Suppl 36):S46–S51

34. Bettencourt A, Pereira C, Carvalho L et al (2008) New insights of HLA class I association to Behçet's disease in Portuguese patients. Tissue Antigens 72:379–382
35. Sano K, Yabuki K, Imagawa Y et al (2001) The absence of disease-specific polymorphisms within the HLA-B51 gene that is the susceptible locus for Behçet's disease. Tissue Antigens 58:77–82
36. Takemoto Y, Naruse T, Namba K et al (2008) Re-evaluation of heterogeneity in HLA-B*510101 associated with Behçet's disease. Tissue Antigens 72:347–353
37. Arber N, Klein T, Meiner Z et al (1991) Close association of HLA-B51 and B52 in Israeli patients with Behçet's syndrome. Ann Rheum Dis 50:351–353
38. Sugisaki K, Saito R, Takagi T et al (2005) HLA-B52-positive vasculo-Behçet's disease: usefulness of magnetic resonance angiography, ultrasound study, and computed tomographic angiography for the early evaluation of multiarterial lesions. Mod Rheumatol 15:56–61
39. Falk K, Rötzschke O, Takiguchi M et al (1995) Peptide motifs of HLA-B51, -B52 and -B78 molecules, and implications for Behçet's disease. Int Immunol 7:223–228
40. Sakaguchi T, Ibe M, Miwa K et al (1997) Predominant role of N-terminal residue of nonamer peptides in their binding to HLA-B* 5101 molecules. Immunogenetics 46:245–248
41. Lemmel C, Rammensee H-G, Stevanovic S (2003) Peptide motif of HLA-B*5101 and the linkage to Behçet's disease. In: Zierhut M, Ohno S (eds) Immunology of Behçet's disease. Swets & Zeitlinger, Lisse, pp 127–137
42. Mizuki N, Inoko H, Ando H et al (1993) Behçet's disease associated with one of the HLA-B51 subantigens, HLA-B* 5101. Am J Ophthalmol 116:406–409
43. Mizuki N, Ota M, Katsuyama Y et al (2002) Sequencing-based typing of HLA-B*51 alleles and the significant association of HLA-B*5101 and -B*5108 with Behçet's disease in Greek patients. Tissue Antigens 59:118–121
44. Pirim I, Atasoy M, Ikbal M et al (2004) HLA class I and class II genotyping in patients with Behçet's disease: a regional study of eastern part of Turkey. Tissue Antigens 64:293–297
45. Kera J, Mizuki N, Ota M et al (1999) Significant associations of HLA-B*5101 and B*5108, and lack of association of class II alleles with Behçet's disease in Italian patients. Tissue Antigens 54:565–571
46. Yabuki K, Ohno S, Mizuki N et al (1999) HLA class I and II typing of the patients with Behçet's disease in Saudi Arabia. Tissue Antigens 54:273–277
47. Yasuoka H, Okazaki Y, Kawakami Y et al (2004) Autoreactive CD8+ cytotoxic T lymphocytes to major histocompatibility complex class I chain-related gene A in patients with Behçet's disease. Arthritis Rheum 50:3658–3662
48. Martin MP, Gao X, Lee J-H et al (2002) Epistatic interaction between *KIR3DS1* and *HLA-B* delays the progression to AIDS. Nat Genet 31:429–434
49. Gül A, Uyar FA, Inanç M et al (2002) A weak association of HLA-B*2702 with Behçet's disease. Genes Immun 3:368–372
50. Duymaz-Tozkir J, Uyar A, Norman PJ et al (2008) Distribution of killer immunoglobulin-like receptor 3DL1/3DS1 alleles in Behçet's disease. Arthritis Rheum 58(Suppl):S855
51. Wildner G, Thurau SR (1994) Cross-reactivity between an HLA-B27-derived peptide and a retinal autoantigen peptide: a clue to major histocompatibility complex association with autoimmune disease. Eur J Immunol 24:2579–2585
52. Kurhan-Yavuz S, Direskeneli H, Bozkurt N et al (2000) Anti-MHC autoimmunity in Behçet's disease: T cell responses to an HLA-B-derived peptide cross-reactive with retinal-S antigen in patients with uveitis. Clin Exp Immunol 120:162–166
53. Hill A, Takiguchi M, McMichael A (1993) Different rates of HLA class I molecule assembly which are determined by amino acid sequence in the alpha 2 domain. Immunogenetics 37:95–101
54. Turner MJ, Sowders DP, DeLay ML et al (2005) HLA-B27 misfolding in transgenic rats is associated with activation of the unfolded protein response. J Immunol 175:2438–2448
55. Takeno M, Kariyone A, Yamashita N et al (1995) Excessive function of peripheral blood neutrophils from patients with Behçet's disease and from HLA-B51 transgenic mice. Arthritis Rheum 38:426–433

56. Sensi A, Gavioli R, Spisani S et al (1991) HLA B51 antigen associated with neutrophil hyper-reactivity. Dis Markers 9:327–331
57. Taurog JD, Maika SD, Satumtira N et al (1999) Inflammatory disease in HLA-B27 transgenic rats. Immunol Rev 169:209–223
58. Gül A, Hajeer AH, Worthington J et al (2001) Evidence for linkage of the HLA-B locus in Behçet's disease, obtained using the transmission disequilibrium test. Arthritis Rheum 44(1):239–240
59. Miretti MM, Walsh EC, Ke X et al (2005) A high-resolution linkage-disequilibrium map of the human major histocompatibility complex and first generation of tag single-nucleotide polymorphisms. Am J Hum Genet 76:634–646
60. Mizuki N, Ota M, Kimura M et al (1997) Triplet repeat polymorphism in the transmembrane region of the MICA gene: a strong association of six GCT repetitions with Behçet's disease. Proc Natl Acad Sci U S A 94:1298–1303
61. Hughes EH, Collins RW, Kondeatis E et al (2005) Associations of major histocompatibility complex class I chain-related molecule polymorphisms with Behçet's disease in Caucasian patients. Tissue Antigens 66:195–199
62. Mizuki N, Meguro A, Tohnai I et al (2007) Association of major histocompatibility complex Class I chain-related Gene A and HLA-B alleles with Behçet's disease in Turkey. Jpn J Ophthalmol 51:431–436
63. Mizuki N, Ota M, Yabuki K et al (2000) Localization of the pathogenic gene of Behçet's disease by microsatellite analysis of three different populations. Invest Ophthalmol Vis Sci 41:3702–3708
64. Mizuki N, Ohno S, Tanaka H et al (1992) Association of HLA-B51 and lack of association of class II alleles with Behçet's disease. Tissue Antigens 40:22–30
65. Mizuki N, Ohno S, Ando H et al (1996) HLA-C genotyping of patient with Behçet's disease in the Japanese population. Hum Immunol 50:47–53
66. Sanz L, González-Escribano F, de Pablo R et al (1998) HLA-Cw*1602: a new susceptibility marker of Behçet's disease in southern Spain. Tissue Antigens 51:111–114
67. Park KS, Park JS, Nam JH et al (2007) HLA-E*0101 and HLA-G*010101 reduce the risk of Behçet's disease. Tissue Antigens 69:139–144
68. Meguro A, Inoko H, Ota M, et al (2009) Genetics of Behçet's disease inside and outside the MHC. Ann Rheum Dis 69:747–754
69. Ahmad T, Wallace GR, James T et al (2003) Mapping the HLA association in Behçet's disease: a role for tumor necrosis factor polymorphisms? Arthritis Rheum 48:807–813
70. Akman A, Sallakci N, Coskun M et al (2006) TNF-alpha gene 1031 T/C polymorphism in Turkish patients with Behçet's disease. Br J Dermatol 155:350–356
71. Park K, Kim N, Nam J et al (2006) Association of TNFA promoter region haplotype in Behçet's disease. J Korean Med Sci 21:596–601
72. Kamoun M, Chelbi H, Houman MH et al (2007) Tumor necrosis factor gene polymorphisms in Tunisian patients with Behçet's disease. Hum Immunol 68:201–205
73. Karasneh J, Hajeer AH, Barrett J et al (2003) Association of specific interleukin 1 gene cluster polymorphisms with increased susceptibility for Behçet's disease. Rheumatology (Oxford) 42:860–864
74. Chang HK, Jang WC, Park SB et al (2005) Association between interleukin 6 gene polymorphisms and Behçet's disease in Korean people. Ann Rheum Dis 64:339–340
75. Lee EB, Kim JY, Zhao J et al (2007) Haplotype association of IL-8 gene with Behçet's disease. Tissue Antigens 69:128–132
76. Wallace GR, Kondeatis E, Vaughan RW et al (2007) IL-10 genotype analysis in patients with Behçet's disease. Hum Immunol 68:122–127
77. Yanagihori H, Oyama N, Nakamura K et al (2006) Role of IL-12B promoter polymorphism in Adamantiades-Behçet's disease susceptibility: an involvement of Th1 immunoreactivity against Streptococcus Sanguinis antigen. J Invest Dermatol 126:1534–1540
78. Jang WC, Nam YH, Ahn YC et al (2008) Interleukin-17F gene polymorphisms in Korean patients with Behçet's disease. Rheumatol Int 29:173–178

79. Lee YJ, Kang SW, Park JJ et al (2006) Interleukin-18 promoter polymorphisms in patients with Behçet's disease. Hum Immunol 67:812–818
80. Mojtahedi Z, Ahmadi SB, Razmkhah M et al (2006) Association of chemokine receptor 5 (CCR5) delta32 mutation with Behçet's disease is dependent on gender in Iranian patients. Clin Exp Rheumatol 24(Suppl 42):S91–S94
81. Ateş O, Dalyan L, Hatemi G et al (2009) Genetic susceptibility to Behçet's syndrome is associated with NRAMP1 (SLC11A1) polymorphism in Turkish patients. Rheumatol Int 29:787–791
82. Kim SK, Jang WC, Park SB et al (2006) SLC11A1 gene polymorphisms in Korean patients with Behçet's disease. Scand J Rheumatol 35:398–401
83. Ben Dhifallah I, Chelbi H, Braham A et al (2009) CTLA-4 +49A/G polymorphism is associated with Behçet's disease in a Tunisian population. Tissue Antigens 73(3):213–217
84. Park KS, Baek JA, Do JE et al (2009) CTLA4 gene polymorphisms and soluble CTLA4 protein in Behçet's disease. Tissue Antigens 74:222–227
85. Wang H, Nakamura K, Inoue T et al (2004) Mannose-binding lectin polymorphisms in patients with Behçet's disease. J Dermatol Sci 36:115–117
86. Park KS, Min K, Nam JH et al (2005) Association of HYPA haplotype in the mannose-binding lectin gene-2 with Behçet's disease. Tissue Antigens 65:260–265
87. Chen X, Katoh Y, Nakamura K et al (2006) Single nucleotide polymorphisms of Ficolin 2 gene in Behçet's disease. J Dermatol Sci 43:201–205
88. Hou S, Yang P, Du L et al (2008) SUMO4 gene polymorphisms in Chinese Han patients with Behçet's disease. Clin Immunol 129:170–175
89. Li K, Zhao M, Hou S, Du L et al (2008) Association between polymorphisms of FCRL3, a non-HLA gene, and Behçet's disease in a Chinese population with ophthalmic manifestations. Mol Vis 14:2136–2142
90. Seo J, Park JS, Nam JH et al (2007) Association of CD94/NKG2A, CD94/NKG2C, and its ligand HLA-E polymorphisms with Behçet's disease. Tissue Antigens 70:307–313
91. Baranathan V, Stanford MR, Vaughan RW et al (2007) The association of the PTPN22 620W polymorphism with Behçet's disease. Ann Rheum Dis 66:1531–1533
92. Gunesacar R, Erken E, Bozkurt B et al (2007) Analysis of CD28 and CTLA-4 gene polymorphisms in Turkish patients with Behçet's disease. Int J Immunogenet 34:45–49
93. Meguro A, Ota M, Katsuyama Y et al (2008) Association of the toll-like receptor 4 gene polymorphisms with Behçet's disease. Ann Rheum Dis 67:725–727
94. Horie Y, Meguro A, Ota M et al (2009) Association of TLR4 polymorphisms with Behçet's disease in a Korean population. Rheumatology (Oxford) 48:638–642
95. Touitou I, Magne X, Molinari N et al (2000) MEFV mutations in Behçet's disease. Hum Mutat 16:271–272
96. Atagunduz P, Ergun T, Direskeneli H (2003) MEFV mutations are increased in Behçet's disease (BD) and are associated with vascular involvement. Clin Exp Rheumatol 21(Suppl 30):S35–S37
97. Imirzalioglu N, Dursun A, Tastan B et al (2005) MEFV gene is a probable susceptibility gene for Behçet's disease. Scand J Rheumatol 34:56–58
98. Rabinovich E, Shinar Y, Leiba M et al (2007) Common FMF alleles may predispose to development of Behçet's disease with increased risk for venous thrombosis. Scand J Rheumatol 36:48–52
99. Ayesh S, Abu-Rmaileh H, Nassar S et al (2008) Molecular analysis of MEFV gene mutations among Palestinian patients with Behçet's disease. Scand J Rheumatol 37:370–374
100. Amoura Z, Dodé C, Hue S et al (2005) Association of the R92Q TNFRSF1A mutation and extracranial deep vein thrombosis in patients with Behçet's disease. Arthritis Rheum 52:608–611
101. Verity DH, Vaughan RW, Kondeatis E et al (2000) Intercellular adhesion molecule-1 gene polymorphisms in Behçet's disease. Eur J Immunogenet 27:73–76
102. Boiardi L, Salvarani C, Casali B et al (2001) Intercellular adhesion molecule-1 gene polymorphisms in Behçet's disease. J Rheumatol 28:1283–1287
103. Kim EH, Mok JW, Bang DS et al (2003) Intercellular adhesion molecule-1 polymorphisms in Korean patients with Behçet's disease. J Korean Med Sci 18:415–418

104. Chmaisse HN, Fakhoury HA, Salti NN, Makki RF (2006) The ICAM-1 469 T/C gene poly-morphism but not 241 G/A is associated with Behçet's disease in the Lebanese population. Saudi Med J 27:604–607
105. Salvarani C, Boiardi L, Casali B et al (2002) Endothelial nitric oxide synthase gene poly-morphisms in Behçet's disease. J Rheumatol 29:535–540
106. Kim JU, Chang HK, Lee SS et al (2003) Endothelial nitric oxide synthase gene polymorphisms in Behçet's disease and rheumatic diseases with vasculitis. Ann Rheum Dis 62:1083–1087
107. Karasneh JA, Hajeer AH, Silman A et al (2005) Polymorphisms in the endothelial nitric oxide synthase gene are associated with Behçet's disease. Rheumatology (Oxford) 44:614–617
108. Ben Dhifallah I, Houman H, Khanfir M, Hamzaoui K (2008) Endothelial nitric oxide synthase gene polymorphism is associated with Behçet's disease in Tunisian population. Hum Immunol 69:661–665
109. Gül A, Ozbek U, Oztürk C et al (1996) Coagulation factor V gene mutation increases the risk of venous thrombosis in Behçet's disease. Br J Rheumatol 35:1178–1180
110. Verity DH, Vaughan RW, Madanat W et al (1999) Factor V Leiden mutation is associated with ocular involvement in Behçet's disease. Am J Ophthalmol 128(3):352–356
111. Mammo L, Al-Dalaan A, Bahabri SS, Saour JN (1997) Association of factor V Leiden with Behçet's disease. J Rheumatol 24:2196–2198
112. Gül A, Aslantas AB, Tekinay T et al (1999) Procoagulant mutations and venous thrombosis in Behçet's disease. Rheumatology (Oxford) 38:1298–1299
113. Ricart JM, Vayá A, Todolí J et al (2006) Thrombophilic risk factors and homocysteine levels in Behçet's disease in eastern Spain and their association with thrombotic events. Thromb Haemost 95(4):618–624
114. Nakao K, Isashiki Y, Sonoda S et al (2007) Nitric oxide synthase and superoxide dismutase gene polymorphisms in Behçet's disease. Arch Ophthalmol 125:246–251
115. Tursen U, Tamer L, Api H et al (2007) Cytochrome P450 polymorphisms in patients with Behçet's disease. Int J Dermatol 46:153–156
116. Yen JH, Tsai WC, Lin CH et al (2004) Cytochrome P450 1A1 and manganese superoxide dismutase gene polymorphisms in Behçet's disease. J Rheumatol 31:736–740
117. Tamer L, Tursen U, Eskandari G et al (2005) N-acetyltransferase 2 polymorphisms in patients with Behçet's disease. Clin Exp Dermatol 30:56–60
118. Karasneh J, Gül A, Ollier WE et al (2005) Whole-genome screening for susceptibility genes in multicase families with Behçet's disease. Arthritis Rheum 52:1836–1842
119. Gül A, Hajeer AH, Worthington J et al (2001) Linkage mapping of a novel susceptibility locus for Behçet's disease to chromosome 6p22-23. Arthritis Rheum 44:2693–2696

Chapter 16
Animal Models of Behçet's Disease

Ehud Baharav, Abraham Weinberger, Felix Mor, and Ilan Krause

Keywords Infectious • Autoimmunity • Herpes simplex • Air pollution • Heat shock proteins • Uveitis

Introduction

Animal models are of great value in the evaluation of pathogenic mechanisms as well as novel and experimental treatments, which cannot be tested directly on patients. The ideal characteristics for an animal model are similarities to the human disease in terms of course, symptomatology, pathophysiology, and response to treatment. In addition, we would like the animal model to show reproducibility: a high rate of response to disease induction in the animals as well as homogeneity of the onset and disease manifestations between the animals. In this chapter, we survey the various experimental models that were introduced for Behçet's disease (BD), and present some of our unpublished experience in this field. Basically, these models can be divided according to the proposed etiological paradigms.

Environmental Pollution Model

Prolonged oral administration of organic chlorides, organo-phosphate (DDT-trichloroethanediyl-bis-chlorobenzene, polychlorated-biphenyl (PCB), Sumithion™ – dimethyl-nitro-phosphorothioate), and inorganic copper to Pitman-Moor swine induced folliculitis, cutaneous nodules, genital ulcers, oral aphthae, and intestinal ulcers [1]. The clinical manifestations and histology resembled BD including changes in vascular endothelium, bleeding, hair follicles, and intestine mucosa necrosis. Microanalysis detected high levels of the above metals and low zinc

I. Krause (✉)
Department of Medicine E, Rabin Medical Center, Beilinson Hospital, Petah-Tiqva 49100, Israel
e-mail: ikrause@post.tau.ac.il

Y. Yazıcı and H. Yazıcı (eds.), *Behçet's Syndrome*,
DOI 10.1007/978-1-4419-5641-5_16, © Springer Science+Business Media, LLC 2010

concentrations in the peripheral neutrophils, infiltrating inflammatory cells and endothelial cells derived from the mucocutaneous lesions [1]. Although a study on BD patients sera had reported low levels of zinc and normal levels of magnesium, an X-ray spectroanalysis of BD skin lesions failed to detect the proposed offending elements [2]. To the best of our knowledge, this experimental model has not been used in further work. Nevertheless, it underlines the fact that prolonged exposure to certain chemical combinations can elicit multisystem inflammatory response.

Infectious Models

Bacterial Infectious Models

In the search for possible infectious causative agents of BD 4, species of the Streptococcus genus (*S. salivarius*, *S. faecalis*, *S. pyogenes* and *S. sanguis*) were isolated from lesions of patients with active BD. It was noted that crude extract of the bacterium and its superantigens induced higher immunoreactivity in BD lymphocytes in comparison to the healthy control immune cells. Animal experiments utilizing the whole bacteria or their capsular lipoteichoic acid induced acute multi organ infectious/inflammatory reactions, septic shock, and noninfiltrative short-term uveitis. The failure to reproduce an experimental model of BD led to search for other bacterial derived components as causative agents in BD. So far, no bacterial model has found uniform recognition [3].

Viral Infectious Models

Hulusi Behçet in his historical description of BD in 1937 proposed that the syndrome might be caused by a viral infection. For many decades, efforts were made to confirm this hypothesis. The results of extensive data collected regarding the significance of herpes simplex virus (HSV) in BD including the detection of anti-HSV antibodies, viral DNA expression, and antiherpetic therapeutic trials were controversial [4]. In 1998, Sohn et al. [5] reported that inoculation of HSV type I at the earlobe of ICR mice produced a BD-like disease in approximately 50% of the animals, including genital and oral ulcers, skin and eye lesions, arthritis, and gastrointestinal involvement. This model was induced in other mice strains including B10.BR (MHC H-2k), B10.RIII (H-2r), C57BL/6 (H-2b), C3H/He (H-2k), and Balb/c (H-2d) [6]. Symptoms developed in 40–50% of B10.BR, B10.RIII, and C57BL/6m but in only 2% of C3H/He and Balb/c. The lack of correlation between H-2 type and disease frequency cannot support the concept that MHC genetic phenotype is involved in the pathogenesis of this model of BD. This model has a high mortality rate; 30% of the infected mice and only 50% of the surviving mice develop some signs resembling BD. The disappointing results of therapeutic trials with antiherpes virus drugs in BD do not support the possibility that BD is a subtype of active chronic HSV infection [4]. This does not rule out the possibility that HSV infection can serve as a trigger to initiate the immunological dysregulation leading to the development of BD. Finally, this model provides extensive data about the inflammatory aspects of BD and serves as an experimental model to assess therapeutic modalities for human disease [7,8].

Autoimmune Models

Heat Shock Proteins

Heat shock proteins (HSP) are intracellular chaperone molecules with scavenger properties that are expressed in cells upon various stress stimuli [9]. The microbial HSP 65 kDa and the animal HSP 60 share a significant homology (over 50%). It was found that various antibodies directed to amino acid sequences of HSP 65 are cross-reactive with the human HSP 60 expressed in active lesions of BD. Moreover, T cells of BD patients from different ethnicity were highly reactive to HSP sequences, and the immunodominance hierarchy of these sequences differed from the pattern in healthy controls. Subcutaneous immunization of rats with human 60-kDa HSP-derived peptide 336-351 induced clinical and/or histological uveitis in 80% of rats. Subsequent experiments to prevent the development of uveitis by oral or nasal administration of the peptide have failed. Instead, uveitis was induced in 75% of rats when given the peptide orally, in 75% when given nasally, and 92% of those administered the peptide by both routes. Examination of mRNA from CD4-enriched splenic cells failed to yield significant differences in Th1 or Th2 cytokines. Treatment with monoclonal antibody (mAb) to CD4 yielded a dose-dependent decrease in uveitis from 82 to 25%. Similarly, treatment with IL-4 significantly decreased the development of uveitis from 68 to 30%. Conversely, treatment of the rats with mAb to CD8 greatly enhanced the onset of uveitis (from about 22 days in the controls to 11 days after immunization) and all the rats developed uveitis by day 24. Thus, CD4+ cells mediate, whereas CD8+ cells suppress the development of uveitis in this model. It was suggested that this experimental mucosal model of induction of uveitis by the human 60-kDa HSP-derived peptide is consistent with the oro-genital onset of BD and the development of uveitis [10]. This model can be categorized as an organ specific auto-immune model for BD.

S-Ag-Induced Uveitis

Retinal S-Ag is an immunologically sequestered protein existing mainly in the photoreceptor region of the retina. It is used for the induction of the classical model of experimental autoimmune uveitis [11]. The sera of BD patients among other patients with uveitis had antibodies directed against S-Ag, and their T cells were recognized and activated by this protein. Of high importance was the finding that an S-Ag epitope (aa 342–355) designated PDS-Ag shared homology to a conserved sequence in the HLA-B molecules (aa 125–138) designated B27PD. Immunization of rats with both peptides caused uveitis [12] supporting the concept of anti-HLA autoimmunity in the pathogenesis of BD. Activation of peripheral CD4+ T cells with these peptides occurred only in HLA B51 positive BD patients with posterior uveitis but not in patients without eye involvement. This implied that the normal tolerance to self-HLA class I epitopes is preserved in BD, and additional conditions are needed for its breakdown and for the development of posterior uveitis.

This model can be categorized together with the HSP model, as an organ specific auto-immune model.

Tropomyosin

Our group has shown that sera of patients with BD contain IgG antibodies directed to α-tropomyosin (TPM) protein, a component of the contractile apparatus of the muscles. Vaccination of Lewis rats with TPM emulsified in complete Freund's adjuvant (CFA) caused an inflammatory disease with involvement of the skin, joints, and eyes. Infusion of an anti-TPM-directed T-cell line derived from the draining lymph node lymphocytes of the TPM-vaccinated rats induced a similar pathology [13]. The cytokine profile of pathogenic cells had a Th1 pattern. The model was used to test the therapeutic effects of lactobacillus GG [14]. In this model, we also analyzed the membranal fatty acids composition induced by probiotic bacteria consumption. We noticed a shift in the ratio of $n-3/n-6$ poly unsaturated fatty acids (PUFA) toward reduction in PUFA that can serve as precursors of pro-inflammatory prostaglandins (submitted for publication).

Transgenic Model

The paradigm of ethnic and genetic predisposition in BD is widely accepted. The discovery of the association between BD and the HLA Class I molecule B51 [15], led Takeno et al. [16] in 1995 to produce a transgenic (Tg) mouse model. The production of Tg was an important step in the attempt to elucidate the role of the genetic marker HLA B51 in the pathogenesis of BD. They inserted the human HLA B*5101 gene into C3H/He mice. The neutrophils of the Tg mice produced excessive superoxide similar to the documented phenomenon in BD patients. However, no clinical signs of the disease developed. Based on these results, it remains unknown whether HLA B51 is just a marker and other gene/s with linkage disequilibrium to its locus are involved in the pathogenesis of BD, whether the HLA B51 molecule is essential but insufficient for the development of BD, or if the mouse strain used was resistant for the development of active disease. We have failed to induce BD-like disease in these mice (Received from Prof. M. Takiguchi, Kumamoto University School of

Medicine, Japan.) by vaccinating some antigens, mentioned above [17], which were proposed to be involved in the autoimmune aspects of BD (unpublished data). One should note that the Tg construct contained only the HLA-B*5101's heavy chain without the coupled binding arm of the molecule, the β_2-microglobulin. Thus, the fact that the Tg mice did not develop a BD like disorder spontaneously or upon antigenic challenges does not refute this hypothesis. The development of Tg mice with the complete molecule is warranted.

In an attempt to combine both assumptions – that BD is an HLA-B51-dependant autoimmune disorder – we used bio-informatic methods to estimate the potential role of B*5101 and the above antigens in the pathogenesis of BD based on the aforementioned animal models. Briefly, it is commonly accepted that the T cells recognize a particular peptide presented by the HLA molecule. For that purpose, three elements are required. Firstly, T-cell receptors (TCR) should have potential binding capacity to the amino acid sequences of the peptide. Secondly, the presented peptides should contain a particular motif that can be anchored by the HLA binding sites, and finally, the three dimensional-structure of the peptide should be recognized by the HLA molecule. Because of its steric structure, the binding sites of HLA class I molecules can bind only short peptides with a length of up to 10 amino acids. We searched for 9-mer peptide candidates for antigenic peptide motifs derived from the antigens proposed to induce experimental BD in animals. For that purpose, we used computerized programs that rank sequences of peptides according to their predicted half-time dissociation coefficient from the HLA and rat MHC class I molecules. The binding capacity of the human HLA-B*5101 and the corresponding rat class I molecule, designated MHC RT1.Al, to the following proteins or peptides, was studied: HSP-65, HSP-65 (aa 336–351), MICA, HLA-B*5101, Retinal S-Antigen, Sort sequence of Retinal S-Antigen (aa 342–355) designates PDS-Ag, short peptide HLA-B27 (aa 125–138) and human-Tropomyosin. In each protein examined, several short sequences with potential high binding capacity were found, with the exception of the short peptide B-27PD that has no binding capacity motif to HLA-B*5101 but only to rat molecule MHC RT1.Al. The peptide designated PDS-Ag has a potential binding capacity to HLA B*5101 but not to MHC RT1.Al. In addition, it was found that the Tropomyosin short peptide T_2 has the highest predicted binding capacity to the human and rat class I molecules compared to the other TPM-derived peptides. This finding is in accordance with the clinical disease severity caused by TPM T_2 in the animal model [13]. On the other hand, this information is still theoretical; in order to prove this concept, it should be tested by immunization of Tg animals bearing the complete HLA-B51molecule with each of the proteins and peptides mentioned above.

Comments (Summarized in Table 16.1)

The environmental pollution model is conceptually interesting since the pigs developed multisystem symptoms similar to BD, but the model has limitations to become utilized as a model for the disease since it is difficult to produce and the onset of

Table 16.1 Comparison summary table

Model	Model characteristics				Hypothetical etiologies				Immunologic characteristics resembling BD
	Similarity	Reproducibility	Homogeneity	Genetic	Environmental	Infectious	Autoimmune	
Environmental pollution	High	Not tested	Low	No	Yes	No	No	Unknown
Streptococcal infectious	Mono symptomatic	High	High	No	No	Yes	Yes	
HSV infection	High	Moderate	Low	No	No	Yes	No	Th1
S-Ag uveitis	Mono symptomatic	High	High	Probable	No	Probable	Yes	T cell, CD_8
Tropomyosin	Oligo symptomatic	High	Moderate	Unknown	No	No	Yes	CD_4, Th1
HLA B51 transgenic	No			Yes	Unknown	Unknown	Unknown	Neutrophil activation

symptoms appears erratically in a wide time range of 4–10 months. Moreover, the failure to show increased levels of the offending pollutants in BD patients raises questions as to its relevance. The Streptococcal models have similarity only to the eye involvement in BD. Eliciting autoreactivity to HSP in the animals contributed to the understanding the potential reactive autoimmune component of BD. This model is simple to induce with high rate of homogeneity. The HSV model has multisystem manifestations resembling BD; it has a moderate reproducibility since 30% of the inoculated mice die upon induction and low homogeneity. The use of human live virus demands special laboratory facilities. The autoimmune model utilizing S-Ag is a monosymptomatic model of BD-like uveitis. This model is easy to induce and extensive studies elucidated some of the immunological characteristics of BD including the paradigm of anti-HLA autoimmunity. The TPM model shares some clinical features of BD. This model has a potential to become a useful autoimmune model for BD. The only published trial to establish a Tg model for BD did not show any significant similarity to the human disease except hyper-responsiveness of neutrophils.

References

1. Hori Y, Miyazawa S, Nishiyama S et al (1979) Experimental Behçet's disease and ultrastructural X-ray microanalysis of pathological tissues. J Dermatol 6:31–37
2. Bang D, Honma T, Saito T et al (1987) Electron microscopic observation on dark endothelial cells in erythema nodosum-like lesions of Behçet's disease with ultrastructural X-ray spectro-analysis. J Toxicol Sci 12:321–328
3. Kaneko F, Oyama N, Nishibu A (1997) Streptococcal infection in the pathogenesis of Behçet's disease and clinical effects of minocycline on the disease symptoms. Yonsei Med J 38:444–454
4. Saenz A, Ausejo M, Shea B, et al. (2000) Pharmacotherapy for Behçet's syndrome. Cochrane Database Syst Rev CD001084 Vol. 2
5. Sohn S, Lee ES, Bang D et al (1998) Behçet's disease-like symptoms induced by the Herpes simplex virus in ICR mice. Eur J Dermatol 8:21–23
6. Sohn S, Lee ES, Lee S (2001) The correlation of MHC haplotype and development of Behçet's disease-like symptoms induced by herpes simplex virus in several inbred mouse strains. J Dermatol Sci 26:173–181
7. Bang D, Choi B, Kwon HJ et al (2008) Rebamipide affects the efficiency of colchicine for the herpes simplex virus-induced inflammation in a Behçet's disease mouse model. Eur J Pharmacol 598:112–117
8. Choi B, Hwang Y, Kwon HJ et al (2008) Tumor necrosis factor alpha small interfering RNA decreases herpes simplex virus-induced inflammation in a mouse model. J Dermatol Sci 52:87–97
9. Javid B, MacAry PA, Lehner PJ (2007) Structure and function: heat shock proteins and adaptive immunity. J Immunol 179:2035–2040
10. Hu W, Hasan A, Wilson A et al (1998) Experimental mucosal induction of uveitis with the 60-kDa heat shock protein-derived peptide 336–351. Eur J Immunol 28:2444–2455
11. de Smet MD, Bitar G, Mainigi S et al (2001) Human S-antigen determinant recognition in uveitis. Invest Ophthalmol Vis Sci 42:3233–3238
12. Kurhan-Yavuz S, Direskeneli H, Bozkurt N et al (2000) Anti-MHC autoimmunity in Behçet's disease: T cell responses to an HLA-B-derived peptide cross-reactive with retinal-S antigen in patients with uveitis. Clin Exp Immunol 120:162–166

13. Mor F, Weinberger A, Cohen IR (2002) Identification of alpha-tropomyosin as a target self-antigen in Behçet's syndrome. Eur J Immunol 32:356–365
14. Baharav E, Mor F, Halpern M et al (2004) Lactobacillus GG bacteria ameliorate arthritis in Lewis rats. J Nutr 134:1964–1969
15. Ohno S, Ohguchi M, Hirose S et al (1982) Close association of HLA-Bw51 with Behçet's disease. Arch Ophthalmol 100:1455–1458
16. Takeno M, Kariyone A, Yamashita N et al (1995) Excessive function of peripheral blood neutrophils from patients with Behçet's disease and from HLA-B51 transgenic mice. Arthritis Rheum 38:426–433
17. Direskeneli H, (2001) Behçet's disease infectious aetiology, new autoantigens, and HLA-B51. Ann Rheum Dis 60:996–1002

Chapter 17
Prognosis in Behçet's Syndrome

Emire Seyahi and Hasan Yazıcı

Keywords Behçet's syndrome • Prognosis • Mortality • Morbidity • Eye disease • Vascular involvement • Neurological involvement • Cancer

Introduction

A good portion of the substance of this chapter on prognosis is mainly based on a survey of a 20-year outcome of an inception cohort of BS patients we published a few years ago [1]. In this survey, we had sought outcome information, after 20 years of their initial visit, on 428 (286 M/142 F) patients who had registered in our multidisciplinary outpatient clinic between 1977 and 1983. Since we were able to collect outcome information on 90.4% of our patients and there were no significant differences between the initial demography and the clinical findings of the 10% lost to follow-up and the remainder of the group, we like to give good credence to our findings.

It is often said that in many patients with Behçet's, especially if they present with skin-mucosa findings, the disease fades away with the passage of time. Even though the due emphasis probably was not given to this in original paper, the findings are at hand to have a good estimate of the proportion of patients in whom this happens [1]. Of the initial cohort of 428 patients, there were 42 that had died and 41 who were lost to follow up at the end 20 years. The survey revealed that only 94 of the remaining 345 (in whom outcome information was available) would have fulfilled O'Duffy's criteria for diagnosis. If one adds these 94 patients to the 42 that had died and 41 lost to follow up, the remaining 251/428 (59%) of the patients could not be identified as Behçet's disease at the end of 20 years [1]. It should also be added this is a rather conservative estimate in that it assumes that all who were lost to follow-up had active disease at the time of survey.

E. Seyahi (✉)
Division of Rheumatology, Department of Medicine, Cerrahpasa Medical Faculty,
University of Istanbul, Istanbul, Turkey
e-mail: eseyahi@yahoo.com

Y. Yazıcı and H. Yazıcı (eds.), *Behçet's Syndrome*,
DOI 10.1007/978-1-4419-5641-5_17, © Springer Science+Business Media, LLC 2010

Although BS affects both genders equally, the disease runs a more severe course among men and among the young as brought up by many studies [1–7]. In particular, the presence and severity of eye disease, vascular involvement, and finally the increased mortality are definitely associated with being male and young.

Mortality

Table 17.1 summarizes the main outcome studies available. In our survey, the mean age of the patients was 31.5 ± 8.3 years and median disease duration was 2.5 years at the time they presented at our clinic [1]. Among these, a total of 42 (39 M/3 F) patients (10%) had died at the time of the survey. The mortality rate was significantly higher in males compared to females (39/286 vs. 3/142, $P = 0.001$). Standardized mortality ratios (SMR's) were specifically increased among young males (14–24 and 25–34 years old age groups), while older males (35–50 year old age) and females had a normal life span (Fig. 17.1). Furthermore, we observed that the mortality rate was highest during the first years (7 years) of disease onset and had a tendency to decrease with time (Fig. 17.1). We demonstrated that patients who had died had significantly more major organ involvement (such as eye, large vessel and CNS) at disease onset compared to those who had been alive [1]. Probable causes of mortality were large vessel disease especially pulmonary artery aneurysms ($n = 17$), parenchymal CNS disease ($n = 5$), neoplasms ($n = 4$), chronic renal failure ($n = 4$), ischemic heart disease ($n = 3$), congestive heart failure/stroke ($n = 3$), suicide ($n = 2$), and a traffic accident ($n = 1$).

In an earlier work, we had reported no increased mortality at 10 years compared to the general population among a smaller group of patients ($n = 152$), of whom 4% (6/152) were dead and 21% (32/152) were lost to follow-up [6]. Kaklamani et al. similarly observed no single death among 64 patients, some of whom had been followed for 30 years [7]. Others had reported lower mortality rates as well [8–10]. Benamour et al. found a mortality rate of 3% (10/316) among a cohort of patients diagnosed between 1981 and 1989 in a university hospital [8]. Yamamoto et al. reported that 22 (1%) died among 2,031 patients from Japan during the course of a single year's follow-up [9]. Similarly, Park et al. observed 7 deaths (0.3%) due to the disease among 2,220 patients in 9 years [10]. Causes of death were defined as intestinal involvement, large vessel disease, valvular heart disease, infection, and cerebrovascular disease [5,8,10]. Methodological differences such as short and uneven follow-up times, the strictly retrospective nature of the analyses, and the geographical variations in disease expression (lower frequency of vascular disease in the Far-East) may explain some of the discrepancies.

A certainly interesting feature of the mortality in our 20-year prognosis survey was the clear trend of the mortality to decrease with the passage of time [1] (Fig. 17.1). This is in striking contrast with other inflammatory diseases like rheumatoid arthritis and systemic lupus where the reverse trend is seen [11,12]. It indicates that the disease indeed fades away in many patients with BS with the passage of time. It also ties with the lack of accelerated atherosclerosis in BS (see Chap. 8) as different from rheumatoid arthritis and systemic lupus [13–16].

Table 17.1 Studies on mortality and general outcome in Behçet's syndrome

Ref. no.	Author (chronological)	N (M/F)	Follow-up time	Mortality	Blindness	Vascular outcome	Neurological outcome
[9]	Yamamoto et al. (1974)	2,031	1 year	22 (1%)	–	–	–
[3]	Chajek et al. (1975)	41 (34 M/7 F)	Mean 8 years	1 (2%)	8/31 (26%) of affected patients	–	Severe neurological deficit in 2 of 12 patients with neurological disease
[8]	Benamour et al. (1990)	316 (224 M/92 F)	–	10 (3.2%)	88/226 (39 %) of affected patients (Bilateral: 17%, unilateral: 22%)	–	Severe motor deficiency in 23 of 50 patients with neurological disease
[10]	Park et al. (1993)	2,200 (M/F not defined)	–	7 (0.3%)	–	–	–
[6]	Yazıcı et al. (1996)	152 (92 M/60 F); lost to follow up: 21%	Mean 10 years	6 (3.9%)	–	–	–
[1]	Seyahi et al. (2003)	428 (286 M/142 F); lost to follow-up: 9.6%	Mean 20 years	42 (10%) (39 M/3 F)	At the end of follow-up: Bilateral (total) : 72/184[a] (39%) (males): 64/146 (44%) (females): 8/38 (21%) Unilateral (total): 48/184 (26%) (males): 38/146 (26%) (females): 10/38 (26%)	At the end of follow-up: Vascular disease mortality: Total: 17/136[b] (13%) Males: 17/129 (13%) Females: 0/7 (0%) Arterial disease mortality[b]: Total: 10/21 (50%) Males: 10/20 (50%) Females: 0/1 (0%) Venous disease mortality: Total: 7/115 (6%) Males: 7/109 (6%) Females: 0/6 (0%)	At the end of follow-up: Neurological disease mortality: Total: 5/41[c] (12%) Males: 5/34 (15%) Females: 0/7 (0%)

[a]There were 184 (146 M/38 F) with eye disease at the end of follow-up

[b]There were 136 (129 M/7 F) patients with vascular disease

[c]There were 41 (34 M/7 F) patients with neurological disease

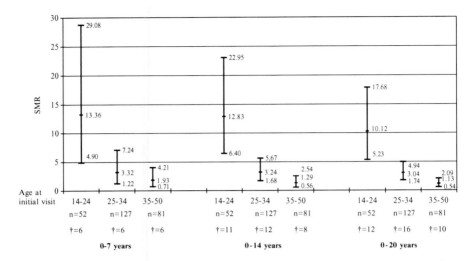

Fig. 17.1 Standardized mortality ratios (SMR's with 95% confidence interval) of a cohort of 260 male patients with Behçet's syndrome. (Reproduced by permission from Kural-Seyahi et al., The Long-Term Mortality and Morbidity of Behçet's Syndrome. Medicine 2003; 82(1):62. © 2003 Lippincott Williams & Wilkins)

Skin-Mucosa Lesions and Arthritis

Skin-mucosa lesions recur in virtually every patient and are the most frequent manifestations. These lesions together with joint involvement rarely lead to serious complications and permanent damage [17–19]. Their frequency and severity tend to abate with time [1]. We had already noted that in about 60% of the patients, the whole clinical picture fades at 20 years. In the same survey, the frequency of each of the skin mucosa manifestations and arthritis decreased considerably during the same time span [1]. Similarly, Shimizu et al. observed a slowing of the attacks after 3–7 years of disease onset in many patients [5].

Eye Disease

Eye involvement is the most serious manifestation and affects about 50% of the patients (males: 55%, females: 30%) [1]. It develops within the first few years of the disease onset and runs its most severe course during these years. Bilateral involvement is observed in 70–80% of patients at the beginning and becomes 90% when followed long-term [1,20]. Male gender, posterior involvement, frequent attacks, strong vitreous opacity, and exudates along side retinal vascular arcade are identified as poor prognostic factors [21,22]. Table 17.2 summarizes some of the largest studies

Table 17.2 Studies specifically addressing eye disease

Ref. no.	Author (chronological)	N	Follow-up time	Blindness	Comments
[24]	Mishima et al. (1979)	152 (121 M/31 F) 272 eyes	5 years	Loss of useful vision in 136/272 (50 %) eyes	Visual prognosis is better in females
[25]	Benezra et al. (1986)	26 (52 eyes)	6–10 years	Loss of useful vision in 39/52 (74%) eyes	Despite intensive follow up and treatment the long term prognosis of eye disease remains very poor
[21]	Sakamoto et al. (1995)	52 (39 M/13 F) 104 eyes	3 years	Loss of useful vision in 35/101 (35%) eyes	The presence of skin lesions, arthritis, posterior attacks increase the risk of visual loss
[29]	Yoshida et al. (2004)	Group A (1980s): 133 (107 M/ 26 F); 261 eyes Group B (1990s): 107 (79 M/ 28 F); 203 eyes	Group A: 2.8 years Group B: 4 years	Loss of useful vision at the end of follow-up: Group A: 129/261 eyes (49%) Group B: 42/203 eyes (21%)	Prognosis of eye disease improved after 1990
[20]	Tugal-Tutkun et al. (2004)	880 (599 M/281 F); 1,567 eyes	Median follow-up approximately 5 years	Risk of useful vision loss: 5 years: 21% for males 10% for females 10 years: 30% for males 17% for females	Better outcome in patients admitted after 1990s
[28]	Cho et al. (2007)	99 (57 M/42 F); 168 eyes	4.8 years	Risk of useful vision loss: 5 years : 17% 10 years: 21%	Long-term prognosis of eye disease is mostly affected by initial visual acuity
[31]	Chung et al. (2008)	Group A (1984–1993): 95 (64 M/31 F); 178 eyes Group B (1994–2003): 132 (76 M/ 56 F); 231 eyes	Group A: 7 years Group B: 2 years	Loss of useful vision at the end of follow-up: Group A: 94/178 eyes (53%) Group B: 49/231 eyes (21%)	Visual prognosis is improved in the recent decade due to increased azathioprine and cyclosporine use

addressing visual prognosis. The prognosis of eye disease has been reported to be very poor in the past. Total blindness was often considered as the eventual outcome in an average of 3 years after the onset of ocular symptoms [23]. Approximately 12% of acquired visual loss in adulthood in Japan was reported to be caused by BS and more than half of the Japanese BS patients were reported to have lost their useful vision within 5 years of disease onset [24]. In a study from Israel, 75% of treated patients were found to have lost useful vision in 6–10 years after the onset of uveitis [25]. In our 20 year survey, 17% (25/146) of males and 10.5% (4/38) of females with eye involvement had bilateral useful vision loss at their initial presentation [1]. After two decades, additional 27% (39/146) of males and 10.5% (4/38) of the females with initially useful vision had lost their eye sight. This added up to a total of 44% (64/146) and 21% (8/38), loss of vision for males and females, respectively. The majority of the bilateral loss of vision among males had already developed at the initial years of follow-up (40%) and during the first 4 years following inception (42%) decreasing substantially thereafter. Furthermore, a quarter of males (38/146) and females (10/38) with eye involvement were found to have unilateral loss of useful vision at the end of survey. It is also to be noted that relatively few of our patients were treated with immunosuppressive agents (systemic corticosteroids: 19%, azathioprine: 15%, cyclophosphamide: 12%, cyclosporine: 3%). Our survey had included patients registered between 1977 and 1983 and the routine use of cyclosporine in our clinic began after 1985 and that of azathioprine after 1990 [1]. The routine and early use of these agents promptly began to change the visual prognosis. In this respect, there was no decrease in mean visual acuity between the beginning and the end of the 2-year period among the azathioprine users in our azathioprine trial [26], and when these patients were reassessed at 8 years [27], blindness developed in 8/20 (40%) of the patients initially allocated to placebo, whereas in 3/24 (13%) of those who initially received azathioprine. It is also worth noting that the outcome of those in whom eye disease develop de novo later during the follow-up was better, since none of the patients in this group developed bilateral loss of useful vision [1].

Tugal-Tutkun et al. also studied the outcome of 880 (599 M/281 F) consecutive patients seen between 1980 and 1998 [20]. At the beginning of the follow-up, 31% of eyes in males and 24% of eyes in females had loss of useful vision (visual acuity of ≤0.1). The risk of having useful vision loss at 5 and 10 years was predicted to be 21 and 30% for males whereas 10 and 17% for females, ($P<0.001$) under conventional immunosuppressive treatment [20]. The number of patients who received immunosuppressive treatment in this study was substantially higher than that was reported in our survey (systemic corticosteroids: 79%, azathioprine: 30%, cyclophosphamide: 28%, cyclosporine: 10%). This was expected in that this survey also included patients who were treated after the beneficial effects of cyclosporine and azathioprine were more widely appreciated. Accordingly, male patients who presented after 1990 were found to have a lower rate of visual loss compared to those who presented in the 1980s [20]. The risk of becoming blind at 1, 5, and 7 years were calculated as 9% vs. 5%, 26% vs. 16%, and 30% vs. 21%, for those admitted in the 1980s and after 1990, respectively [20]. Comparable to the study of Tugal-Tutkun et al. [20], in a Korean study in which hospital records of 99 BS patients seen between 1995 and 2005 were analyzed, loss of useful vision was observed in 20% (34/168) of eyes at the beginning of follow-up and occurred in only 11% (15/134) of the eyes during a mean follow-up of 5 years [28]. The risk of becoming blind at 5 and 10 years was calculated as 17 and 21%, respectively [28]. Similarly Yoshida et al. investigated clinical records of 240 (186 M/54 F) patients followed-up at the uveitis clinic of University of Tokyo Hospital between 1980 and 1999 [29]. They observed a significant decrease in the number of ocular attacks per year and the percentage of patients with poor visual acuity among patients seen in the 1990s compared to those seen in 1980s. It is clear that the recent studies describe a more favorable outcome [20,28–32]. We believe that the outcome of eye disease will get even better with the more wide-spread use of new biological agents such as tumor necrosis factor blockers and interferon-alpha in daily practice.

A recent international effort found that a poor visual outcome is still prevalent in many regions [33] with 30% of patients in Japan and Iran still losing useful vision. On the other hand, there is evidence to suggest that widespread use of the drugs we have been mentioning as distinctly useful in managing eye disease are, for some reason, underused in these regions. In a comparative study, it was recently reported that the use of immunosuppressives for BS was less in Japan compared to USA [34]. These observations we believe underline the need for urgent implementation research in Behçet's to see if our patients are getting the due treatment.

Vascular Disease

Vascular disease develops in up to 25–35% of the patients and has a definite male preponderance [1–5,35–42]. Its frequency could be up to 49% among males when followed for 20 years [1]. Venous involvement is more common than arterial disease (75% vs. 25%) and lower extremity deep vein thrombosis (DVT) is the most frequent manifestation [1,38]. Vena cava thrombosis, pulmonary artery aneurysms (PAA), Budd–Chiari syndrome, peripheral artery aneurysms, dural sinus thrombosis, and abdominal aorta aneurysms were the other manifestations as listed in decreasing frequency [1,38]. DVT is an early finding occurring usually within the first few years of disease onset [38]. Similarly, PAA and Budd–Chiari syndrome are also reported to occur early [38]. Dural sinus thrombosis also seems to occur early since it is the most preferred manifestation among juvenile BS patients [38,43,44]. However, vena cava thrombosis and aneurysms other than PAA are late findings. We had reported that vena cava thrombosis develops in a median of 5 years whereas abdominal aorta and peripheral arterial aneurysms develop in a median of 7 years [1]. Arterial disease is manifested mostly in the form of aneurysms [1,35,38]. Arterial occlusions are seldom seen and reported to have a better prognosis than that of the arterial aneurysms [35].

Table 17.3 summarizes some of the major outcome studies on vascular involvement. Among all type of venous involvement, Budd–Chiari syndrome has the worse outcome [1,39]. Bayraktar et al. investigated the frequency and outcome of Budd–Chiari syndrome in 493 patients with BS seen in Ankara, Turkey during a

Table 17.3 Studies specifically addressing vascular disease

Ref. no.	Author (chronological)	N	Follow-up time	Mortality	Major cause of mortality	Comments
[35]	Hamza et al. (1987)	10 (9 M/1 F) with arterial disease out of 450 patients	Median 2 years	3 (33.3%)	Hepatic failure due to Budd–Chiari syndrome ($n=1$); abdominal aorta surgery complication ($n=1$); heart failure due to intracardiac thrombosis ($n=1$)	Arterial disease generally occurs in the late stage of the disease. Prognosis of arterial occlusion was better than that of the arterial aneurysm
[40]	Hamuryudan et al. (1994)	24 M with PAA out of 2,179 patients	Mean 2 years	12 (50%)	Hemoptysis due to rupture of pulmonary arterial aneurysm	High short term mortality despite treatment (50% died after 9.5±11 months after the onset of hemoptysis)
[39]	Bayraktar et al. (1997)	14 (12 M/2 F) with Budd–Chiari syndrome out of 493 patients	Mean 3 years	10 (71.2%)	Hepatic failure due to Budd–Chiari syndrome	Behçet's syndrome is a common cause of Budd–Chiari syndrome.
[41]	Hamuryudan et al. (2004)	26 (25 M/ 1 F) with PAA out of 2,200 patients Lost to follow-up: 15% (4/26)	Mean 4 years	6 (23%)	Hemoptysis due to rupture of pulmonary arterial aneurysm	Improvement in prognosis is due to to earlier recognition and aggressive treatment
[42]	Tüzün et al. (1997)	24 (all males) with aneurysms other than PAA Lost to follow-up: 17% (4/24)	Mean 4 years	4 (17%)	Gastrointestinal/mediastinal bleeding or hemoptysis due to abdominal aorta and peripheral artery aneurysms	Ligation is the suggested way of surgery in aneurysms limited to the extremities. Abdominal aortic aneurysms could be treated with tube graft insertions

PAA pulmonary artery aneurysms

8-year period from 1985 to 1994 [39]. There were 14 (26%) patients with Budd–Chiari syndrome out of 53 patients with large vessel thrombosis. Of these 14 patients, 10 (60%) died with a mean survival of 10 months [39]. In our 20 year survey, all three patients with Budd–Chiari syndrome had died during the follow-up [1].

PAA is another serious complication, leading to death by massive hemoptysis. We reported in 1994 that 12 patients with PAA out of 24 (all men) died after a mean of 10 months after the onset of haemoptysis [40]. A decade later in 2004, we updated the outcome of PAA with 26 BS patients who had been followed between 1992 and 2002 [41]. There were significantly less deaths (6/26, 23%) during a mean of 4 years in the recent group attributed mainly to earlier recognition and prompt treatment.

Aortic and peripheral arterial aneurysms are also major causes of death because of the risk of rupture. Twenty-four patients (all male) with either abdominal aorta or peripheral artery aneurysms were identified between 1977 and 1996 at the thoracic and cardiovascular surgery department of Cerrahpasa Medical Faculty in a study by Tüzün et al. [42]. Four patients were lost to follow-up, another 4 (17%) had died. Ligations were defined as the preferred choice of surgical treatment for aneurysms localized in the extremities while, abdominal aortic aneurysms were treated better with graft insertions [42]. It has been also suggested that immunosuppressive treatment should be given to prevent recurrences.

Neurological Disease

There are mainly two types of neurological disease in BS: parenchymal CNS disease, which is the most common (75–80%) and dural sinus thrombosis (10–20%) [45,46]. The frequency of all type of neurological involvement has been reported to be around 5% in cross-sectional studies [45,46]. However, this rate doubles when a same cohort is followed for two decades [1].

Parenchymal CNS disease is usually a late manifestation, developing after 5–10 years of the disease onset. Brainstem involvement is the most characteristic type of involvement [45,46]. Spinal cord and hemispheric involvement are rarely observed. Pyramidal signs, hemiparesis, behavioral –cognitive changes and sphincter disturbances, and/or impotence are the main clinical manifestations. Parenchymal CNS disease is a serious morbidity of BS leading often to disability or mortality. We had identified CNS disease as the second most common cause of mortality in our long-term survey [1]. The two most important studies on neurological outcome are summarized in Table 17.4. Siva et al. showed that the disease may follow relapsing remitting course and will progress to severe disability in approximately 50% of the cases in 10 years [46]. Akman –Demir et al. reported that 22 of 200 patients (11%) with neurological involvement died 4 years after neurological onset and almost 60% of patients with parenchymal involvement became either dead or dependant on another person 10 years after onset of neurological disease [45]. Factors that may play significant role in the poor prognosis were defined as abnormal cerebrospinal fluid, having parenchymal involvement, frequent attacks, and being dependant

Table 17.4 Studies specifically addressing neurological disease

Ref. no.	Author (chronological)	N	Follow-up time	Mortality	Major reported morbidity	Comments
[45]	Akman-Demir et al. (1999)	200 (155 M/45 F)	Median 5 years	22 deaths (20M/2F)	28 patients become dependent	Non-parenchymal CNS involvement is associated with a better prognosis than parenchymal CNS involvement. Polymorphonuclear pleocytosis in cerebrospinal fluid and parenchymal involvement are typical findings for bad prognosis
[46]	Siva et al. (2001)	164 (130 M/34 F)	Mean 2.9 ± 3.2 years	9 deaths	45.1% moderate to severe neurological disability, by 10 years after the onset of neurological symptom	Cerebellar symptoms and progressive course are unfavorable whereas onset with headache and having venous sinus thrombosis are favorable

M male, *F* female, *CNS* central nervous system

on others at admission [45,46]. Normal CSF findings, disease course limited to single episode, nonparenchymal (dural sinus) type of involvement, and independence at admission were good prognostic factors. Finally, it should be added that Akman–Demir group recently presented data suggesting that the prognosis might be improving in CNS disease, as well [47].

Dural sinus thrombosis has a significantly favorable outcome than parenchymal type and is usually associated with other types of venous disease [1,45–48]. Thrombosis of the venous sinuses may present with symptoms of increased intracranial pressure such as severe headache, papilloedema, sixth nerve palsy, and rarely with fever. Dural sinus thrombosis is also the predominant type of neurological involvement in juvenile BS patients. We had observed 9 boys (mean age: 13 ± 2 year) with dural sinus thrombosis (7%) whereas 1 with parenchymal neurological disease (0.8%) among 121 juvenile patients with BS (61 boys/60 girls) in a cross-sectional survey [43]. Similarly, another study identified 16 pediatric cases with dural sinus thrombosis and 3 with parenchymal involvement among a group of 19 juvenile BS patients attending a neurological outpatient clinic [44].

Development of De Novo Major Organ Complications During Follow-Up

Male patients with BS may still develop serious morbidities at long term even when they have no major organ involvement during the early years of their disease. Hamuryudan et al. recently assessed the long-term prognosis of 96 male patients with BS who had no significant major organ involvement at the time when they had taken part in a randomized controlled trial of thalidomide between October 1993 and April 1996 [49]. Seventeen patients (18%) were lost to follow-up; 4 (4%) had died. A total of 39 patients out of 91 (43%) developed major organ complications such as eye disease ($n=16$), vascular ($n=14$), and CNS ($n=4$) involvement during a mean follow-up of 12 years [49]. Those who developed new organ involvement were significantly younger than who did not (mean age: 22 vs. 27, $P<0.001$). In this line, in a multicenter study, Alpsoy et al. observed a significant increase in the mean clinical severity scores (CSS) of 661 patients with BS followed for a mean of 3.7 ± 3.4 years (4.0 ± 0.1 vs. 4.6 ± 0.1, at first visit and at the end of follow-up, respectively $P<0.001$) [50]. It was seen that the total CSS calculated at the end of the study, was significantly higher in patients whose age at disease onset was <40 years ($CSS=5.0 \pm 0.1$) compared to those >40 years ($CSS=4.3 \pm 0.2$) ($P=0.004$) [50].

Cancer

The frequency of cancer in BS does not seem to be increased compared to that found in the general population. In our long-term prognosis study, we had observed 8 patients with cancer among a cohort of 387 BS patients followed for two decades [1].

Annual incidence rate of cancer in our study ($103/10^5$) was not found to be different than that reported in Turkey ($158/10^5$) [51]. More recently, Kaklamani et al. found a lower – albeit not statistically significant – age standardized rate of cancer in a cohort of BS patients ($160/10^5$: two cancer cases in a cohort of 128 patients during a median of 10 years) compared to that of general population living in Greece ($273/10^5$) [52].

References

1. Kural-Seyahi E, Fresko I, Seyahi N et al (2003) The long-term mortality and morbidity of Behçet's syndrome: a 2-decade outcome survey of 387 patients followed at a dedicated center. Medicine (Baltimore) 82:60–76
2. Yazici H, Tüzün Y, Pazarli H et al (1984) Influence of age of onset and patient's sex on the prevalence and severity of manifestations of Behçet's syndrome. Ann Rheum Dis 43: 783–789
3. Chajek T, Fainaru M (1975) Behçet's disease. Report of 41 cases and a review of the literature. Medicine (Baltimore) 54:179–196
4. Mishima Y, Ishikawa K, Ueno A (1973) Arterial involvement in Behçet's disease. Jpn J Surg 3:52–60
5. Shimizu T, Ehrlich GE, Inaba G, Hayashi K (1979) Behçet's disease (Behçet's syndrome). Semin Arthritis Rheum 8:223–260
6. Yazici H, Başaran G, Hamuryudan V et al (1996) The ten-year mortality in Behçet's syndrome. Br J Rheumatol 35:139–141
7. Kaklamani VG, Vaiopoulos G, Kaklamanis PG (1998) Behçet's disease. Semin Arthritis Rheum 27:197–217
8. Benamour S, Zeroual B, Bennis R, Amraoui A (1990) Bettal S [Behçet's disease. 316 cases]. Presse Med 19:1485–1489
9. Yamamoto S, Toyokawa H, Matsubara J et al (1974) A nation-wide survey of Behçet's disease in Japan, 1. Epidemiological survey. Jpn J Ophthalmol 18:282–290
10. Park KD, Bang D, Lee ES, Lee SH, Lee S (1993) Clinical study on death in Behçet's disease. J Korean Med Sci 8:241–245
11. Urowitz MB, Bookman AA, Koehler BE, Gordon DA, Smythe HA, Ogryzlo MA (1976) The bimodal mortality pattern of systemic lupus erythematosus. Am J Med 60:221–225
12. Wolfe F, Mitchell DM, Sibley JT et al (1994) The mortality of rheumatoid arthritis. Arthritis Rheum 37:481–494
13. Manzi S, Meilahn EN, Rairie JE et al (1997) Age-specific incidence rates of myocardial infarction and angina in women with systemic lupus erythematosus: comparison with the Framingham study. Am J Epidemiol 145:408–415
14. del Rincón I, Freeman GL, Haas RW, O'Leary DH, Escalante A (2005) Relative contribution of cardiovascular risk factors and rheumatoid arthritis clinical manifestations to atherosclerosis. Arthritis Rheum 52:3413–3423
15. Chung CP, Oeser A, Raggi P et al (2005) Increased coronary-artery atherosclerosis in rheumatoid arthritis: relationship to disease duration and cardiovascular risk factors. Arthritis Rheum 52:3045–3053
16. Van Doornum S, McColl G, Wicks IP (2002) Accelerated atherosclerosis: an extraarticular feature of rheumatoid arthritis? Arthritis Rheum 46:862–873
17. Hamza M (1993) Juvenile Behçet's disease. In: Wechsler B, Odeau PG (eds) Behçet's disease. Excerpta Medica, Amsterdam, pp 377–380
18. Mansur AT, Kocaayan N, Serdar ZA, Alptekin F (2005) Giant oral ulcers of Behçet's disease mimicking squamous cell carcinoma. Acta Derm Venereol 85:532–534

19. Almoznino G, Ben-Chetrit E (2007) Infliximab for the treatment of resistant oral ulcers in Behçet's disease: a case report and review of the literature. Clin Exp Rheumatol 25(4 Suppl 45):S99–S102
20. Tugal-Tutkun I, Onal S, Altan-Yaycioglu R (2004) Huseyin Altunbas H, Urgancioglu M. Uveitis in Behçet's disease: an analysis of 880 patients. Am J Ophthalmol 138:373–380
21. Sakamoto M, Akazawa K, Nishioka Y, Sanui H, Inomata H, Nose Y (1995) Prognostic factors of vision in patients with Behçet's disease. Ophthalmology 102:317–321
22. Takeuchi M, Hokama H, Tsukahara R, Kezuka T, Goto H, Sakai J, Usui M (2005) Risk and prognostic factors of poor visual outcome in Behçet's disease with ocular involvement. Graefes Arch Clin Exp Ophthalmol 243:1147–1152
23. Mamo JG, Baghdassarian A (1964) Behçet's disease. Arch Ophthalmol 71:38–48
24. Mishima S, Masuda K, Izawa Y, Mochizuke M, Namba K (1979) Behçet's disease in Japan: ophthalmological aspects. Tr Am Ophthalmol Soc 77:225–279
25. Benezra D, Cohen E (1986) Treatment and visual prognosis in Behçet's disease. Br J Ophthalmol 70:589–592
26. Yazici H, Pazarli H, Barnes CG et al (1990) A controlled trial of azathioprine in Behçet's syndrome. N Engl J Med 322:281–285
27. Hamuryudan V, Ozyazgan Y, Hizli N et al (1997) Azathioprine in Behçet's syndrome: effects on long-term prognosis. Arthritis Rheum 40:769–774
28. Cho YJ, Kim WK, Lee JH et al (2008) Visual prognosis and risk factors for Korean patients with Behçet's uveitis. Ophthalmologica 222:344–350
29. Yoshida A, Kawashima H, Motoyama Y et al (2004) Comparison of patients with Behçet's disease in the 1980s and 1990s. Ophthalmology 111:810–815
30. Ando K, Fujino Y, Hijikata K, Izawa Y, Masuda K (1999) Epidemiological features and visual prognosis of Behçet's disease. Jpn J Ophthalmol 43:312–317
31. Chung YM, Lin YC, Tsai CC, Huang DF (2008) Behçet's disease with uveitis in Taiwan. J Chin Med Assoc 71:509–516
32. Kump LI, Moeller KL, Reed GF, Kurup SK, Nussenblatt RB, Levy-Clarke GA (2008) Behçet's disease: comparing 3 decades of treatment response at the National Eye Institute. Can J Ophthalmol 43:468–472
33. Kitaichi N, Miyazaki A, Iwata D, Ohno S, Stanford MR, Chams H (2007) Ocular features of Behçet's disease: an international collaborative study. Br J Ophthalmol 91:1579–1582
34. Kobayashi T, Kishimoto M, Tokuda Y et al (2009) Disease manifestations and treatment differences among Behçet's patients in the United States and Japan. Ann Rheum Dis 68(Suppl 3): 609
35. Hamza M (1987) Large artery involvement in Behçet's disease. J Rheumatol 14:554–559
36. Koc Y, Gullu I, Akpek G et al (1992) Vascular involvement in Behçet's disease. J Rheumatol 19:402–410
37. Düzgun N, Ateş A, Aydintuğ OT, Demir O, Olmez U (2006) Characteristics of vascular involvement in Behçet's disease. Scand J Rheumatol 35:65–68
38. Melikoglu M, Ugurlu S, Tascilar K et al (2008) large vessel involvement in Behçet's syndrome: a retrospective survey. Ann Rheum Dis 67(Suppl II):67
39. Bayraktar Y, Balkanci F, Bayraktar M, Calguneri M (1997) Budd–Chiari syndrome: a common complication of Behçet's disease. Am J Gastroenterol 92:858–862
40. Hamuryudan V, Yurdakul S, Moral F et al (1994) Pulmonary arterial aneurysms in Behçet's syndrome: a report of 24 cases. Br J Rheumatol 33:48–51
41. Hamuryudan V, Er T, Seyahi E et al (2004) Pulmonary artery aneurysms in Behçet's syndrome. Am J Med 117:867–870
42. Tüzün H, Besirli K, Sayin A, Yazici H et al (1997) Management of aneurysms in Behçet's syndrome: an analysis of 24 patients. Surgery 121:150–156
43. Seyahi E, Ozdogan H, Ugurlu S et al (2004) The outcome children with Behçet's syndrome. Clin Exp Rheumatol 22(Suppl 34):116
44. Akman-Demir G, Saip S, Uluduz D et al (2008) Pediatric neuro- Behçet's syndrome. Clin Exp Rhematol 26(Suppl 50):S32

45. Akman-Demir G, Serdaroglu P, Tasci B (1999) Clinical patterns of neurological involvement in Behçet's disease: evaluation of 200 patients. The Neuro-Behçet's Study Group. Brain 122: 2171–2182

46. Siva A, Kantarci OH, Saip S, Altintas A, Hamuryudan V, Islak C, Kocer N, Yazici H (2001) Behçet's disease: diagnostic and prognostic aspects of neurological involvement. J Neurol 248:95–103

47. Kurtuncu M, Tüzün E, Mutlu M et al (2008) Clinical patterns and course of neuro-Behçet's disease: analysis of 354 patients comparing cases presented before and after 1990. Clin Exp Rheumatol 26(4 Suppl 50):S17

48. Tunc R, Saip S, Siva A, Yazici H (2004) Cerebral venous thrombosis is associated with major vessel disease in Behçet's syndrome. Ann Rheum Dis 63:1693–1694

49. Hamuryudan V, Hatemi G, Tascilar K et al (2008) The long term prognosis of Behçet's syndrome among men with skin-mucosa involvement at onset: re-evaluation of a cohort of patients enrolled in a controlled trial. Ann Rheum Dis 67(Suppl II):354

50. Alpsoy E, Donmez L, Onder M et al (2007) Clinical features and natural course of Behçet's disease in 661 cases: a multicentre study. Br J Dermatol 157:901–906

51. Fidaner C, Eser SY, Parkin DM (2001) Incidence in Izmir in 1993–1994: First results from Izmir Cancer Registry. Eur J Cancer 37:83–92

52. Kaklamani VG, Tzonou A, Kaklamanis PG (2005) Behçet's disease associated with malignancies. Report of two cases and review of the literature. Clin Exp Rheumatol 23(4 Suppl 38):S35–S41

Chapter 18
Disease Assessment in Behçet's Disease

Gonca Mumcu, Yusuf Yazıcı, and M. Anne Chamberlain

Keywords Behçet's disease • Disease activity • Indices • Measurement • Oral health • Quality of life

Behçet's disease (BD) remains without a diagnostic or laboratory marker, and until recently, there was no measure that would help us in deciding whether the disease was active or responding to treatment. Recently, however, there has been clarification of our thinking about the disease and its sequelae and development of some measurement tools to assess disease activity in Behçet's disease. Also, new drugs with much promise are available. There is now a handful of fully validated measures for disease activity and quality of life (QoL), and these are widely used. They are specific to the disease and valid.

BD starts early and may last a long time so that the whole of the working life and the family can be compromised by the disease process. Sometimes, it may burn out in the middle age, but on the other hand, there are some markers of severe disease (starting early, in young men, with eye or thrombotic episodes), which indicate that the prognosis may then be poor. Fluctuant chronic disorders, such as BD, multiple sclerosis, and rheumatoid arthritis, are notoriously difficult for patients and their doctors to manage. Also, in many countries, expensive but more effective drugs will not be an option, which will mean that some patients will not get access to them and that they and their physicians will have to choose whether the expense will be worth the sacrifices to families [1]. Good advice rests on good information, and this itself can rest on the observations from repeated measurement of disease activity using a reliable measure.

Y. Yazıcı (✉)
New York University School of Medicine, NYU Hospital for Joint Diseases, New York, NY, USA
e-mail: yusuf.yazici@nyumc.org

Y. Yazıcı and H. Yazıcı (eds.), *Behçet's Syndrome*,
DOI 10.1007/978-1-4419-5641-5_18, © Springer Science+Business Media, LLC 2010

Principles of Measurement

First, we have to be clear about what we are trying to measure and for what purpose.

For a disease activity measure, we have to use signs of activity, which can change and hopefully diminish. We also have to distinguish these signs of activity from damage, which is permanent. Next, we have to have a framework of thought, which allows us to distinguish the activity of disease at either the different organ systems, such as eye or joints, or the whole body level, from the activities and functioning of the person, which may be compromised as a result of the disease. On the other hand, the disease activity is not the only determinant of this impaired function. We all know people who manage all their tasks (such as daily living ones) either because they are alone, or they are ingenious or they have dependent children when others would have given up or sought aid. Similarly, when considering roles in the family, the workplace, or the wider society, there are those (few) who still perform very well in the presence of a major disease. The International Classification of Function provides a globally accepted and comprehensive framework for us.

ICF Model of Disease

WHO's international classification of functioning, disability, and health (2001), also known as ICF, helps us to understand the impact of a disease on a person, their functioning, and their life. The information obtained from the ICD (International classification of disease 1980) is more limited. Thus the following:

Pathology leads to disease which in turn leads to changes in the physiological and psychological functions of body systems.

Activity is the execution of a task or action by an individual and represents the individual perspective of functioning. Documentation can be made of the tasks the person cannot do and which are important to their functioning so that consideration can be given as to how to meet this need.

Participation is involvement in a life situation and represents the societal perspective of functioning. It is concerned with the role of the person. It is important to be aware of this possible effect of disease on the individual.

Contextual factors include those environmental and personal factors, which impact on the person's living. Environmental factors make up the physical, social, and attitudinal environments in which people live and conduct their lives. Personal factors relate to an individual's life and living situation that are not part of the health condition i.e., gender, age, race, fitness, lifestyle, habits, and social background. All these factors may act positively or negatively to determine the outcome for the individual.

This model highlights the need for interventions at more than the level of disease. Its routine use as a framework for clinical decision-making will bring considerable benefits to patients as well as a clarity of thought, which will aid research and help guide social policy.

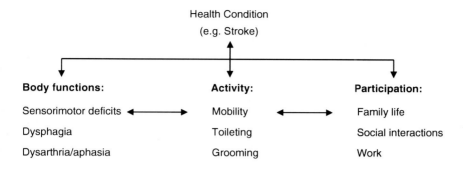

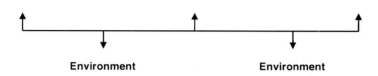

An Example

A receptionist suffered a stroke with a mild right hemiplegia and dysphasia. She found difficulty with conversation and using the telephone, activities of daily living, and with walking. All these affected her ability to look after her children and her elderly parents, her interaction with her husband, and her job.

Rehabilitation can be directed not only to her performance but also to her reintegration. Personality has a major influence on this as do the physical and psychological environments. Environmental and personal factors, if identified, can be modified, and adaptations can be utilized.

Choosing a Measure

We have to consider what the proposed measure is to be used for: Is this for routine clinical use or research? If for research, the measure must be able to be criticized and accepted by the research community worldwide and must be capable of supporting the evidence base we all need.

Is the measure to monitor changes in disease activity or in the person's function? Or are we aiming to assess a change in one organ, such as the eye, in which instance we will need markers for the eye, both for change and damage?

Are we more interested in patient's general health or QoL, which in turn will depend on what the patient wants of life? This last issue demands serious attention when we utilize the same QoL measures across the globe. Is the measure sensitive to the changes known to occur in the situation in which it is to be used? Does it perform well over the whole of the range?

Finally, is the measure acceptable or not to the patient, and should not just an extra piece of paper in an already overburdened clinic needs to be assessed?

Rasch Analysis

This is increasingly used in medicine having been brought from the education field. It enables a test developer to produce a unidimensional linear measurement scale based on additive numbers (as numbers on a ruler). It refines a wealth of data to a parsimonious linear set and, as a ruler, items are chosen as points at equal intervals. One can test the goodness of fit of the proposed items and select the best, one often acting as a proxy for several. It can indicate where a particular item fails to fit, perhaps for a particular country or patient subgroup. It can thus handle data obtained worldwide and have applicability for many countries.

It has been used to produce some of the more modern scales for BD (the Behçet's Disease Current Activity Form (BDCAF) and the BD QoL.

Individual Tests and Assessment in BD

Disease Activity: The Whole Person Assessments

In some diseases such as rheumatoid arthritis, there are a few salient measures that can easily and reliably quantify the changing disease activity. The much utilized Disease Activity Score (DAS) is one such measure [2]. In BD, on the other hand, there is no single dominant organ, and similarly, there are no laboratory tests or radiologic markers that accurately reflect disease activity and damage.

Consequently, we use tools which assess clinical disease activity, derived from the observed signs and symptoms. One issue is that it is not always clear whether these tools effectively separate the signs of disease activity from permanent damage. Another issue is that these tools are usually not on an interval, but on an ordinal scale. For example, as is sometimes done, we might decide to call any patient with eye or major vessel disease as having Stage 4 disease on a scale where numerically smaller stages stand for lesser degrees of major organ involvement. It is obvious on such a scheme that there is no arithmetically quantifiable distance between the various stages; thus, the distance between stages 2 and 3 will probably not be the same as between stages 3 and 4. For example, a clinical activity index was developed in

Istanbul to study the influence of age of onset and patient's sex on severity and prevalence of BD manifestations [3]. This was based on a numerical sum of clinical features related to the eye, skin, vascular involvement, arthritis, and neurological involvement (Fig. 18.1).

Total Clinical Activity Index

Eye

0   normal

1   cells in vitreous and/or anterior chamber only

2   vision 50%

3   vision 30%

4   able to see few feet

5   blind

Skin

1   aphthae

1   erythema nodosum

1   genital ulcers

Vascular involvement

5   thrombosis of vena cava superior (vcs) and vena cava inferior (vci) and/or arterial occlusion

4   thrombosis of vcs or vci

3   calf vein thrombosis (cvt) and/or superficial thrombophlebitis (st)

2   bilateral cvt and/or st

1   unilateral cvt and /or st

Arthritis

1   each joint

Neurological involvement

2   intracranial hypertension

4   multiple-sclerosis-/ like syndrome

5   pyramidal and/or cerebellar involvement

Fig. 18.1   Total clinical activity index

It is apparent that the problem mentioned above with ordinal scales noted above was present also in this clinical activity index. Another important issue is that there is usually no uniformity as to whether the patient complaints or clinical observations that make up these scales relate to a single point in time or a time span and whether this time span is short enough to allow of reliable recall.

The Behçet's Disease Current Activity Form

This was produced for the International Scientific Committee on BD with the participation of investigators in five countries. It is based on data from 524 persons. The questions have been honed down to the minimum number (14), which will reliably give a unidimensional scale, and each is dichotomized [4], (Fig. 18.2).

The questions are easy to ask, by a physician or an evaluator, and follow the order of the clinic interview. They ask for events only in the previous month, a time frame which most patients can manage. The data have a good fit to the Rasch model and can be used with confidence as the index will show changes in disease activity of importance. However, the number of patients with the rarer symptoms, such as gastrointestinal and neurological impairments, available for the production of the index was relatively few, so the results here have to be interpreted with caution. Data can be compared from country to country, but this requires that Rasch analysis is employed using the original data, the exceptions being data from Turkey, Korea, and the UK that can be compared directly, in that cross-cultural validity information is available between these countries. The index has been translated into several languages correctly using the guidelines for the process of cross-cultural adaptation of self-report measures [5–8].

The Behçet's Syndrome Activity Scale (BSAS)

BSAS was derived from the Multi Dimensional Health Assessment Questionnaire as a model for patient reported outcome measure collection tool. The aim was to develop an assessment tool completed by patients only, as physician-completed forms have been found to be difficult to implement in the busy clinic settings. Also, at least in the case of RA, patient derived outcomes are as good as, if not better, than physician derived measures. Ten questions are scored 0–10 each for a total score of 0–100 (Fig. 18.3). The questionnaire asks about various symptoms over the previous month before the clinic visit and is completed by the patient at the time of visit. It is strongly correlated with the BDCAF and less so with QoL assessments, as would be expected [9].

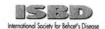

BEHÇET'S DISEASE CURRENT
ACTIVITY FORM 2006

International Society for Behcet's Disease

Date: Name: Sex: M/F
Centre: Telephone   Date of birth:
Country:
Clinician: Address:

> **All** scoring depends on the symptoms present over the **4 weeks** prior to assessment.
> **Only** clinical features that the **clinician feels are due to Behçet's Disease** should be scored.

PATIENT'S PERCEPTION OF DISEASE ACTIVITY
(Ask the patient the following question:)

**"Thinking about your Behçet's disease only, which of
these faces expresses how you have been feeling over
the last four weeks? "(Tick one face)**

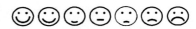

HEADACHE, MOUTH ULCERS, GENITAL ULCERS, SKIN LESIONS, JOINT INVOLVEMENT AND GASTROINTESTINAL SYMPTOMS

Ask the patient the following questions and fill in the related boxes **"Over the past 4 weeks have you had?"**

(please tick one box per line)

	not at all	Present for up to 4 weeks
Headache		
Mouth Ulceration		
Genital Ulceration		
Erythema		
Skin Pustules		
Joints - Arthralgia		
Joints - Arthritis		
Nausea/vomiting/abdominal pain		
Diarrhoea+altered/frank blood per rectum		

EYE INVOLVEMENT
(Ask questions below)

		(please circle)		
		Right Eye		Left Eye
"Over the last 4 weeks have you had?" a red eye	No	Yes	No	Yes
a painful eye	No	Yes	No	Yes
blurred or reduced vision	No	Yes	No	Yes

If any of the above is present: "Is this new"?   No   Yes
(circle the correct answer)

Fig. 18.2 Behçet's disease current activity form 2006

NERVOUS SYSTEM INVOLVEMENT (include intracranial vascular disease)

New Symptoms in nervous system and major vessel involvement are defined as those not previously documented or reported by the patient
(Ask questions below)

Over the last 4 weeks have you had any of the following?	*please circle*		tick if <u>new</u>
blackouts	No	Yes	
difficulty with speech	No	Yes	
difficulty with hearing	No	Yes	
blurring of/double vision	No	Yes	
weakness/loss of feeling of face	No	Yes	
weakness/loss of feeling of arm	No	Yes	
weakness/loss of feeling of leg	No	Yes	
memory loss	No	Yes	
loss of balance	No	Yes	

Is there any evidence of <u>new</u> active nervous system involvement?   No   Yes

MAJOR VESSEL INVOLVEMENT(exclude intracranial vascular disease)
(Ask question below)

"Over the last 4 weeks have you had any of the following?"	*please circle*		tick if <u>new</u>
had chest pain	No	Yes	
had breathlessness	No	Yes	
coughed up blood	No	Yes	
had pain/swelling/discolouration of the face	No	Yes	
had pain/swelling/discolouration of the arm	No	Yes	
had pain/swelling/discolouration of the leg	No	Yes	

Is there evidence of new active major vessel inflammation?   No   Yes

CLINICIAN'S OVERALL PERCEPTION OF DISEASE ACTIVITY

Tick one face that expresses how you feel the patient's disease has been over the last 4 weeks.   ☺ ☺ ☺ ☺ ☹ ☹ ☹

BEHÇET'S DISEASE ACTIVITY INDEX

Add up all the scores which are highlighted in <u>blue</u> (front page items, one tick = score of 1 on index, all other items score 'yes' = 1. You should now have a score out of 12 which is the patient's Behçet's Disease Activity Index Score.

SCORE

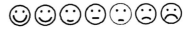

Patients index score	0	1		2	3		4	5	6	7	8	9	10	11	12
Transformed index score on interval scale	0	3		5	7		8	9	10	11	12	13	15	17	20

©University of Leeds UK   06.03.06

Explanation to doctor completing the form;

1. Use your clinical judgment recording only those features you believe are due to Behcet's disease.

2. Please explain to the patient the meaning of the words used, if necessary.

3. If there is <u>pain</u> in a joint (whether or not there is swelling etc) score 'arthralgia'.

4. If there is swelling or inflammation of a joint score 'arthritis'. Thus you can score 'arthralgia' <u>and</u> 'arthritis'.

5. The form concerns the impairments relating to Disease Activity. It is produced by Rasch analysis and is psychometrically robust. It is not measuring the <u>impact</u> of the disease activity.

Fig. 18.2 (continued)

Behçet's Syndrome Activity Scale (BSAS)

Your name   : _____   Date of Birth: _____   Today's Date: _____

Your: SEX: ☐ Female   ETHNIC ☐ Asian ☐ Hispanic ☐ Other _____
              ☐ Male   GROUP: ☐ Black ☐ White

1. How much have **ulcers in your mouth** bothered you over the last 4 weeks? Please indicate below

NO ULCERS ○○○○○○○○○○○○○○○○○○○○○ **ULCERS WERE A MAJOR PROBLEM**

0 0.5 1 1.5 2 2.5 3 3.5 4 4.5 5 5.5 6 6.5 7 7.5 8 8.5 9 9.5 10

2. How many **ulcers (new or old)** did you have in your **mouth** over the last 4 weeks?
    0   ☐
    1-3   ☐
    More than 3 ☐

3. How much has **ulcers in genital area** bothered you over the last 4 weeks? Please indicate below

NO ULCERS ○○○○○○○○○○○○○○○○○○○○○ **ULCERS WERE A MAJOR PROBLEM**

0 0.5 1 1.5 2 2.5 3 3.5 4 4.5 5 5.5 6 6.5 7 7.5 8 8.5 9 9.5 10

4. How many **ulcers (new or old)** did you have in your **genital area** over the last 4 weeks?
    0   ☐
    1-3   ☐
    More than 3 ☐

5. How much has **acne or acne like skin lesions (new or old)** bothered you over the last 4 weeks? Please indicate below

NO SKIN LESIONS ○○○○○○○○○○○○○○○○○○○○○ **SKIN LESIONS WERE A MAJOR PROBLEM**

0 0.5 1 1.5 2 2.5 3 3.5 4 4.5 5 5.5 6 6.5 7 7.5 8 8.5 9 9.5 10

6. How many **acne or acne like skin lesions (new or old)** did you have over the last 4 weeks?
    0   ☐
    1-5   ☐
    More than 5 ☐

7. Have you had **abdominal pain and diarrhea** lasting most of the day for most days of the week over the last 4 weeks?
    ☐ No   ☐ Yes

8. Did you have **painful or red eyes and/or blurred or reduced vision** over the last 4 weeks?
    ☐ No   ☐ Yes

9. Did you have any **swelling/discoloration of your lower extremities, or a blood clot** over the last 4 weeks?
    ☐ No   ☐ Yes

10. In terms of your **Behcet's activity, (oral ulcers, genital ulcers, skin problems, joint pains, eye, neurologic problems),** how active would you say your condition has been over the last 4 weeks?

NOT ACTIVE AT ALL ○○○○○○○○○○○○○○○○○○○○○ **EXTREMELY ACTIVE**

0 0.5 1 1.5 2 2.5 3 3.5 4 4.5 5 5.5 6 6.5 7 75. 8 8.5 9 9.5 10

Scoring:

Questions 1, 3, 5, and 10 are scored 0-10

Questions 2, 4, 6, are scored 0, 5 or 10 depending on which of the 3 are checked

Questions 7, 8, 9 are scored 0 or 10

For a total score of 100

Fig. 18.3 Behçet's Syndrome Activity Scale (BSAS)

The Iranian BD Dynamic Measure

This is used by Iranian physicians and consists of many items noticed by the patient between one visit to the clinic and the next. Areas that are covered include oral, genital ulcers, skin lesions, eye involvement, joint, central nervous system, vascular, gastrointestinal involvement, epididymitis, and pathergy positivity. Most areas are scored differently depending on the severity and extent of involvement and the items are added up to produce the final score [10].

In addition to the measures mentioned above, Simsek et al. looked at the accuracy of recall of patients with BD using a daily diary over 2 months and comparing this with the original BDCAF and the slightly modified IBDDAM, done twice a month. The correlation over this limited time, and accepting that there were few patients with GI complaints and headache, was good [11].

Biological Markers in Disease Activity

Many but not all patients with what is obviously active disease have a raised ESR or a usually modestly raised CRP; hence these have limited use in assessing disease activity [12].

The same also holds true for various cytokine levels [13–15].

There are suggestions that the activity of the vascular endothelium may relate to the overall disease activity or its commencement [16]. Cekmen et al. looked at the Vascular Endothelial Growth Factor (VEGF), a cytokine, in a case-controlled study in BD. Patients were described as having active or inactive disease, not based on a standard clinical assessment, but on a battery of acute phase reactants and a correlation was shown. It is unclear how this related to the clinical findings.

A study of the potential importance of regulatory T cells (TREG) in disease activity by Nanke et al. suggests that these may be predictive of ocular attacks in BD. However, the numbers studied were small, and the evidence of a correlation with disease activity was difficult to determine [17]. On the other hand, Pay et al. used the BDCAF to determine the correlation between Serum MMP-2 and MMP-9 in BD patients and found that the levels of these were significantly higher in those patients with active disease [18].

Measurement of Visual Activity

The assessment of visual activity is very important and relies mostly on the accurate examination of the eye. While visual acuity is the functional end point for the patient, it does not necessarily correlate with the amount of eventual damage. In BD, the clinical signs which are most useful in terms of indicating the need for such treatment are in the posterior chamber (see Chap. 5). While visual acuity is a good and easily obtained measure of the impairment of function in the patient, measures of posterior chamber disease activity have been devised.

Recently a physicians group has been established, called the Uveitis Working Group. This has been looking at the scoring for dual fluorescein and ICG inflammatory angiography signs. They concluded that the score may help in the estimation of the magnitude of retinal versus choroidal inflammation and in the monitoring of disease progression but more work has to be done to further develop the measure [19]. It is best to treat the patient with the co-operation and, ideally in the presence, of the rheumatologist and/or internist, along with the ophthalmologist in the clinic so that the patient's eye condition can be treated in conjunction with the general condition and one may inform the other (as has been done in Leeds since 1983 and Istanbul since 1977). This approach has probably resulted in better, earlier treatment with more preservation of vision. The presence of visual symptoms may precede or parallel the onset of serious symptom in other systems and the use of the BDCAF may increase the awareness of these relationships both in the first few years of the disease and where there are threatened recurrences.

Mouth Ulcers

Oral ulcer activity as a part of the disease spectrum can be evaluated in the context of the general activity indices including Behçet's Disease Current Activity Form and Total Activity Index [3, 4]. In BDCAF, the duration of the oral ulcer is the main criterion for oral ulcer activity. Oral ulcer activity is scored 1–4 in the global activity score. This form was revised (2006) and scoring was dichotomized (0 vs. 1 in a 28-day period) [4]. The Total Activity Index evaluates the numerical sum of each patient's clinical features. The oral ulcer is coded as present or absent in this activity form. In the BSAS, numbers of oral ulcers and the severity of these as reported by the patient are graded [9].

A Composite Index for Oral Ulcer Activity in Behçet's Disease

The oral ulcer is an unpredictable but a cardinal clinical condition in patients with BD. The number of oral ulcers, the healing period of oral ulcers, ulcer-related pain, and complete remission of oral ulcers are important outcomes in taking care of BD patients in clinical practice [20].

In order to assess the impact of oral ulcers on functional status, a composite index has been developed. Oral ulcer-related pain and functional disability are its main components. The patients without oral ulcers have "0" points, whereas the score of active patients can be from 1 to 10. The index is simple to use, reliable, valid, acceptable, and amenable to statistical analysis [21].

Assessment of Oral Health Related QoL in Clinical Practice

Traditionally, dentists dealing with diagnosis, prevention, and treatment of oral health problems use clinical indices. Most objective measurements of disease activity provide little information about the effects of oral health problems and therapies on a patient's life. Recently, the term "oral health-related quality of life" has attracted considerable attention in dentistry. Oral Health Quality of Life (OHQoL) is a patient-centered outcome scale that includes subjectively perceived physical, psychological, and social functions as making up the well-being of the patient. Oral Health Impact Profile (OHIP-14) and Oral Health Related Quality of Life measurement (OHQoL-UK) are used in oral medicine and in BD [22, 23]. OHIP-14 is a 14 item measurement tool which evaluates negative impact of oral health on QoL. The seven dimensions addressed are functional limitation, pain, psychological discomfort, physical disability, psychological disability, social disability, and handicap. Responses to these items are coded with a Likert scale (never, hardly ever, occasionally, fairly often, very often) during a specific period selected by the dentist according to the clinical condition. OHIP-14 score indicates the severity of the problems described by items. Scores can be from zero (no impact) to 56 (problems occur very often). A high score indicates a poor oral QoL. The OHQoL-UK attempts to assess the positive and negative aspects in each of 16 areas. Physical, social, and psychological dimensions are evaluated by this questionnaire. Response categories range from "very bad effect," "bad effect," "no effect," "good effect" to "very good effect." Scores range from 16 (worst) to 80 (best score). A lower overall score reflects poorer OHRQoL in OHQoL-UK. Questionnaires are completed by patients [24].

Oral Ulcer Treatment Modalities and OHQoL

While the success of treatment in oral ulcers is measured by biomedical/clinical end points such as recurrence-free survival and relapses, patients' self-assessed QoL status is influenced by different treatments in clinical practice, especially in chronic disease such as BD. This measure is also responsive to change [25] where the presence of oral ulcers and poor oral health are associated to impaired OHRQoL status in BD [25]. OHQoL is a "dynamic construct" that can change with the patient's clinical condition and treatment modalities. OHQoL is usually measured by the OHIP-14 in BD patients [22, 23].

The presence of oral ulcers is not a life-threatening condition compared to major organ involvement, such as vascular disease in BD. Therefore, topical treatment protocols and effective oral hygiene are commonly used as the first choice in oral ulcers of BD [26]. Elimination of oral infections may also prevent flare-ups of oral ulcers in the 6-month time period [27]. Although colchicine is used commonly in clinical practice, it has only a limited role in oral ulcer treatment based on randomized clinical trials [26]. Immunosuppressive medications are used mainly for major organ involvement; however, they also eliminate oral ulcers effectively [26].

As related with these clinical effects of various treatment modalities, the OHIP-14 score and psychological subscale score of OHIP-14 are better in patients treated with immunosuppressive medications compared to colchicine [23]. It is also to be remembered that different factors could lead to a poor OHRQoL in different patient groups, although similar impairment of OHQoL status may be observed as we have recently observed in formally comparing oral ulceration and its impact between patients from the UK and Turkey [28].

A crucial component of OHRQoL is gender. Poor OHRQoL status is observed mainly among female patients [29]. Moreover, subscale scores of OHIP-14 structured by factor analysis in patients with active oral ulcers are significantly worse in females compared to males [23].

Overall, the results suggest that oral health related QoL is an important domain of the health related QoL status in patients with BD.

Nervous System

There are no diseases activity measurements specifically developed for BD, as they relate to the nervous system. There is also little consensus as to which other tests are best to use in BD. We need to ask which area of the brain is known to be affected and hence which tests are likely to be needed or conversely which types of difficulties the patient has been experiencing and thus which tests are most appropriate.

A quick and reliable screening test is of value. Traditionally, this has usually been the Minimental State Examination produced to screen for dementia but used much more widely; however, this does not show the deficits resultant on frontal lobe lesions. The Addenbrooke's Cognitive examination revised (ACE-R) promises to be better [30]. This is comprehensively validated and reliability is good. It includes tests of executive function and is reasonably quick to perform. Also Siva et al. used [31] the Extended Disability Status Scale (EDSS) to assess disability due to central nervous system disease. The EDSS is again an ordinal scale primarily designed for multiple sclerosis. The authors adapted this to Behçet's by excluding the eye disease assessment as they reasoned, perhaps with justification, that the eye disease in Behçet's was mainly due to uveitis rather than central nervous system pathology.

Joint Involvement

The joints in BD are rarely damaged so that the measures of erosion are not needed.

The Multidimensional Health Assessment Questionnaire – MDHAQ, which is short and simple to use, has recently been used in both BD and RA. It measures disability as well as pain and fatigue. BD patients with arthritis compared to early RA patients had similar levels of functional disability and pain. This suggests that there may be unrecognized functional problems in BD particularly when the joints are affected [32].

Disability and Participation Measures

These areas of the ICF are not specifically covered for BD. Where there is disability and this needs to be measured, the HAQ for RA and the generic Barthel index may be of use. There is also the Rivermead Activities Index of Daily Living and the Nottingham Extended Activities of Daily Living Index but both of these are usually used in neurological disorders. The AMPS is a valid occupational therapy battery, but this is time-consuming. The measure that promises to be of considerable importance is the WHODAS. This also covers participation.

QoL Assessments

Many of our patients find that their lives are changed, sometimes catastrophically, as a result of a diagnosis of BD. Since this, lifestyle, is the level on which they will gauge our interventions, it is important that treatments are assessed with the disease assessment measure which most closely reflects the main brunt of their disease. The overall effect on their life and that of the family also needs to be known and quantified. This is true for each individual, but it is also necessary information for those who wish to provide the best, often expensive, treatment for their patients, for research, for health economics, and for funding. Funding bodies will want to know also whether the cost of medication is balanced by the benefits, whether these are measured using a QoL measure, in cost benefit terms, or in the days lost from work.

There has been considerable research and a great number of new QoL measures have been introduced in the last few decades. It is now common to find these included as outcome measures in clinical trials. QoL Measures derive from politics but also reflect a critique of classical clinical end points. There is an acknowledged lack of theory behind much of what is produced and considerable difficulty in defining QoL.

Measures may be generic or specific to a disease. The former are useful when it is important to compare the effect of one disease against another in terms of benefit and in relation to costs of treatment. The latter are more closely related to the disease in question, particularly when derived from patient experience and will be more useful within a specialty or disease focused research community.

An interesting study was done by Boder et al. [33] in which disease activity, as measured by the BDCAF (Turkish version), was found to be correlated with the QoL and psychological well-being as measured by the Nottingham Health Profile (NHP) and life satisfaction index (LS). The greatest correlation was between fatigue, joint involvement and oral ulcers, and the physical domains of the NHP. Joint involvement and genital ulcers were the most related activity measures to the psychosocial domains of the NHP. The LS was most correlated with the patient and physician impressions of the disease.

BD-Specific QoL Measure

This was produced by the Psychometric Group of the Academic Department of Rehabilitation Medicine Department of Leeds University in response to a request for it from the International Study Group for BD [34]. It was produced using a standard qualitative needs-based approach, the measure deriving from semistructured interviews of patients with BD with all severities covered and with the brunt of the disease falling on different systems. Many items were identified, and these were used in a postal questionnaire to test its scaling properties, reliability, internal consistency, and validity. The findings were subjected to Rasch analysis. Then, a second, shorter questionnaire was derived from this and similarly tested so that the 71 items were reduced to 30. These 30 items emerged free of gender and age bias and fit to the Rasch model was excellent. In the second postal survey, the test–retest reliability was 0.84.

The test answers are dichotomized, and the questionnaire is easy to complete, enjoyed by patients, and done in 3 min. It has high internal consistency and test–retest reliability.

Conclusions

A vast number of general disease assessment measures are available and only a few have been studied in BD and their utility is not clear. Tools that have been developed specifically for BD are few, and most lack coverage for some manifestations of the disease, which may be seen with different frequencies in different parts of the world, such as gastrointestinal and neurological involvement. Finally, eye involvement, the main cause of morbidity, still lacks good and easy to use assessment tools.

References

1. Sut N, Seyahi E, Yurdakul S, Senocak M, Yazici H (2007) A cost analysis of Behçet's syndrome in Turkey. Rheumatology (Oxford) 46:678–682
2. Prevoo ML, Van't Hof MA, Kuper HH, van Leeuwen MA, van de Putte LB, van Riel PL (1995) Modified disease activity scores that include twenty-eight-joint counts. Development and validation in a prospective longitudinal study of patients with rheumatoid arthritis. Arthritis Rheum 38:44–48
3. Yazici H, Tuzun Y, Pazarli H, Yurdakul S, Ozyazgan Y, Ozdogan H, Serdaroglu S, Ersanli M, Ulkü BY, Müftüoğlu AU (1984) Influence of age of onset and patient's sex on the prevalence and severity of manifestations of Behçet's syndrome. Ann Rheum Dis 43:783–789

4. Lawton G, Bhakta BB, Chamberlain MA, Tennant A (2004) The Behçet's disease activity index. Rheumatology (Oxford) 43:73–78
5. Beaton DE (2000) Understanding the relevance of measured change through studies of responsiveness. Spine 25:3192–3199
6. Lee ES, Kim HS, Bang D, Yu HG, Chung H, Shin DH, Song YW, Park YB, Lee SK, Shin SK, Kim WH, Choi J, Park BJ, Lee S (2003) Development of clinical activity form for Korean patients with Behçet's disease. Adv Exp Med Biol 528:153–156
7. Neves FS, Moraes JC, Kowalski SC, Goldenstein-Schainberg C, Lage LV, Gonçalves CR (2007) Cross-cultural adaptation of the Behçet's Disease Current Activity Form (BDCAF) to Brazilian Portuguese language. Clin Rheumatol 26:1263–1267
8. Hamuryudan V, Fresko I, Direskeneli H, Tenant MJ, Yurdakul S, Akoglu T, Yazici H (1999) Evaluation of the Turkish translation of a disease activity form for Behçet's syndrome. Rheumatology (Oxford) 38:734–736
9. Forbess C, Swearingen C, Yazici Y (2008) Behçet's Syndrome Activity Score (BSAS): a new disease activity assessment tool, composed of patient-derived measures only, is strongly correlated with The Behçet's Disease Current Activity Form (BDCAF). Ann Rheum Dis 67(SII):360
10. Shahram F, Khabbazi A, Nadji A, Ziaie N, Banihashemi AT, Davatchi F (2009) Comparison of existing disease activity indices in the follow-up of patients with Behçet's disease. Mod Rheumatol 19(5):536–541
11. Simsek I, Meric C, Erdem H, Pay S, Kilic S, Dinc A (2008) Accuracy of recall of the items included in disease activity forms of Behçet's disease: comparison of retrospective questionnaires with a daily telephone interview. Clin Rheumatol 27:1255–1260
12. Bang D, Kim HS, Lee ES, Lee S (2000) The significance of laboratory test in evaluating the clinical activity of Behçet's disease. In: Proceedings of the 9th international conference in Behçet's disease held in Seoul, Korea, 27–29 May
13. Deuter CME, Kotter I, Gunaydin I, Zierhut M, Stubiger N (2004) Ocular involvement in Behçet's disease: first 5-year-results for visual development after treatment with interferon alfa-2a. Ophthalmologe 101:129–134
14. Amberger M, Groll S, Günaydin I, Deuter C, Vonthein R, Kötter I (2007) Intracellular cytokine patterns in Behçet's disease in comparison to ankylosing spondylitis – influence of treatment with interferon-alpha2a. Clin Exp Rheumatol 25(Suppl 45):S52–S57
15. Kötter I, Koch S, Vonthein R, Rückwaldt U, Amberger M, Günaydin I, Zierhut M, Stübiger N (2005) Cytokines, cytokine antagonists and soluble adhesion molecules in patients with ocular Behçet's disease treated with human recombinant interferon-alpha2a. Results of an open study and review of the literature. Clin Exp Rheumatol 23(Suppl 38):S20–S26
16. Cekmen M, Evereklioglu C, Er H, Inaloz HS, Doganay S, Yurkoz Y, Ozerol IH (2003) Vascular endothelial growth factor levels are increased and associated with disease activity in patients with Behçet's syndrome. Int J Dermatol 42(11):870–875
17. Nanke Y, Kotake S, Goto M, Ujihara H, Matsubara M, Kamatani N (2008) Decreased percentages of regulatory T cells in peripheral blood of patients with Behçet's disease before ocular attack: a possible predictive marker of ocular attack. Mod Rheumatol 18(4):354–358
18. Pay S, Abbasov T, Erdem H, Musabak U, Simsek I, Pekel A, Akdogan A, Sengul A, Dinc A (2007) Serum MMP-2 and MMP-9 in patients with Behçet's disease: do their higher levels correlate to vasculo-Behçet's disease associated with aneurysm formation? Clin Exp Rheumatol 25(Suppl 45):S-70–S-75
19. Tugal-Tutkun I, Herbort CP, Khairallah M (2008) The Angiography Scoring for Uveitis Working Group (ASUWOG). Scoring of dual fluorescein and ICG inflammatory angiographic signs for the grading of posterior segment inflammation (dual fluorescein and ICG angiographic scoring system for uveitis). Int Ophthalmol Sep 16. [Epub ahead of print]
20. Mumcu G, Ergun T, Inanc N, Fresko I, Atalay T, Hayran O, Direskeneli H (2004) Oral health is impaired in Behçet's disease and is associated with disease severity. Rheumatology (Oxford) 43:1028–1033

21. Mumcu G, Sur H, Inanç N, Karacayli U, Cimilli H, Sisman N, Ergun T, Direskeneli H (2009) A composite index for determining the impact of oral ulcer activity in Behçet's disease and recurrent aphthous stomatitis. J Oral Pathol Med 38:785–791

22. Mumcu G, Inanc N, Ergun T, Ikiz K, Gunes M, Islek U, Yavuz S, Sur H, Atalay T, Direskeneli H (2006) Oral health related quality of life is affected by disease activity in Behçet's disease. Oral Dis 12:145–151

23. Mumcu G, Hayran O, Ozalp Do, Inanc N, Yavuz S, Ergun T, Direskeneli H (2007) The assessment of oral health related quality of life by factor analysis in patients with Behçet's disease and recurrent apthous stomatitis. J Oral Pathol Med 36:147–152

24. McGrath C, Hegarty AM, Hodgson TA, Porter SR (2003) Patient-centered outcome measures for oral mucosal disease are sensitive to treatment. Int J Oral Maxillofac Surg 32:334–336

25. Mumcu G (2008) Behçet's disease: a dentist's overview. Clin Exp Rheumatol 26(Suppl 50): S121–S124

26. Hatemi G, Silman A, Dang B, Bodaghi B, Chamberlain AM, Gul A, Houman MH, Kötter I, Olivieri I, Salvarani C, Sfikakis PP, Siva A, Stanford MR, Stübiger N, Yurdakul S, Yazici H (2008) EULAR recommendation for the management of Behçet's disease. Ann Rheum Dis 67:1656–1662

27. Karacayli U, Mumcu G, Simsek I, Pay S, Kose O, Erdem H, Direskeneli H, Gunaydin Y, Dinc A (2009) The close association between dental and periodontal treatments and oral ulcer course in Behçet's disease: a prospective clinical study. J Oral Pathol Med 38:410–415

28. Mumcu G, Niazi S, Stewart J, Hagi-Pavli E, Gokani B, Seoudi N, Ergun T, Yavuz S, Stanford MR, Fortune F, Direskeneli H (2009) Oral health and related quality of life status in patients from UK and Turkey: a comparative study in Behçet's disease. J Oral Pathol Med 38:406–409

29. Mumcu G, Inanc N, Ergun T, Islek U, Yavuz S, Fresko I, Sur H, Atalay T, Direskeneli H (2004) Gender effects quality of life in Behçet's disease. Clin Exp Rheumatol 22(Suppl 34):S-86

30. Mioshi E, Dawson K, Mitchell J, Arnold R, Hodges JR (2006) The Addenbrooke's Cognitive Examination Revised (ACE-R): a brief cognitive test battery for dementia screening. Int J Geriatr Psychiatry 21:1078–1085

31. Siva A, Kantarci OH, Saip S, Altintas A, Hamuryudan V, Islak C, Kocer N, Yazici H (2001) Behçet's disease: diagnostic and prognostic aspects of neurologic involvement. J Neurol 248:95–103

32. Moses Alder N, Fisher M, Yazici Y (2008) Behçet's syndrome patients have high levels of functional disability, fatigue and pain as measured by a Multi-dimensional Health Assessment Questionnaire (MDHAQ). Clin Exp Rheumatol 26(Suppl 50):S110–S113

33. Bodur H, Borman P, Ozdemir Y, Atan C, Kural G (2006) Quality of life and life satisfaction in patients with Behçet's disease: relationship with disease activity. Clin Rheumatol 25:329–333

34. Gilworth G, Chamberlain MA, Bhakta B, Haskard D, Silman A, Tennant A (2004) Development of the Behçet's disease quality of life, a quality of life measure specific to Behçet's disease. J Rheumatol 31:931–937

Chapter 19
Medical Management of Behçet's Syndrome

Vedat Hamuryudan and Ina Kötter

Keywords Azathioprine • Biologic agents • Colchicine • EULAR guidelines
• Immunosuppressives • Interferon alpha • Management • Stem cell transplantation
• TNF antagonists • Treatment • Uveitis • Vasculitis

The current treatment of Behçet's syndrome (BS) is largely directed at the suppression of symptoms to prevent organ damage. BS, for many patients, is a disease that impairs the quality of life by frequently relapsing mucocutaneous manifestations. However, there are also many who carry an increased risk of significant morbidity or even mortality as a consequence of vital organ involvement. Many factors need to be considered when planning treatment for a patient with BS (Table 19.1). The patient's sex, age of disease onset, and the disease duration greatly influence the disease course [1]. Additionally, the site and severity of symptoms as well as the frequency of recurrences affect the treatment decisions. For example, a young male patient at the initial years of his disease is usually treated more aggressively because of his increased risk of developing serious complications. However, in most instances, only reassurance would be sufficient for an older female patient. Indeed, a two-decade outcome survey indicated that many patients could be managed without using systemic medications [2].

Several different groups of drugs are used in the treatment of BS. The efficacy of some has been shown in controlled trials with the primary efficacy measures being mainly eye involvement or mucocutaneous manifestations. No controlled evidence is available for the treatment of vascular, neurological, and gastrointestinal manifestations of BS (Table 19.2). There are data to indicate a more favorable long-term outcome when treatment with azathioprine is initiated in male patients early in their disease course [3]. The use of azathioprine may be consid-

V. Hamuryudan (✉)
Division of Rheumatology, Department of Medicine, Cerrahpasa Medical Faculty,
University of Istanbul, Istanbul, Turkey
e-mail: vhamuryudan@yahoo.com

Y. Yazıcı and H. Yazıcı (eds.), *Behçet's Syndrome*,
DOI 10.1007/978-1-4419-5641-5_19, © Springer Science+Business Media, LLC 2010

Table 19.1 Factors that need to be considered when planning treatment for BS

Factor	Comment
Patient's sex	Male sex is associated with more severe disease course
Patient's age at the onset of BS	Developing the disease at younger age (24 years or below) is associated with more severe disease course
Disease duration	The burden of BS is highest during the early years and tends to abate with the passage of time
Severity of symptoms	Intensive treatment may not be necessary for mild symptoms
Frequency of recurrences	Frequent attacks can result in earlier irreversible organ damage

ered before the emergence of organ involvement in selected patients with poor prognostic factors, but more formal information is needed to recommend its routine prophylactic use. An approach to the treatment of various manifestations of BS is given in Table 19.3.

Recently, a group of experts developed nine recommendations for the management of BS by combining the current evidence from controlled trials [4]. The development of these recommendations was endorsed by the European League against Rheumatism (EULAR), which aims to help all clinicians involved in the treatment of BS. In this chapter, medical treatment of BS is summarized by giving the current available data on individual drugs. An overview of the EULAR recommendations is also presented in relevant drug sections.

Colchicine

Colchicine is an alkaloid that acts by inhibiting leukocyte function [5]. A beneficial effect of colchicine in BS was first reported in 1975 in an open study of 12 patients [6]. Shortly thereafter, a controlled trial attempting to compare colchicine with nonsteroid anti-inflammatory drugs (indomethacine or flufenamic acid) was stopped because of severe ocular attacks in the control group [7].

The first randomized double-blind placebo-controlled study of colchicine enrolled 35 BS patients with mainly mucocutaneous manifestations to receive 1.5 mg colchicine per day or placebo for 24 weeks [8]. Colchicine was found to be superior to placebo in treating erythema nodosum and, to some degree, joint manifestations only. A more recent double-blind, randomized-controlled study of 2 years duration compared colchicine (1–2 mg/day adjusted according to body weight) with placebo in a larger group of BS patients with active mucocutaneous manifestations [9]. Colchicine was not superior to placebo for treating oral ulcers and follicular lesions in either sex. However, it was effective for genital ulcers, erythema nodosum, and arthritis in women and only for arthritis among men. The more favorable effect of colchicine among women was interpreted as a reflection of the less severe disease course of BS in this sex.

Table 19.2 List of drugs tested in randomized controlled trials for the treatment of BS

Drug	Comparator	Patient number	Duration	Primary outcome	Result
Acyclovir 800 mg/day [57]	Placebo	44	3 months	Oral and genital ulcers	Negative result
Azapropazone 900 mg/day [66]	Placebo	63	3 weeks	Acute arthritis	Negative result
Azathioprine 2.5 mg/kg/day [11]	Placebo	73	104 months	Ocular	Azathioprine is effective in maintaining visual acuity and preventing the development of new eye disease
Benzathine penicillin 1.2 MU every 3 weeks plus colchicine 1.5 mg/day [46]	Colchicine 1.5 mg/day	107	24 months	Arthritis	Combination therapy is effective in reducing the frequency of arthritis attacks
Benzathine penicillin 1.2 MU every 3 weeks plus colchicine 1.5 mg/day [47]	Colchicine 1.5 mg/day	154	24 months	Mucocutaneous	Combination therapy is more effective in improving mucocutaneous manifestations
Colchicine 1.5 mg/day [8]	Placebo	35	6 months	Mucocutaneous	Colchicine is effective for erythema nodosum
Colchicine 1–2 mg/day [9]	Placebo	116	48 months	Mucocutaneous	Colchicine is effective for genital ulcers, erythema nodosum in women, for arthritis in men and women
Cyclosporin A 5–10 mg/kg/day [16]	Conventional treatment with Corticosteroids or chlorambucil	40	104 months	Ocular	Cyclosporin improves eye disease but this effect diminishes during follow-up
Cyclosporin A 10 mg/kg/day [19]	Colchicine 1 mg/day	96	4 months	Ocular	Cyclosporin A is superior to colchicine for eye disease and mucocutaneous lesions. This effect is sustained during follow-up
Cyclosporin A 5 mg/kg/day [18]	Cyclophosphamide 1 gm/month	23	12 months	Ocular	Cyclosporin is effective for uveitis but this effect diminishes during follow-up
Cyclosporine A (topical) [59]	Placebo	24	2 months	Oral ulcers	Negative result
Daclizumab 1 mg/kg bw every 2 weeks for 6 weeks, then every 4 weeks, conventional immunosuppressives continued [103]	Placebo	17	15 months (median)	Ocular	Not better than placebo, even more flares in the daclizumab group

(continued)

Table 19.2 (continued)

Drug	Comparator	Patient number	Duration	Primary outcome	Result
Dapsone 100 mg/day [52]	Placebo	20	3 months	Oral and genital ulcers	Dapsone effectively reduces oral and genital ulcer parameters
Etanercept 25 mg 2×/week [87]	Placebo	40	4 weeks	Mucocutaneous and arthritis	Significant decrease of mucocutaneous symptoms and arthritis in etanercept group. No effect of etanercept on pathergy reaction
Interferon (topical) alpha [61]	Placebo	63	6 months	Oral ulcers	Negative result
Interferon alpha2b 3 million units every other day plus Benzathine penicillin 1.2 MU every 3 weeks plus colchicine 1.5 mg/day [69] retracted	Benzathine penicillin 1.2 MU every 3 weeks plus colchicine 1.5 mg/day	135	6 months/12 months	All except active ocular	Combination with IFN alpha is significantly superior for number of ocular attacks, visual acuity, mucocutaneous and arthritis
Interferon alpha 2a 6 million units 3×/week [71]	Placebo	50	3 months	Mucocutaneous and arthritis	Significant decrease of oral ulcers, genital ulcers in IFN group, decrease of erythema nodosum, arthritis attacks and thrombophlebitis. Significantly more responders in IFN group
Methylpredisolone acetate 40 mg/every 3 weeks [37]	Placebo	86	7 months	Mucocutaneous	Methylprednisolone injections are effective for erythema nodosum
Rebamipide300 mg/day [53]	Placebo	35	6 months	Oral ulcers	Rebamipide is effective in decreasing the numbers and pain of oral ulcers
Sucralfate (topical) [54]	Placebo	40	3 months	Oral and genital ulcers	Sucralfate is effective for pain, healing time of oral and genital ulcers
Thalidomide 100 or 300 mg/day [34]	Placebo	96	6 months	Mucocutaneous	Thalidomide is effective in suppressing mucocutaneous manifestations except nodular lesions

Table 19.3 Treatment of various manifestations of BS

Mucocutaneous manifestations	Topical creams may provide symptomatic relief
	Colchicine may be used for mild – moderately severe manifestations especially for erythema nodosum and genital ulcers
	Depot methylprednisolone injections are useful for erythema nodosum
	Azathioprine is effective in controlling frequent recurrences of oral and genital ulcers
	Thalidomide is effective in treating large and painful oral and genital ulcers; short term use is recommended because of its side effects
	TNF α inhibitors or IFNα can be useful in selected patients with refractory manifestations
Arthritis	Nonsteroids may provide symptomatic relief
	Colchicine may be effective in most cases
	Azathioprine may suppress long lasting and frequently recurring arthritis
	TNFα inhibitors or IFNα may be used in more refractory cases
Uveitis	Azathioprine is the first line immunosuppressive. It can be combined with topical and systemic corticosteroids especially during attacks
	In case of retinal involvement and/or drop of visual acuity azathioprine should be combined with cyclosporine A or infliximab in addition to corticosteroids
	IFNα with or without corticosteroids is also a good alternative for severe eye disease
Deep vein thrombosis	The efficacy of anticoagulants for acute or chronic thrombophlebitis is not known. They can be hazardous in the presence of arterial aneurysms
	Azathioprine, corticosteroids, cyclosporin A, IFNα or cyclophosphamide can be used. The choice of these agents depends on the extent and severity of the involvement
Arterial involvement	Pulmonary aneurysms should be treated intensively with cyclophosphamide and high dose corticosteroids
	Endovascular embolization may be life saving in abundant hemoptysis. In addition to surgery or endovascular repair, peripheral aneurysms should be managed with cyclophosphamide and corticosteroids
Gastrointestinal involvement	Sulfasalazine, azathioprine, corticosteroids, thalidomide, infliximab should be tried
	In emergent cases, surgery requiring large resections of bowel segments may not be avoidable
Central nervous system involvement	Dural sinus thrombosis and acute attacks of parenchymal involvement may respond to high dose corticosteroids
	Azathioprine, cyclophosphamide, TNFα inhibitors may be used for parenchymal treatment

Colchicine is still widely used in the treatment of almost all manifestations of BS in some countries like Japan, but there is no formal evidence for its efficacy in the systemic complications of BS. In the EULAR recommendations, the use of colchicine is advised for arthritis and mucocutaneous manifestations of BS especially when the dominant lesion is erythema nodosum.

Finally, there is still the concern that a small proportion of patients with BS might indeed respond to colchicine and that the number of patients studied in either of the double-blind studies was not large enough to show this. In this context, a controlled withdrawal study with colchicine might still be needed.

Azathioprine

Azathioprine is a prodrug of 6-mercaptopurine and is in use for the treatment of BS for more than four decades [10]. The efficacy of azathioprine in BS was shown with a randomized, double blind, placebo controlled study in 1990 [11]. This 2 year study enrolled only male patients divided in two groups. The first group consisted of 25 patients under the age of 40 years and less than 2 years disease duration with no history of uveitis. The second group consisted of 48 patients of any age and disease duration and with uveitis. The patients randomly received either azathioprine 2.5 mg/kg/day or placebo tablets. Corticosteroid treatment was available to all patients. At the end, azathioprine was found to be effective in decreasing the attacks of hypopyon uveitis (NNT=4; 95%CI=2.1–16.3) and in preserving visual acuity [12]. Azathioprine also prevented the development of new eye disease among patients without eye involvement (NNT=2; 95%CI=1.2–4.4). There was also an improvement in the development of genital ulcers (NNT=4; 95%CI=7.5–43), arthritis (NNT=6; 95%CI=3.3–35.7), and thrombophlebitis (NNT=8; 95%CI=2.1–30.3). The trial patients were re-evaluated after an average of 8 years after completing the trial [3]. There was less blindness (NNT=4; 95%CI=1.9–43.9) and less development of new eye disease (NNT=3; 95%CI=1.3–3.3) among patients allocated to azathioprine during the trial. Also, vascular and neurologic involvements occurred less among patients allocated to azathioprine. Interestingly, at the end of the survey, the length of immunosuppressive use was similar between placebo and azathioprine groups. Furthermore, the most favorable results were seen among patients who received azathioprine earlier during their disease course. This study opened the question of prophylactic azathioprine treatment among young men which still awaits its answer.

Azathioprine is the most frequently prescribed immunosuppressive in BS today. Its usual dose is 2.5 mg/kg/day (not exceeding 200 mg/day) and an average of 3 months is required for its effect to start. According to the EULAR recommendations [4], azathioprine should be used in any BS patient having inflammatory eye disease with posterior segment involvement. In the case of severe eye disease, which is defined as the presence of retinal disease and/or more than two lines drop in the visual acuity on a ten scale chart, it is recommended to combine azathioprine with cyclosporin A or infliximab in addition to corticosteroids. The combination of azathioprine with interferon α should be avoided because of the increased risk of myelosuppression [13]. Azathioprine is also recommended for the management of acute deep vein thrombosis, gastrointestinal, central nervous system, and resistant mucocutaneous involvement. A beneficial effect of azathoprine on thrombophlebitis was also present in the double-blind trial [11]. As in other vasculitides, azathioprine is used in the maintenance treatment of severe complications of BS like pulmonary artery aneurysms after initial therapy aiming for remission with cyclophosphamide [14].

Cyclosporin A

Several uncontrolled and three controlled trials have shown the efficacy of cyclosporin A in the treatment of BS [15]. In a single blind trial, cyclosporin A 5–10 mg/kg/day was compared to "conventional treatment" consisting of corticos-teroids and chlorambucil [16]. Cyclosporin A markedly decreased the number of ocular attacks and caused a rapid improvement in visual acuity, but there was no difference between the groups 2 years later [17]. A single blind trial compared cyclosporin A 5 mg/kg/day with monthly pulses of cyclophosphamide [18]. Cyclosporin A showed a rapid and significant improvement in visual acuity but this improvement did not persist during the subsequent follow-up approaching 24 months. In a randomized, double-blind study of 16 weeks duration, 10 mg/kg/day of cyclosporin A was found to be superior to 1 mg/day of colchicine in suppressing the ocular manifestations of BS as well as the oral ulcers, genital ulcers, and dermal lesions [19]. In contrast to the other trials, the efficacy of cyclosporin A did not dampen during the open extension phase lasting for a mean of 44 weeks. However, the dose of cyclosporin A in this study was 10 mg/kg which is not used today because of toxic effects. In an open study on seven patients, treatment with cyclosporin A resulted in complete resolution of venous thrombosis in the lower extremities within 2 months [20].

In summary, cyclosporin A is a rapidly acting and effective drug in the treatment of severe eye disease. It is also recommended for the treatment of acute deep vein thrombosis in the EULAR recommendations but there is no formal evidence on efficacy. Patients should be followed-up closely when attempting to stop cyclosporin A since relapses of uveitis have been reported following the cessation of cyclosporin A [21]. The dose of cyclosporin A should be adjusted to no higher and usually lower than 5 mg/kg/day and the patients should be monitored closely for side effects with special emphasis on nephrotoxicity. According to one survey, cyclosporin A toxicity was the reason for end-stage renal failure in two of the 17 BS patients undergoing dialysis [22]. Neurotoxicity is another important side effect. Four case-control studies have reported the more frequent occurrence of central nervous system involvement in BS patients using cyclosporin A for eye disease [23–26]. It is currently still not very clear whether this finding is the result of cyclosporin neurotoxicity or simply reflects the more common occurrence of central nervous system disease among patients with severe uveitis for whom this medication had been prescribed in the first place. Until more information is available, it is recommended to avoid cyclosporin A in patients with central nervous system involvement unless absolutely necessary for intraocular inflammation [4].

Thalidomide

Thalidomide is a derivative of glutamic acid, which was put on the market as an over-the-counter sedative in the 1950s [27]. With an apparent good safety profile, it became popular among pregnant women for reducing morning sickness. However, thalidomide was withdrawn from the market in 1961 since its use during pregnancy was subsequently found to be associated with severe birth defects. In 1965, a fortuitous discovery led to the rebirth of thalidomide as an immunomodulatory drug that is today used in the treatment of various diseases including BS. It is believed that thalidomide exerts its effect largely by TNFα blockade and NF-κb inhibition [28].

In uncontrolled studies, thalidomide, in doses up to 400 mg/day has been found to be effective mainly for the mucocutaneous manifestations of BS [29–31]. The effect of thalidomide on other manifestations of BS has not been formally studied, but improvement in arthritis [32], gastrointestinal manifestations [33], and uveitis [32] has been reported in case reports.

In the only double-blind randomized trial, two different doses of thalidomide (100 mg/day and 300 mg/day) were compared with placebo in 96 male BS patients having active mucocutaneous manifestations but no major organ involvement [34]. This 24-week trial showed that thalidomide is not only effective in treating the oral ulcers, genital ulcers, and follicular lesions of BS, but it can also prevent the occurrence of new oral and genital ulcers. The effect of thalidomide started rapidly and persisted throughout the trial but symptoms recurred shortly after stopping thalidomide. There was no significant difference between the two doses of thalidomide regarding efficacy but sedation was more frequent at the higher dose. Interestingly, an increase in the frequency of nodular skin lesions was seen in patients allocated to thalidomide. Since no biopsies were done in this trial, it is not clear whether these lesions were erythema nodosum or superficial thrombophlebitis, perhaps triggered by the thrombophilic potential of thalidomide, which is well recognized today [35].

Thalidomide is one of the most powerful drugs for the treatment of oral and genital ulcers of BS. According to EULAR recommendations, it may also be tried in the management of gastrointestinal involvement before surgery, but another position paper from Japan did not reach a consensus on this issue [36]. Important side effects, especially teratogenesis and polyneuropathy, which can be irreversible and more common in the elderly, restrict the use of thalidomide only to carefully selected patients only for a short period of time.

Corticosteroids

Systemic corticosteroids are mainly used in combination with immunosuppressives for almost every manifestation of BS, but formal data on their efficacy are lacking. The dosage is empirically adjusted according to the severity of symptoms. Topical application of corticosteroid containing creams is believed to have a palliative effect on oral and genital ulcers. Intra-articular steroid injections may be useful for swollen joints with large effusions. Pulsed steroids are usually given as induction treatment of major complications such as central nervous system involvement and pulmonary aneurysms.

Until now, only one randomized, placebo-controlled trial assessed the efficacy of low-dose intramuscular methylprednisolone injections (40 mg every 3 weeks for 27 weeks) on the mucocutaneous manifestations of BS [37]. This trial showed a beneficial effect of corticosteroid treatment only for erythema nodosum and that among females only. This is obviously reminiscent of the gender difference in the effect of colchicine as discussed above. On the other hand, the low dose of corticosteroids used in this study, as well as a Type II error due to the limited number of patients enrolled, might also have played a role in the negative results.

In the EULAR recommendations, corticosteroids are advised as part of immunosuppressive treatment in any patient with uveitis affecting the posterior segment as well as in patients having severe uveitis. Corticosteroids are also recommended for acute deep vein thrombosis, pulmonary and peripheral artery aneurysms, gastrointestinal and central nervous system involvement [4].

Cyclophosphamide

Previous experience with cyclophosphamide was mostly on eye involvement of BS [18]. However, the introduction of less toxic and effective agents like azathioprine and cyclosporine A has today limited the use of this alkylating drug mainly to severe and life-threatening complications such as pulmonary aneurysms [14]. In this situation, cyclophosphamide is usually combined with high dose corticosteroids. Monthly intravenous pulses of 1 gm cyclophosphamide, with concomitant use of Mesna to prevent bladder toxicity, are preferred to continuous oral cyclophosphamide treatment because of lower toxicity. EULAR recommendations advise the use of cyclophosphamide for large vessel disease and parenchymal central nervous system involvement [4].

Other Immunosuppressives

In uncontrolled studies, chlorambucil appeared to be beneficial in the treatment of parenchymal central nervous system involvement and uveitis of BS [38, 39]. Today, the use of chlorambucil as a first line agent is not recommended because it may induce chromosome abnormalities and hematological maliganancies [40, 41]. Methotrexate and tacrolimus also have been found to be beneficial in uncontrolled studies [42, 43]. An open study with mycophenolate mofetil was interrupted because of the inefficacy of this drug in treating the mucocutaneous manifestations of BS [44].

Antibiotics

The possible role of infectious agents, especially streptococci, in the etiology of BS (see Chap. 14) has led some investigators to try antibiotics in the treatment of BS [45]. A randomized trial assessed the efficacy of the combination of benzathine penicillin and colchicine with colchicine alone in 120 BS patients [46]. The duration and severity of arthritis attacks were not found to be different between the two groups but the combination treatment significantly reduced the frequency of arthritis attacks and prolonged the duration of arthritis free periods. By using similar methodology, the same group reported better results with the combination of colchicine and benzathine penicillin in controlling the mucocutaneous lesions of BS [47]. Two open trials with small number of patients also reported successful results with azithromycine and minocycline [48, 49]. More data from properly designed trials are needed to recommend the use of antibiotics in BS.

Anticoagulants

Data evaluating the place of anticoagulants in BS are very limited. A retrospective study on 95 BS patients suggests that immunosuppressive treatment is more effective than anticoagulation in reducing the risk of recurrent deep vein thrombosis [50]. A second retrospective study on 37 BS patients reported similar results [51]. Until more data are available, the use of anticoagulants is not recommended in BS. The risk of bleeding from coexisting aneurysms is another limitation for anticoagulation treatment.

Miscellaneous

Dapsone, a sulfon used to treat leprosy, was effective for mucocutaneous manifestations of BS in a controlled trial with small number of patients [52]. Rebamipide, a gastric mucosa protecting agent, was found to be beneficial for oral ulcers in a randomized controlled trial [53]. Topical application of sucralfate, a cytoprotective agent, was effective for oral and genital ulcers in a randomized controlled trial [54]. Levamisole, an anthelmintic with immunomodulatory effects and transfer factor are not used today [55, 56]. Acyclovir, an antiviral agent, has failed to show efficacy in orogenital ulceration in a double blind placebo controlled cross-over trial [57]. Lactobacilli containing lozenges decreased oral ulcers in an open study [58]. Topical application of orobase containing cyclosporin was not found to be superior to simple topical orobase for oral ulcers in a double blind controlled trial [59]. Topical pimecrolimus cream combined with colchicine was effective in shortening the pain duration of genital ulcers [60]. Topical application of interferon alpha (IFN alpha) was also not better than placebo for oral ulcers in a double blind trial [61]. Oral rinse with granulocyte colony stimulating factor containing suspension was beneficial for oral and genital ulcers in an open trial [62]. Pentoxyfilline, an agent used for peripheral vascular disease, is used anecdotally in BS [63]. Beneficial results with indomethacine and oxaprozin have been reported in open studies [64, 65] but the only controlled trial failed to show a beneficial effect of azapropazone – an NSAID that is no longer in the market – in the treatment of acute arthritis of BS [66].

Biologic Agents and Stem Cell Transplantation Used for the Treatment of BS

Interferon Alpha

IFN alpha is a pleiotropic cytokine with immunomodulatory, antiviral, and antiproliferative properties. It is approved for the treatment of viral hepatitis C and some hematological and solid malignancies such as hairy cell leukemia, chronic myelogenous leukemia, follicular and cutaneous lymphoma, Kaposi sarcoma, renal cell carcinoma, or malignant melanoma. Two recombinant isotypes, alpha 2a and alpha 2b, differ in one aminoacid only. There are also consensus interferon and pegylated forms, but no reports are available on their use in BS.

In 1986, Tsambaos et al. [67] introduced IFN alpha for the treatment of severe, treatment resistant BS, postulating that BS was caused by herpes viruses (see Chap. 14). They treated three patients with high dosages of 9–12 million units intramuscularly on a daily basis for 11–16 days. Complete remission was achieved in all except for ocular manifestations in one patient. In 1994, Hamuryudan et al. published an open trial with 20 patients on IFN alpha 2b for mucocutaneous symptoms and arthritis (5 million units three times a week for 6 weeks, followed by 5 million units once a week for 10 weeks) [68]. IFN alpha 2b significantly reduced the mean number of arthritis attacks, their mean duration and ESR; mucocutaneous lesions showed a tendency to decrease, too. Since then, only two randomized studies have been published. The first one appeared in 2000 but was retracted later by the editor of the Lancet [69, 70]. In 2002, Alpsoy et al. [71] published a randomized, placebo-controlled trial on interferon-alpha 2a, including 50 patients without active ocular disease. The dosage of IFN was 6 million units six times per week subcutaneously for 3 months. Here a significant superiority of IFN alpha – in this case over placebo – was shown. IFN significantly decreased duration and pain of oral aphthous ulcers, frequency of genital ulcers and papulopustular lesions. A nonsignificant improvement was seen in erythema nodosa, thrombophlebitis, arthritis, and the frequency of ocular attacks.

The first large retrospective case series on 50 patients with BS was published in 2003 [72]. Here, patients with severe, treatment resistant ocular manifestations, mainly retinal vasculitis, were treated with IFN alpha 2a according to an algorithm, starting with 6 million units daily and tapering to a maintenance dosage of 3 million units three times per week as a maintenance dosage. Prednisolone was given at a maximum dosage of 10 mg. In 40%, IFN could be discontinued without relapse, the rate of complete remissions was 98% and even disappearance of macular edema and retinal neovascularisations were observed. Time to response defined as 50% improvement of retinal inflammation was 2 weeks. In 2004, Kötter et al. [73] did a meta-analysis of all publications on IFN alpha for the treatment of BS. Until then, 405 patients treated with IFN alpha, 216 of these with ocular manifestations, had been published. They concluded that IFN alpha was very effective for all manifestations of BS, especially for ocular disease with retinal vasculitis. IFN alpha 2a appeared to be superior to IFN alpha 2b, but this was probably due to different number of patients treated with either IFN isotype producing a type II error. The percentage of complete remissions appeared to be higher when higher IFN dosages were used at initiation of treatment and was not associated with longer treatment durations. The rate of complete remissions was lower for other manifestations of BS, with the lowest rate for oral aphthous ulcers [74]. Recently, several groups published their retrospective and long-term data on IFN alpha 2a for ocular disease in series of 44, 45, 32, and 9 patients, respectively, and reported complete remissions of ocular disease in 85–95% of their cases, with long-term remissions without relapse after discontinuation of IFN in 20–88% [75–78]. Discontinuation of IFN without relapse was possible in 20% [79] to 68 % [76, 80]. The treatment regimens in these retrospective studies were quite different, with lower initial IFN dosages in the series of Krause and Gueudry (3–6 million units weekly; 3 million units three times per week) than in those by Tugal-Tutkun and Deuter (6 million units per day). This could be the reason for the different rates of complete remissions and treatment-free intervals. Furthermore, in the groups by Krause and Gueudry, prednisolone was given in combination to IFN for a longer period of time and in higher dosages. It has been postulated that glucocorticosteroids may antagonize the effects of IFN alpha [81]. There have been two reports on the treatment of pediatric BS with IFN alpha. In 2007, Guillaume-Czitrom et al. reported on seven children with BS-associated uveitis, where they observed marked steroid-sparing effects; in three children, IFN could be discontinued without relapse [82]. However, there were two major side effects (retinal vein thrombosis and depression). Another report was on two children with CNS vasculitis due to BS, both achieving complete remission [83].

Adverse effects of IFN alpha are frequent, but clearly dose dependent [84]. In the studies on IFN alpha for BS, they mainly consisted of fever at the initiation of IFN treatment (80%), leukopenia (40%), depression(8%), alopecia (10%), arthralgia/fibromyalgia (10%), loss of weight (10%), reddening at the site of injection (10%), development of autoantibodies (16%), or even manifest autoimmune diseases (mostly thyroiditis) and psoriasis (4–6%). A combination of IFN alpha 2b with azathioprine was effective in an open uncontrolled trial with ten patients with retinal vasculitis, but it caused severe myelosuppression normally not seen with either agent alone and cannot be recommended [13].

In conclusion, IFN alpha is effective especially for severe ocular manifestations of BS; it acts rapidly and in 20% to over 80% of patients, long-term remissions of ocular disease without treatment are possible. Higher dosages appear to be more effective than lower dosages, and the combination with glucocorticosteroids remains a matter of discussion, as they may antagonize the effects of IFN alpha. IFN alpha has become the standard treatment for azathioprine resistant or fulminant cases of severe ocular BS in many centers, which also is reflected in the EULAR expert recommendations [4].

TNF-Antagonists

TNF-alpha is a major proinflammatory cytokine, and the antagonists block its effects. The first publication on the use of TNF-antagonists in BS appeared in 2001 [85]. Five patients with severe ocular disease were treated with infliximab (5 mg/kg bw) in combination with prednisolone and their ineffective immunosuppressive (cyclosporin A, azathioprine). Complete remissions were seen after 7 days. This report led to a number of case reports and case series, with at maximum 13 cases per series and maximum observation periods of 36 months [86]. Most case reports to date are on infliximab, followed by etanercept and adalimumab. Most of the publications focused on ocular disease. There is one randomized trial of etanercept versus placebo in 40 male patients with mucocutaneous manifestations of BS and / or arthritis [87]. They received etanercept 2×25 mg/week or placebo for 4 weeks. Patients with ocular disease were excluded from the study. There was a significant improvement of mucocutaneous lesions in the etanercept group. In 2008, Tabbara et al. [88] did a retrospective comparative analysis of 33 patients, comparing conventional treatment (cyclosporin A, azathioprine, methotrexate) with infliximab (ten patients, 5 mg/kg bw). After a median observation period of 36 months, visual acuity was significantly better in the infliximab treated patient group with less relapses and longer durations of remissions.

Several case reports show the efficacy of different TNF antagonists for treatment resistant CNS manifestations of BS [89–93].

Perhaps in contrast to IFN alpha, long-term remissions after discontinuation of the TNF antagonists are not common. In almost all case series, in case of discontinuation of the TNF antagonist, relapses occurred within approximately 8 weeks [94–97]. As prospective and controlled studies on this issue are lacking, it is still unclear if discontinuation of TNF antagonists may be possible when using a conventional immunosuppressive as maintenance treatment and the TNF antagonist as the "remission inducing agent." Adverse effects of TNF antagonists mainly are infectious complications and reactivation of latent tuberculosis. An SLE-like autoimmune disease may occur, and paradoxical development of psoriasis has been described. There also have been some cases of leukencephalopathy and in multiple sclerosis, TNF antagonists are contraindicated because of MS exacerbations. In 2007, expert recommendations on the use of TNF antagonists in BS were published [98]. The recommendation is not to use TNF antagonists as the primary treatment for other manifestations than severe, sight threatening ocular disease. TNF antagonists may be used for other refractory manifestations. In the EULAR recommendations, TNF antagonists are recommended for severe ocular disease and they may also be used for treatment resistant other manifestations [4]. Today the recommendation would be to preferentially use infliximab, as most data are available for this TNF antagonist, in a dosage of 5 mg/kg bw, exclusively for sight threatening retinal vasculitis or refractory other manifestations of BS. As etanercept was described to be less effective than the other TNF antagonists for inflammatory bowel disease and uveitis associated to spondyloarthropathies and juvenile idiopathic arthritis [99–101], it should be used with caution if at all for similar manifestations of BS (ocular, gastrointestinal).

Other Biologic Agents

Alemtuzumab (Campath 1-H)

Alemtuzumab is a humanized monoclonal antibody against CD 52, a surface antigen which is present on lymphocytes and macrophages; it predominantly depletes CD4+ T-cells, which do not recover for a long period of time and often recover only incompletely. It is presently approved for the treatment of B-CLL. Lockwood et al. [102] treated 18 patients with severe active BS with Campath 1-H (total dose134 mg, escalating from 10 to 40 mg daily intravenously). By 6 months, 13 (72%) had entered remission, and prednisolone was significantly reduced. At follow-up after 37 months, seven patients had relapsed after an average of 25 months. There were five moderate infusion related adverse effects and two cases of hypothyroidism. CD4+ T-cells remained depressed for 1 year. The authors discuss alemtuzumab as remission inducing agent, further studies have not been published since 2003.

Daclizumab

Daclizumab is a humanized monoclonal antibody against CD25, the IL-2 receptor alpha chain. It was approved in Europe for the treatment of graft rejection after organ transplantation, but the approval was withdrawn by the pharmaceutical company in January 2009. There also are ongoing studies for the treatment of inflammatory bowel diseases, uveitis, and multiple sclerosis. A randomized, placebo-controlled, double-masked trial in uveitis associated with BS was performed in 2007 by Buggage et al. [103]. Seventeen patients with BS and ocular involvement with at least two prior flares requiring immunosuppressive treatment received daclizumab 1 mg/kg bw intravenously every 2 weeks for 6 weeks, then every 4 weeks while continuing their standard immunosuppressive treatment. Median follow-up was 15 months. Visual acuity remained stable in all patients, but six in the daclizumab group versus four in the placebo group experienced flares under treatment. The median ocular attack rate was greater in the daclizumab than in the placebo group. Hence, daclizumab does not appear to be better than placebo when added to conventional immunosuppressants.

Rituximab

Rituximab is a chimeric monoclonal antibody directed against the surface molecule CD20, which is exclusively expressed on B lymphocytes. It depletes B lymphocytes for an average of 6 months from the peripheral blood. It is approved for the treatment of rheumatoid arthritis in a dosage of 1,000 mg day 1 and 15. There is one case report about a patient with retinal vasculitis resistant to glucocorticoids, azathioprine, and etanercept (the latter was discontinued due to adverse effects) where rituximab finally induced remission of the retinal vasculitis [104].

Il-1-Receptor Antagonist (Anakinra)

The IL-1 receptor antagonist anakinra is approved for the treatment of rheumatod arthritis. To date, it is used preferentially for the treatment of autoinflammatory syndromes, which are IL1-mediated. One patient with severe vascular and gastro-intestinal BS with fever and neutrophilia resistant to azathioprine, methotrexate, prednisolone, colchicine, and infliximab finally entered remission with anakinra 100 mg/day subcutaneously [105].

Stem Cell Transplantation

Autologous and allogeneic peripheral blood or bone marrow transplantations are performed for the treatment of selected hematological malignancies. In the last decade, autologous (and, rarely, also allogeneic) stem cell transplantations have also been applied for treatment resistant autoimmune diseases, mainly multiple sclerosis and systemic sclerosis, postulating a "reset" of the immune system. There are several case reports on patients with treatment-resistant and life-threatening manifestations of BS (such as CNS vasculitis or pulmonary aneurysms) who have been successfully treated with stem cell transplantation. De Cata et al. reported on two patients with severe progressive neurological BS, who after autologous periph-eral blood stem cell transplantation entered complete remission, not requiring treat-ment after the procedure anymore [106], and Rossi et al. on a patient with refractory intestinal BS [107]. Maurer et al. reported on two patients with pulmonary aneu-rysms resistant to conventional immunosuppressives, who after autologous trans-plantation still were in remission after 5 years [108]. There are three reports on allogeneic and one even on haploidentical transplantations resulting in long-term remissions (these were performed for additional hematological malignancies or myelodysplastic syndromes) [109–111]. Three patients with BS are registered in the EULAR/EBMT data base, the data of which were summarized by Daikeler et al. in 2007 [112]. In general, in this analysis of stem cell transplantation for vasculitides, the rates of complete and partial responses were 96% each. However, the transplantation related mortality for autoimmune diseases is high (7% for autologous, 22% for allogeneic), and the procedure is aggressive as well as expensive and should be reserved for life threatening and treatment resistant manifestations of BS.

In summary, newer treatment options have added significantly to our therapeutic repertoire for BS. Especially concerning severe ocular disease, progress has been made with the introduction of IFN alpha and TNF antagonists, leading to improvement of visual prognosis. To date, even life threatening manifestations of BS, such as CNS vasculitis can be managed better with biologic agents (TNF antagonists and IFN alpha). Stem cell transplantation as a last option may also be helpful in individual, refractory cases. However, none of these newer agents and modalities is approved for the treatment of BS, and randomized trials are sparse or even lacking. This is especially the case for ocular disease and IFN alpha or TNF antagonists, but both are used very frequently for this manifestation and their use is even recommended by international experts.

References

1. Yurdakul S, Yazici H (2008) Behçet's syndrome. Best Pract Res Clin Rheumatol 22:793–809
2. Kural-Seyahi E, Fresko I, Seyahi N, Ozyazgan Y, Mat C, Hamuryudan V, Yurdakul S, Yazici H (2003) The long-term mortality and morbidity of Behçet's syndrome: a 2-decade outcome survey of 387 patients followed at a dedicated center. Medicine (Baltimore) 82:60–76
3. Hamuryudan V, Ozyazgan Y, Hizli N, Mat C, Yurdakul S, Tuzun Y, Senocak M, Yazici H (1997) Azathioprine in Behçet's syndrome: effects on long-term prognosis. Arthritis Rheum 40:769–774
4. Hatemi G, Silman A, Bang D, Bodaghi B, Chamberlain AM, Gul A, Houman MH, Kotter I, Olivieri I, Salvarani C et al (2008) EULAR recommendations for the management of Behçet's disease. Ann Rheum Dis 67:1656–1662
5. Ben-Chetrit E, Levy M (1998) Colchicine: 1998 update. Semin Arthritis Rheum 28:48–59
6. Matsumura N, Mizushima Y (1975) Leucocyte movement and colchicine treatment in Behçet's disease. Lancet 2:813
7. Mizushima Y, Matsumura N, Mori M, Shimizu T, Fukushima B, Mimura Y, Saito K, Sugiura S (1037) Colchicine in Behçet's disease. Lancet 1977:2
8. Aktulga E, Altac M, Muftuoglu A, Ozyazgan Y, Pazarli H, Tuzun Y, Yalcin B, Yazici H, Yurdakul S (1980) A double blind study of colchicine in Behçet's disease. Haematologica 65:399–402
9. Yurdakul S, Mat C, Tuzun Y, Ozyazgan Y, Hamuryudan V, Uysal O, Senocak M, Yazici H (2001) A double-blind trial of colchicine in Behçet's syndrome. Arthritis Rheum 44:2686–2692

10. Rosselet E, Saudan Y, Zenklusen G (1968) Effects of azathioprine ("Imuran") in Behçet's disease. Preliminary therapeutic results. Ophthalmologica 156:218–226

11. Yazici H, Pazarli H, Barnes CG, Tuzun Y, Ozyazgan Y, Silman A, Serdaroglu S, Oguz V, Yurdakul S, Lovatt GE et al (1990) A controlled trial of azathioprine in Behçet's syndrome. N Engl J Med 322:281–285

12. Hatemi G, Silman A, Bang D, Bodaghi B, Chamberlain AM, Gul A, Houman MH, Kotter I, Olivieri I, Salvarani C et al (2009) Management of Behçet's disease: a systematic literature review for the EULAR evidence based recommendations for the management of Behçet's disease. Ann Rheum Dis 68:1528–1534

13. Hamuryudan V, Ozyazgan Y, Fresko Y, Mat C, Yurdakul S, Yazici H (2002) Interferon alfa combined with azathioprine for the uveitis of Behçet's disease: an open study. Isr Med Assoc J 4:928–930

14. Hamuryudan V, Er T, Seyahi E, Akman C, Tuzun H, Fresko I, Yurdakul S, Numan F, Yazici H (2004) Pulmonary artery aneurysms in Behçet's syndrome. Am J Med 117:867–870

15. Kaklamani VG, Kaklamanis PG (2001) Treatment of Behçet's disease–an update. Semin Arthritis Rheum 30:299–312

16. BenEzra D, Cohen E, Chajek T, Friedman G, Pizanti S, de Courten C, Harris W (1988) Evaluation of conventional therapy versus cyclosporine A in Behçet's syndrome. Transplant Proc 20:136–143

17. Saenz A, Ausejo M, Shea B, Wells G, Welch V, Tugwell P (2000) Pharmacotherapy for Behçet's syndrome. Cochrane Database Syst Rev (2) CD001084

18. Ozyazgan Y, Yurdakul S, Yazici H, Tuzun B, Iscimen A, Tuzun Y, Aktunc T, Pazarli H, Hamuryudan V, Muftuoglu A (1992) Low dose cyclosporin A versus pulsed cyclophosphamide in Behçet's syndrome: a single masked trial. Br J Ophthalmol 76:241–243

19. Masuda K, Nakajima A, Urayama A, Nakae K, Kogure M, Inaba G (1989) Double-masked trial of cyclosporin versus colchicine and long-term open study of cyclosporin in Behçet's disease. Lancet 1:1093–1096

20. Cantini F, Salvarani C, Niccoli L, Padula A, Arena AI, Bellandi F, Macchioni P, Olivieri I (1999) Treatment of thrombophlebitis of Behçet's disease with low dose cyclosporin A. Clin Exp Rheumatol 17:391–392

21. Muftuoglu AU, Pazarli H, Yurdakul S, Yazici H, Ulku BY, Tuzun Y, Serdaroglu S, Altug E, Bahcecioglu H, Gungen G (1987) Short term cyclosporin A treatment of Behçet's disease. Br J Ophthalmol 71:387–390

22. Akpolat T, Diri B, Oguz Y, Yilmaz E, Yavuz M, Dilek M (2003) Behçet's disease and renal failure. Nephrol Dial Transplant 18:888–891

23. Kotake S, Higashi K, Yoshikawa K, Sasamoto Y, Okamoto T, Matsuda H (1999) Central nervous system symptoms in patients with Behçet's disease receiving cyclosporine therapy. Ophthalmology 106:586–589

24. Kato Y, Numaga J, Kato S, Kaburaki T, Kawashima H, Fujino Y (2001) Central nervous system symptoms in a population of Behçet's disease patients with refractory uveitis treated with cyclosporine A. Clin Exp Ophthalmol 29:335–336

25. Kotter I, Gunaydin I, Batra M, Vonthein R, Stubiger N, Fierlbeck G, Melms A (2006) CNS involvement occurs more frequently in patients with Behçet's disease under cyclosporin A (CSA) than under other medications–results of a retrospective analysis of 117 cases. Clin Rheumatol 25:482–486

26. Akman-Demir G, Ayranci O, Kurtuncu M, Vanli EN, Mutlu M, Tugal-Tutkun I (2008) Cyclosporine for Behçet's uveitis: is it associated with an increased risk of neurological involvement? Clin Exp Rheumatol 26:S84–S90

27. Perri AJ 3rd, Hsu S (2003) A review of thalidomide's history and current dermatological applications. Dermatol Online J 9:5

28. Direskeneli H, Ergun T, Yavuz S, Hamuryudan V, Eksioglu-Demiralp E (2008) Thalidomide has both anti-inflammatory and regulatory effects in Behçet's disease. Clin Rheumatol 27:373–375

29. Saylan T, Saltik I (1982) Thalidomide in the treatment of Behçet's syndrome. Arch Dermatol 118:536
30. Jorizzo JL, Schmalstieg FC, Solomon AR Jr, Cavallo T, Taylor RS 3rd, Rudloff HB, Schmalstieg EJ, Daniels JC (1986) Thalidomide effects in Behçet's syndrome and pustular vasculitis. Arch Intern Med 146:878–881
31. Denman AM, Graham E, Howe L, Denman EJ, Lightman S (1993) Low dose thalidomide treatment of Behçet's syndrome. In: Wechsler B, Godeau P (eds) Behçet's disease. Proceedings of the 6th international conference on Behçet's disease. Excerpta Medica, Amsterdam, pp 649–653
32. Hamza MH (1986) Treatment of Behçet's disease with thalidomide. Clin Rheumatol 5:365–371
33. Brik R, Shamali H, Bergman R (2001) Successful thalidomide treatment of severe infantile Behçet's disease. Pediatr Dermatol 18:143–145
34. Hamuryudan V, Mat C, Saip S, Ozyazgan Y, Siva A, Yurdakul S, Zwingenberger K, Yazici H (1998) Thalidomide in the treatment of the mucocutaneous lesions of the Behçet's syndrome. A randomized, double-blind, placebo-controlled trial. Ann Intern Med 128:443–450
35. Zangari M, Anaissie E, Barlogie B, Badros A, Desikan R, Gopal AV, Morris C, Toor A, Siegel E, Fink L et al (2001) Increased risk of deep-vein thrombosis in patients with multiple myeloma receiving thalidomide and chemotherapy. Blood 98:1614–1615
36. Kobayashi K, Ueno F, Bito S, Iwao Y, Fukushima T, Hiwatashi N, Igarashi M, Iizuka BE, Matsuda T, Matsui T et al (2007) Development of consensus statements for the diagnosis and management of intestinal Behçet's disease using a modified Delphi approach. J Gastroenterol 42:737–745
37. Mat C, Yurdakul S, Uysal S, Gogus F, Ozyazgan Y, Uysal O, Fresko I, Yazici H (2006) A double-blind trial of depot corticosteroids in Behçet's syndrome. Rheumatology (Oxford) 45:348–352
38. O'Duffy JD, Robertson DM, Goldstein NP (1984) Chlorambucil in the treatment of uveitis and meningoencephalitis of Behçet's disease. Am J Med 76:75–84
39. Mudun BA, Ergen A, Ipcioglu SU, Burumcek EY, Durlu Y, Arslan MO (2001) Short-term chlorambucil for refractory uveitis in Behçet's disease. Ocul Immunol Inflamm 9:219–229
40. Palmer RG, Dore CJ, Denman AM (1984) Chlorambucil-induced chromosome damage to human lymphocytes is dose-dependent and cumulative. Lancet 1:246–249
41. Tabbara KF (1983) Chlorambucil in Behçet's disease. A reappraisal. Ophthalmology 90:906–908
42. Sakane T, Mochizuki M, Inaba G, Masuda K (1995) A phase II study of FK506 (tacrolimus) on refractory uveitis associated with Behçet's disease and allied conditions. Ryumachi 35:802–813
43. Davatchi F, Shahram F, Chams H, Jamshidi AR, Nadji A, Chams C, Akbarian M, Gharibdoost F (2003) High dose methotrexate for ocular lesions of Behçet's disease. Preliminary short-term results. Adv Exp Med Biol 528:579–584
44. Adler YD, Mansmann U, Zouboulis CC (2001) Mycophenolate mofetil is ineffective in the treatment of mucocutaneous Adamantiades-Behçet's disease. Dermatology 203:322–324
45. Mumcu G, Inanc N, Yavuz S, Direskeneli H (2007) The role of infectious agents in the pathogenesis, clinical manifestations and treatment strategies in Behçet's disease. Clin Exp Rheumatol 25:S27–S33
46. Calguneri M, Kiraz S, Ertenli I, Benekli M, Karaarslan Y, Celik I (1996) The effect of prophylactic penicillin treatment on the course of arthritis episodes in patients with Behçet's disease. A randomized clinical trial. Arthritis Rheum 39:2062–2065
47. Calguneri M, Ertenli I, Kiraz S, Erman M, Celik I (1996) Effect of prophylactic benzathine penicillin on mucocutaneous symptoms of Behçet's disease. Dermatology 192:125–128
48. Mumcu G, Ergun T, Elbir Y, Eksioglu-Demiralp E, Yavuz S, Atalay T, Direskeneli H (2005) Clinical and immunological effects of azithromycin in Behçet's disease. J Oral Pathol Med 34:13–16
49. Kaneko F, Oyama N, Nishibu A (1997) Streptococcal infection in the pathogenesis of Behçet's disease and clinical effects of minocycline on the disease symptoms. Yonsei Med J 38:444–454

50. Kahraman O, Celebi-Onder S, Kamali S (2003) Long term course of deep vein thrombosis in patients with Behçet's disease. In: Proceedings of the American College of Rheumatology 67th annual meeting, Orlando, FL, Wiley, NJ, p S385

51. Ahn JK, Lee YS, Jeon CH, Koh EM, Cha HS (2008) Treatment of venous thrombosis associated with Behçet's disease: immunosuppressive therapy alone versus immunosuppressive therapy plus anticoagulation. Clin Rheumatol 27:201–205

52. Sharquie KE, Najim RA, Abu-Raghif AR (2002) Dapsone in Behçet's disease: a double-blind, placebo-controlled, cross-over study. J Dermatol 29:267–279

53. Matsuda T, Ohno S, Hirohata S, Miyanaga Y, Ujihara H, Inaba G, Nakamura S, Tanaka S, Kogure M, Mizushima Y (2003) Efficacy of rebamipide as adjunctive therapy in the treatment of recurrent oral aphthous ulcers in patients with Behçet's disease: a randomised, double-blind, placebo-controlled study. Drugs R D 4:19–28

54. Alpsoy E, Er H, Durusoy C, Yilmaz E (1999) The use of sucralfate suspension in the treatment of oral and genital ulceration of Behçet's disease: a randomized, placebo-controlled, double-blind study. Arch Dermatol 135:529–532

55. de Merieux P, Spitler LE, Paulus HE (1981) Treatment of Behçet's syndrome with levamisole. Arthritis Rheum 24:64–70

56. Wolf RE, Fudenberg HH, Welch TM, Spitler LE, Ziff M (1977) Treatment of Bechcet's syndrome with transfer factor. JAMA 238:869–871

57. Davies UM, Palmer RG, Denman AM (1988) Treatment with acyclovir does not affect orogenital ulcers in Behçet's syndrome: a randomized double-blind trial. Br J Rheumatol 27:300–302

58. Tasli L, Mat C, De Simone C, Yazici H (2006) Lactobacilli lozenges in the management of oral ulcers of Behçet's syndrome. Clin Exp Rheumatol 24:S83–S86

59. Ergun T, Gurbuz O, Yurdakul S, Hamuryudan V, Bekiroglu N, Yazici H (1997) Topical cyclosporine-A for treatment of oral ulcers of Behçet's syndrome. Int J Dermatol 36:720

60. Kose O, Dinc A, Simsek I (2009) Randomized trial of pimecrolimus cream plus colchicine tablets versus colchicine tablets in the treatment of genital ulcers in Behçet's disease. Dermatology 218:140–145

61. Hamuryudan V, Yurdakul S, Rosenkaimer F, Yazici H (1991) Inefficacy of topical alpha interferon alpha interferon in the treatment of oral ulcers of Behçet's syndrome: a randomized, double blind trial. Br J Rheumatol 30:395–396

62. Bacanli A, Yerebakan Dicle O, Parmaksizoglu B, Yilmaz E, Alpsoy E (2006) Topical granulocyte colony-stimulating factor for the treatment of oral and genital ulcers of patients with Behçet's disease. J Eur Acad Dermatol Venereol 20:931–935

63. Yasui K, Ohta K, Kobayashi M, Aizawa T, Komiyama A (1996) Successful treatment of Behçet's disease with pentoxifylline. Ann Intern Med 124:891–893

64. Simsek H, Dundar S, Telatar H (1991) Treatment of Behçet's disease with indomethacin. Int J Dermatol 30:54–57

65. Takeuchi A, Mori M, Hashimoto A, Chihara T (1984) Efficacy of oxaprozin in the treatment of articular symptoms of Behçet's disease. Clin Rheumatol 3:397–399

66. Moral F, Hamuryudan V, Yurdakul S, Yazici H (1995) Inefficacy of azapropazone in the acute arthritis of Behçet's syndrome: a randomized, double blind, placebo controlled study. Clin Exp Rheumatol 13:493–495

67. Tsambaos D, Eichelberg D, Goos M (1986) Behçet's syndrome: treatment with recombinant leukocyte alpha-interferon. Arch Dermatol Res 278:335–336

68. Hamuryudan V, Moral F, Yurdakul S, Mat C, Tuzun Y, Ozyazgan Y, Direskeneli H, Akoglu T, Yazici H (1994) Systemic interferon alpha 2b treatment in Behçet's syndrome. J Rheumatol 21:1098–1100

69. Demiroglu H, Ozcebe OI, Barista I, Dundar S, Eldem B (2000) Interferon alfa-2b, colchicine, and benzathine penicillin versus colchicine and benzathine penicillin in Behçet's disease: a randomised trial. Lancet 355:605–609

70. Horton R (2000) Retraction: interferon alfa-2b...in Behçet's disease. Lancet 356:1292

71. Alpsoy E, Durusoy C, Yilmaz E, Ozgurel Y, Ermis O, Yazar S, Basaran E (2002) Interferon alfa-2a in the treatment of Behçet's disease: a randomized placebo-controlled and double-blind study. Arch Dermatol 138:467–471

72. Kotter I, Zierhut M, Eckstein AK, Vonthein R, Ness T, Gunaydin I, Grimbacher B, Blaschke S, Meyer-Riemann W, Peter HH et al (2003) Human recombinant interferon alfa-2a for the treatment of Behçet's disease with sight threatening posterior or panuveitis. Br J Ophthalmol 87:423–431

73. Kotter I, Gunaydin I, Zierhut M, Stubiger N (2004) The use of interferon alpha in Behçet's disease: review of the literature. Semin Arthritis Rheum 33:320–335

74. Kotter I, Vonthein R, Zierhut M, Eckstein AK, Ness T, Gunaydin I, Grimbacher B, Blaschke S, Peter HH, Stubiger N (2004) Differential efficacy of human recombinant interferon-alpha2a on ocular and extraocular manifestations of Behçet's disease: results of an open 4-center trial. Semin Arthritis Rheum 33:311–319

75. Tugal-Tutkun I, Guney-Tefekli E, Urgancioglu M (2006) Results of interferon-alfa therapy in patients with Behçet's uveitis. Graefes Arch Clin Exp Ophthalmol 244:1692–1695

76. Gueudry J, Wechsler B, Terrada C, Gendron G, Cassoux N, Fardeau C, Lehoang P, Piette JC, Bodaghi B (2008) Long-term efficacy and safety of low-dose interferon alpha2a therapy in severe uveitis associated with Behçet's disease. Am J Ophthalmol 146:837–844, e831

77. Krause L, Altenburg A, Pleyer U, Kohler AK, Zouboulis CC, Foerster MH (2008) Longterm visual prognosis of patients with ocular Adamantiades-Behçet's disease treated with interferon-alpha-2a. J Rheumatol 35:896–903

78. Deuter CM, Kotter I, Gunaydin I, Zierhut M, Stubiger N (2004) Ocular involvement in Behçet's disease: first 5-year-results for visual development after treatment with interferon alfa-2a. Ophthalmologe 101:129–134

79. Krause L, Kohler AK, Altenburg A, Papoutsis N, Zouboulis CC, Pleyer U, Stroux A, Foerster MH (2009) Ocular involvement in Adamantiades-Behçet's disease in Berlin, Germany. Graefes Arch Clin Exp Ophthalmol 247:661–666

80. Deuter C, Kotter I, Mohle A, Vonthein R, Stubiger N, Zierhut M (2009) Long-term observations of vision and relapse-free intervals in patients with severe uveitis due to Behçet's disease treated with interferon alfa. ARVO Abstract 2009 No. 2694

81. Deuter CM, Kotter I, Wallace GR, Murray PI, Stubiger N, Zierhut M (2008) Behçet's disease: ocular effects and treatment. Prog Retin Eye Res 27:111–136

82. Guillaume-Czitrom S, Berger C, Pajot C, Bodaghi B, Wechsler B, Kone-Paut I (2007) Efficacy and safety of interferon-alpha in the treatment of corticodependent uveitis of paediatric Behçet's disease. Rheumatology (Oxford) 46:1570–1573

83. Kuemmerle-Deschner JB, Tzaribachev N, Deuter C, Zierhut M, Batra M, Koetter I (2008) Interferon-alpha – a new therapeutic option in refractory juvenile Behçet's disease with CNS involvement. Rheumatology (Oxford) 47:1051–1053

84. Hauschild A, Kahler KC, Schafer M, Fluck M (2008) Interdisciplinary management recommendations for toxicity associated with interferon-alfa therapy. J Dtsch Dermatol Ges 6:829–837, 829–838

85. Sfikakis PP, Theodossiadis PG, Katsiari CG, Kaklamanis P, Markomichelakis NN (2001) Effect of infliximab on sight-threatening panuveitis in Behçet's disease. Lancet 358:295–296

86. Benitez-del-Castillo JM, Martinez-de-la-Casa JM, Pato-Cour E, Mendez-Fernandez R, Lopez-Abad C, Matilla M, Garcia-Sanchez J (2005) Long-term treatment of refractory posterior uveitis with anti-TNFalpha (infliximab). Eye 19:841–845

87. Melikoglu M, Fresko I, Mat C, Ozyazgan Y, Gogus F, Yurdakul S, Hamuryudan V, Yazici H (2005) Short term trial of etanercept in Behçet's disease: a double blind, placebo controlled study. J Rheumatol 32:98–105

88. Tabbara KF, Al-Hemidan AI (2008) Infliximab effects compared to conventional therapy in the management of retinal vasculitis in Behçet's disease. Am J Ophthalmol 146:845–850, e841

89. Ribi C, Sztajzel R, Delavelle J, Chizzolini C (2005) Efficacy of TNF alpha blockade in cyclophosphamide resistant neuro-Behçet's disease. J Neurol Neurosurg Psychiatry 76:1733–1735

90. Sarwar H, McGrath H Jr, Espinoza LR (2005) Successful treatment of long-standing neuro-Behçet's disease with infliximab. J Rheumatol 32:181–183

91. Alty JE, Monaghan TM, Bamford JM (2007) A patient with neuro-Behçet's disease is successfully treated with etanercept: further evidence for the value of TNFalpha blockade. Clin Neurol Neurosurg 109:279–281

92. Belzunegui J, Lopez L, Paniagua I, Intxausti JJ, Maiz O (2008) Efficacy of infliximab and adalimumab in the treatment of a patient with severe neuro-Behçet's disease. Clin Exp Rheumatol 26:S133–S134

93. Kikuchi H, Aramaki K, Hirohata S (2008) Effect of infliximab in progressive neuro-Behçet's syndrome. J Neurol Sci 272:99–105

94. Sfikakis PP, Kaklamanis PH, Elezoglou A, Katsilambros N, Theodossiadis PG, Papaefthimiou S, Markomichelakis N (2004) Infliximab for recurrent, sight-threatening ocular inflammation in Adamantiades-Behçet's disease. Ann Intern Med 140:404–406

95. Ohno S, Nakamura S, Hori S, Shimakawa M, Kawashima H, Mochizuki M, Sugita S, Ueno S, Yoshizaki K, Inaba G (2004) Efficacy, safety, and pharmacokinetics of multiple administration of infliximab in Behçet's disease with refractory uveoretinitis. J Rheumatol 31:1362–1368

96. Tugal-Tutkun I, Mudun A, Urgancioglu M, Kamali S, Kasapoglu E, Inanc M, Gul A (2005) Efficacy of infliximab in the treatment of uveitis that is resistant to treatment with the combination of azathioprine, cyclosporine, and corticosteroids in Behçet's disease: an open-label trial. Arthritis Rheum 52:2478–2484

97. Tognon S, Graziani G, Marcolongo R (2007) Anti-TNF-alpha therapy in seven patients with Behçet's uveitis: advantages and controversial aspects. Ann N Y Acad Sci 1110:474–484

98. Sfikakis PP, Markomichelakis N, Alpsoy E, Assaad-Khalil S, Bodaghi B, Gul A, Ohno S, Pipitone N, Schirmer M, Stanford M et al (2007) Anti-TNF therapy in the management of Behçet's disease–review and basis for recommendations. Rheumatology (Oxford) 46:736–741

99. Song IH, Appel H, Haibel H, Loddenkemper C, Braun J, Sieper J, Rudwaleit M (2008) New onset of Crohn's disease during treatment of active ankylosing spondylitis with etanercept. J Rheumatol 35:532–536

100. Lim LL, Fraunfelder FW, Rosenbaum JT (2007) Do tumor necrosis factor inhibitors cause uveitis? A registry-based study. Arthritis Rheum 56:3248–3252

101. Foeldvari I, Nielsen S, Kummerle-Deschner J, Espada G, Horneff G, Bica B, Olivieri AN, Wierk A, Saurenmann RK (2007) Tumor necrosis factor-alpha blocker in treatment of juvenile idiopathic arthritis-associated uveitis refractory to second-line agents: results of a multinational survey. J Rheumatol 34:1146–1150

102. Lockwood CM, Hale G, Waldman H, Jayne DR (2003) Remission induction in Behçet's disease following lymphocyte depletion by the anti-CD52 antibody CAMPATH 1-H. Rheumatology (Oxford) 42:1539–1544

103. Buggage RR, Levy-Clarke G, Sen HN, Ursea R, Srivastava SK, Suhler EB, Altemare C, Velez G, Ragheb J, Chan CC et al (2007) A double-masked, randomized study to investigate the safety and efficacy of daclizumab to treat the ocular complications related to Behçet's disease. Ocul Immunol Inflamm 15:63–70

104. Sadreddini S, Noshad H, Molaeefard M, Noshad R (2008) Treatment of retinal vasculitis in Behçet's disease with rituximab. Mod Rheumatol 18:306–308

105. Botsios C, Sfriso P, Furlan A, Punzi L, Dinarello CA (2008) Resistant Behçet's disease responsive to anakinra. Ann Intern Med 149:284–286

106. De Cata A, Intiso D, Bernal M, Molinaro F, Mazzoccoli G, D'Alessandro V, Greco A, Curci S, Sperandeo M, Frusciante V et al (2007) Prolonged remission of neuro-Behçet's disease following autologous transplantation. Int J Immunopathol Pharmacol 20:91–96

107. Rossi G, Moretta A, Locatelli F (2004) Autologous hematopoietic stem cell transplantation for severe/refractory intestinal Behçet's disease. Blood 103:748–750

108. Maurer B, Hensel M, Max R, Fiehn C, Ho AD, Lorenz HM (2006) Autologous haematopoietic stem cell transplantation for Behçet's disease with pulmonary involvement: analysis after 5 years of follow up. Ann Rheum Dis 65:127–129

109. Tomonari A, Tojo A, Takahashi T, Iseki T, Ooi J, Takahashi S, Nagamura F, Uchimaru K, Asano S (2004) Resolution of Behçet's disease after HLA-mismatched unrelated cord blood transplantation for myelodysplastic syndrome. Ann Hematol 83:464–466

110. Marmont AM, Gualandi F, Piaggio G, Podesta M (2006) Teresa van Lint M, Bacigalupo A, Nobili F: allogeneic bone marrow transplantation (BMT) for refractory Behçet's disease with severe CNS involvement. Bone Marrow Transplant 37:1061–1063

111. Nonami A, Takenaka K, Sumida C, Aizawa K, Kamezaki K, Miyamoto T, Harada N, Nagafuji K, Teshima T, Harada M (2007) Successful treatment of myelodysplastic syndrome (MDS)-related intestinal Behçet's disease by up-front cord blood transplantation. Intern Med 46:1753–1756

112. Daikeler T, Kotter I, Bocelli Tyndall C, Apperley J, Attarbaschi A, Guardiola P, Gratwohl A, Jantunen E, Marmont A, Porretto F et al (2007) Haematopoietic stem cell transplantation for vasculitis including Behçet's disease and polychondritis: a retrospective analysis of patients recorded in the European bone marrow transplantation and European league against rheumatism databases and a review of the literature. Ann Rheum Dis 66:202–207

Index